Here's How to Treat Childhood Apraxia of Speech

Third Edition

"Here's How"

Series Editor
Thomas Murry, PhD

Here's How to Treat Childhood Apraxia of Speech

Third Edition

Margaret Fish, MS, CCC-SLP
Amy Skinder-Meredith, PhD, CCC-SLP

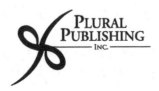

PLURAL
PUBLISHING
INC.

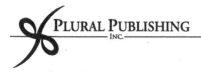

5521 Ruffin Road
San Diego, CA 92123

e-mail: information@pluralpublishing.com
Website: http://www.pluralpublishing.com

Typeset in 10.75/14 Stone Informal by Flanagan's Publishing Services, Inc.
Printed in the United States of America by Integrated Books International

Library of Congress Cataloging-in-Publication Data:
Names: Fish, Margaret A., 1959- author. | Skinder-Meredith, Amy, author.
Title: Here's how to treat childhood apraxia of speech / Margaret Fish, Amy Skinder-Meredith.
Other titles: Here's how series
Description: Third edition. | San Diego, CA : Plural Publishing, Inc., 2022. | Series: Here's how | Includes bibliographical references and index.
Identifiers: LCCN 2022019111 (print) | LCCN 2022019112 (ebook) | ISBN 9781635502831 (paperback) | ISBN 1635502837 (paperback) | ISBN 9781635502848 (ebook)
Subjects: MESH: Apraxias--therapy | Speech Disorders--therapy | Speech Therapy--methods | Child
Classification: LCC RJ496.A63 (print) | LCC RJ496.A63 (ebook) | NLM WL 340.1 | DDC 618.92/855--dc23/eng/20220727
LC record available at https://lccn.loc.gov/2022019111
LC ebook record available at https://lccn.loc.gov/2022019112

Contents

This note icon will be found throughout the text to bring added attention to key points.

Foreword

The clinical practice and especially the science associated with childhood apraxia of speech (CAS) are relatively new compared to many other communicative disorders. In the last 20 years, there has been an explosion of work in this area, in terms of both basic science and clinical assessment tools and treatment strategies. This third edition of *Here's How to Treat Childhood Apraxia of Speech* adds to that literature in a very practical way. It is not always easy to bridge the gap between research and the application of that research to clinical practice. The authors are excellent clinicians who have brought that broad experience to this book. They reviewed a great deal of the science and evidence base in a way that practicing clinicians will appreciate and be able to use. Further, the authors recognize that every child brings individual challenges with respect to severity, personality, previous experience with therapy, comorbidities, and parent involvement, and they provide ways to approach these challenges.

The 13 chapters of this edition cover a wide range of topics. Chapter 1 discusses the nature of CAS, the neurological implications, genetic variants associated with the disorder, the core characteristics, and many associated disorders that may occur with CAS. Chapter 2 focuses on assessment strategies leading to differential diagnosis of CAS. Here the authors provide a framework for assessment in general and strategies for evaluation that covers cognition and language as well as speech. They provide some direction for assessing children for whom English is not their first language and give specific strategies for different ages, encouraging clinicians to use clinical thinking when devising assessment protocols for individual children. There are many tables and worksheets that clinicians may find helpful for assessing children with CAS, as well as many children with other types of speech sound disorders. Chapter 3 focuses on the fundamentals of treatment, with special attention to the principles of motor learning, the application of which is essential in the treatment of CAS. In addition to providing a broad description of several important principles to incorporate into treatment, the authors provide many practical tasks to allow for the repetitive practice often required in treating CAS. Further, they describe different activities that may apply to a variety of children and contexts.

The authors discuss both external and internal evidence to inform treatment decisions in Chapter 4. They describe the different published treatment methods and the evidence that has been shown for their efficacy. Chapter 5 focuses on treatment strategies for vowel accuracy and natural prosody, both which are common areas of difficulty for children with CAS. This book, however, goes beyond treatment specific to CAS. For example, Chapter 6 focuses on activities for minimally verbal children including children at risk for CAS or any child who may need very early speech-language intervention. Parents and caregivers will appreciate tables related to developmental milestones as well as activities that support early language and speech development.

While Chapter 7 addresses early literacy in CAS, the treatment strategies suggested would likely be appropriate for many children with speech sound disorders who are having trouble learning to read. The authors provide a thorough discussion of the types of phonological awareness and early literacy challenges as well as suggestions for working with these challenges in the context of speech sensorimotor planning treatment. Likewise, clinicians will appreciate Chapter 8 in which strategies for supporting the needs of older children are discussed. These strategies addressing residual articulation errors, persistent phonological patterns, cluster reduction, and reduced comprehensibility will be extremely helpful for older children with CAS as well as children with other speech sound disorders. While the authors discussed many ways to facilitate expressive language development in younger children in Chapter 6, this chapter provides information in treating ongoing language issues. Strategies for improving vocabulary, grammar, conversational skills, and use of language in social interactions will be widely appreciated by clinicians.

Two important additional chapters appear in this edition: treating children with concomitant disorders and considerations of treatment via telepractice. Many children with CAS present with a large variety of co-occurring disorders. Expressive language impairment and phonological disorders are very common, and practical suggestions for addressing these linguistic deficits are presented throughout the book. Described in Chapter 9 are treatment strategies for those children who also exhibit dysarthria, attention deficit hyperactivity disorder, autism, and developmental coordination disorder. Also discussed is how to improve social interaction skills for children with social-emotional difficulties and/or anxiety around communication. Parents as well as clinicians will appreciate the practical suggestions in this chapter. Given the COVID-19 pandemic, more treatment has been and will likely continue to be offered via telepractice. In Chapter 10, the authors give recommendations for telepractice for speech and language in general as well as specific suggestions for children with CAS. This is a timely and important issue.

Chapters 11 and 12 focus on how to address changing needs of the child over time and how to address that in therapy as well as writing meaningful goals and collecting data. While this certainly pertains to treating CAS, the issues discussed will be helpful to clinicians working with a variety of children with speech and language disorders. Importantly, the authors also provide helpful information regarding home practice and working with parents.

The breadth of this book is large and will therefore be of interest to a variety of audiences. Students and clinicians will find many of the practical strategies and worksheets provided to be extremely helpful in their clinical practice. Parents will find it useful for understanding the nature of their child's speech problem and feel empowered by the authors' emphasis on including parents in the management of their child's speech problems.

Margaret Fish and Amy Skinder-Meredith are experienced, excellent clinicians. They have spent many years specializing in the assessment and treatment of children with severe speech sound disorders. They have a great deal of experience in treating CAS, providing courses and workshops on the management of CAS for both students and practicing clinicians, and volunteering many hours to support families of children with CAS. This rich experience is evident throughout this book. Students and clinicians will appreciate the many intervention ideas based on best practice. The authors' desire to bring the literature to clinical application is evident in this book. I know them to have a passion for helping children with speech and language deficits, especially CAS, and it shows. They are enthusiastic in their endeavors to educate students and clinicians in pediatric motor speech disorders. This book continues that work. The scope of the strategies presented for assessment and treatment is wide ranging, clearly written, and clinically applicable. Management of CAS is complicated, challenging, and rewarding. This book provides guidance and support that will be appreciated by many.

Edythe A. Strand, PhD, CCC-SLP
Emeritus Professor, Mayo College of Medicine
Emeritus Consultant, Department of Neurology,
    Mayo Clinic
Rochester, Minnesota
Affiliate Professor, University of Washington
Department of Speech and Hearing Sciences
Seattle, Washington

Acknowledgments

We have so many colleagues to thank who supported us in myriad ways throughout the writing of this book. We would first like to thank Dr. Edythe Strand (Edy) for paving the way for us to have a better understanding of CAS back when we started this journey over 20 years ago. Edy's vast knowledge of pediatric motor speech disorders is matched by her warmth and compassion, which she generously shares with her clients, families, students, and colleagues. Her willingness to write the Foreword was truly an honor. We would also like to thank Nancy Potter, who read through and edited chapters, in addition to being a sounding board about what should be included in the book over many miles of cross-country skiing, hiking, biking, and office conversations.

Many of our colleagues were incredibly generous with their time in responding to our questions about their research, by engaging in professional dialogue, sharing information and resources, reading through early drafts, and provided much needed encouragement and ongoing support. We are grateful for the work they do for children with CAS and their families. Thanks to Angela Morgan, Aravind Namasivayam, Beate Peter, Deb Hayden, Edwin Mass, Heather Rusiewicz, Jan Norris, Jenya Iuzzini-Seigel, Jonathan Preston, Laura Moorer, Megan Hodge, Megan Overby, Christina Gildersleeve-Neumann, Nancy Kaufman, Nancy Tarshis, Pamela Williams, Patricia McCabe, Ruth Stoeckel, Sharynne McLeod, Shelly Velleman, and Susan Caspari, for sharing their expertise throughout our writing process.

We would also like to thank the founder of Childhood Apraxia of Speech of North America (CASANA), Sharon Gretz. If it wasn't for Sharon and the original CASANA team with Kathy Hennessey and Mary Sturm (three fearless mothers of children with CAS), many of us would not have met each other and forged the collaborations across the country and world we have today to support children and families with CAS. We are grateful for the Executive Director of Apraxia Kids (formerly known as CASANA), Angela Grimm, for continuing the mission to improve the lives of children with CAS and help each child with CAS find their voice.

This book wouldn't have been possible without the support of our talented and dedicated team at Plural Publishing. Thanks to Emily Pooley, Valerie Johns, Lori Asbury, Jessica Bristow, and Kristin Banach who were responsive to our many questions over the past several months. They have been instrumental in keeping the production on track and refining the manuscript.

Last, but not least, we are eternally grateful for the children and the families we have worked with, who are our greatest teachers. We are appreciative of their resilience, patience, hard work, tenacity, stories, and humor.

For John, Jackie, and Michael, who fill my world with joy.

MAF

For Todd, Alisher, and Jasmine, who have made life an amazing adventure.

ASM

1

Understanding Childhood Apraxia of Speech

In 2007, the American Speech-Language-Hearing Association's (ASHA) technical report on childhood apraxia of speech (CAS) provided a definition of this complex neurological pediatric motor speech disorder that impacts both articulatory accuracy and prosody. The report provided three core characteristics observed in CAS that help the clinician differentiate it from other speech sound disorders and a list of frequently co-occurring challenges. The quest to fully understand CAS, however, keeps researchers and speech-language pathologists (SLPs) in a constant state of investigation and learning. The purpose of this chapter is to provide an overview of the journey of our understanding of CAS—from the initial discovery in the 1950s to what we currently know based on behavioral, acoustic, kinematic, genetic, and brain imaging research.

What Is CAS?

CAS falls under the umbrella of speech sound disorders (SSDs) as shown in Figure 1–1. SSDs can be due to motor-based articulation challenges, structural differences, sensory deficits, or linguistically based phonological issues. A child with an SSD could have a combination of factors making speech production difficult. For example, a child could have speech impacted by hearing loss and cleft lip and palate, in addition to CAS.

History of CAS

The history of apraxia of speech in children is an interesting one. It was first noted by Morley, Court, and Miller in 1954 in the United Kingdom. In 1950, these authors proposed a taxonomy to classify childhood speech disorders. They used the following five broad categories: deafness, defective articulation or dysarthria, retarded development of language or

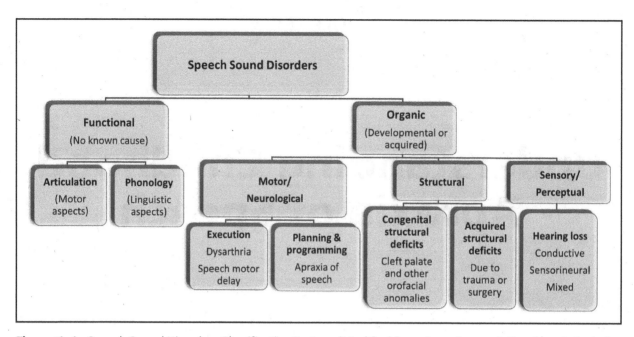

Figure 1–1. Speech Sound Disorders Classification System. (Modified from *Speech sound disorders: Articulation and phonology* [Practice portal] by American Speech-Language-Hearing Association, n.d., https://www.asha.org/Practice-Portal/Clinical-Topics/Articulation-and-Phonology/. Reproduced with permission from ASHA.)

dysphasia, dyslalia, and stammering. When they further examined the children with dysarthria in their 1954 paper, they noted that there was a subgroup of children whose lips, tongue, and palate appeared normal on voluntary movements but clumsy and awkward when they attempted the more complex and rapid movements required of speech. They labeled the disorder, "dyspraxic dysarthria" or "articulatory dyspraxia." In the United States, researchers Rosenbek and Wertz (1972) were bringing attention to a set of speech characteristics observed in children with SSDs that, in many ways, resembled the apraxia of speech affecting adults following stroke or brain injury. These children appeared to have the strength and structural integrity of the speech mechanism to be capable of speaking clearly; however, they demonstrated significant difficulty in speech production, including difficulty with phoneme sequencing, inconsistent errors, groping for sounds, difficulty imitating oral movements, difficulty imitating sounds and words, and atypical stress and intonation patterns. These children did not respond as expected to traditional types of speech therapy, often making very slow progress. Given the similarities of the nature of the speech difficulties of these children to adults with acquired apraxia, researchers began to label these children as apraxic or dyspraxic. Over the years, terms such as developmental apraxia of speech, childhood verbal apraxia, developmental verbal apraxia, developmental verbal dyspraxia, and CAS have been used to describe these types of speech characteristics in children. The term *childhood apraxia of speech* (CAS) was recommended by ASHA in 2007 as the classification term for children who demonstrate certain types of speech characteristics (e.g., inconsistent articulation errors, disordered prosody, and poor coarticulation). These characteristics are detailed in the following section. CAS is estimated to occur in approximately one to two children per thousand (Shriberg et al., 1997a), with a higher prevalence occurring in children with certain syndromes or types of genetic deviations.

Defining CAS

To provide greater clarity for SLPs working with children with CAS, ASHA formed a committee (Ad Hoc Committee on Apraxia of Speech in Children) to review the available scientific research related to CAS. The committee also described current trends in professional management of CAS and made recommendations related to assessment, treatment, and future research. In its report (ASHA, 2007a), the committee proposed the following definition of CAS:

> *Childhood apraxia of speech (CAS)* is a neurological childhood (pediatric) speech sound disorder in which the precision and consistency of movements underlying speech are impaired in the absence of neuromuscular deficits (e.g., abnormal reflexes, abnormal tone). CAS may occur as a result of known neurological impairment, in association with complex neurobehavioral disorders of known or unknown origin, or as an idiopathic neurogenic speech sound disorder. The core impairment in planning and/or programming spatiotemporal parameters of movement sequences results in errors in speech sound production and prosody. (ASHA Position Statement, 2007, para. 3)

There is a lot of information packed in this definition, so let us break it down:

> CAS is a **neurological** childhood speech sound disorder in which the **precision and consistency of movements underlying speech** are impaired in the **absence of neuromuscular deficits**.

What Do We Know About the Neurological Component?

Although some children with CAS may have a history of clear neurological involvement, such as an intrauterine stroke, infections that attack the brain, epilepsy, or trauma, the majority do not. However, this does not rule out a neurological component. Brain imaging and genetic studies over the past two decades have revealed more insight into the neurological differences of children with CAS. This has not been an easy or straightforward discovery. Unlike adults with acquired apraxia of speech, children with CAS do not typically present with a focal brain lesion in the left hemisphere. The *heterogeneity* of the disorder also caused challenges when using neuroimaging studies that looked only at the brain morphology. Studies prior to the completion of the human genome project (1990–2003) and availability of more sophisticated neuroimaging tools, like functional magnetic resonance imaging (fMRIs) and *diffusion tensor imaging*, limited researchers in their ability to better understand the genetics and neural correlates that correspond with motor planning and sequencing for speech and the other characteristics frequently associated with CAS, such as language and literacy impairments. Advancements in neuroimaging and genetic testing methods have put us on an exciting trajectory of learning more about these children we care so deeply about.

No story illustrates the evolution of genetic and neurological discoveries better than the account of the KE family. In the late 1980s, the KE family caught the attention of a special educator in Brentford, England. The teacher, Ms. Auger, noticed she had several members of the same family that presented with motor speech and language disorders. Assuming these traits were heritable, she contacted Jane Hurst, a geneticist and researcher (Fowler, 2017). When examining three generations of the KE family, they discovered that the grandmother, four of her five children, and 11 of her 23 grandchildren had CAS in addition to other challenges, showing this to be an *autosomal dominant monogenic trait* (Hurst et al., 1990). With the advancements made in genetics (e.g., *semiautomatic genotyping*), Fisher and colleagues (1998) were able to localize the gene responsible, *FOXP2* (*SPCH1*) on the chromosomal band 7q31. To investigate the neural correlates, the team did brain imaging on affected and unaffected family members (Vargha-Khadem et al., 1998). In the areas of speech, language, and orofacial praxis development, all the affected family members were significantly more impaired than the unaffected members. By analyzing the results produced by positron-emission tomography (PET) activation scans during a word repetition task and magnetic resonance imaging (MRI) scans, the authors found that affected family members had functional and structural abnormalities. PET scan results revealed reduced activity in the *left supplementary motor area* (SMA), the *left cingulate cortex*, and the *left preSMA/cingulate cortex*. Overactive regions included the head and tail of the *left caudate nucleus*, the *left premotor cortex with a ventral extension into Broca area*, and the *left ventral prefrontal cortex*. Consistent with these findings, the MRI scans of affected members revealed significantly more gray matter in the *lentiform nucleus* (*putamen and globus pallidus*) and *angular gyrus* bilaterally and less gray matter in the *preSMA/cingulate cortex Broca area*, and the *caudate nucleus* bilaterally than the unaffected members. Authors speculated that the bilateral reduction in the volume of the *caudate nucleus* may explain the orofacial dyspraxia and verbal apraxia. A follow-up study using fMRIs during a nonsense word repetition task confirmed and added to these findings. Results showed that the affected members had significantly reduced activity in the *premotor, supplementary*, and *primary motor cortices*, as well as in the *cerebellum* and *basal ganglia* (Liégeois et al., 2011). See Figure 1–2 for the neural correlates. These findings led to more research on the *FOXP2* gene, yet it was found that this gene only accounted for a small number of cases of CAS. As brain imaging and genetic analysis have become more sophisticated, more neurological and genetic links to CAS are being discovered.

Chilosi and colleagues (2015) examined 32 Italian children with idiopathic CAS for genetic and brain morphology differences. Although 70% of the children with CAS had parents or relatives with language disorders, dyslexia, or both, only six of the children had a known genetic alteration, where three of the genetic abnormalities were inherited from a parent and one was a *de novo genetic alteration*. De novo refers to a new mutation, one not inherited from either parent. Interestingly, the parents who passed on the gene did not present with a history of CAS and appeared phenotypically normal with none of the gene alterations involved the *FOXP2* gene. Findings from conventional MRI images of the 32 participants did not show significant visible neuroanatomical abnormalities and suggested CAS may be due to microstructural alterations in the brain. A follow-up study using *diffusion tensor imaging* (DTI) (Fiori et al., 2016) found differences in the structural connectivity of speech and language networks. Using this approach, researchers were able to determine three *intrahemispheric* and *interhemispheric subnetworks* that had reduced connectivity when compared to controls. When one thinks about reduced connectivity of a neural pathway, it helps to conceptualize these connections as ranging from slow and inefficient, like a hard-to-find path that has you bushwhacking through the forest, to a superhighway that allows you to move quickly. When a child has CAS, they may lack some of the superhighways that provide rapid connections for effortless acquisition of speech, language, and literacy skills. See Table 1–1 for a summary of the results of Fiori and colleagues (2016).

From a theoretical basis, connectivity issues discovered by Fiori and colleagues (2016) correlate with deficits in the areas presented in Table 1–2.

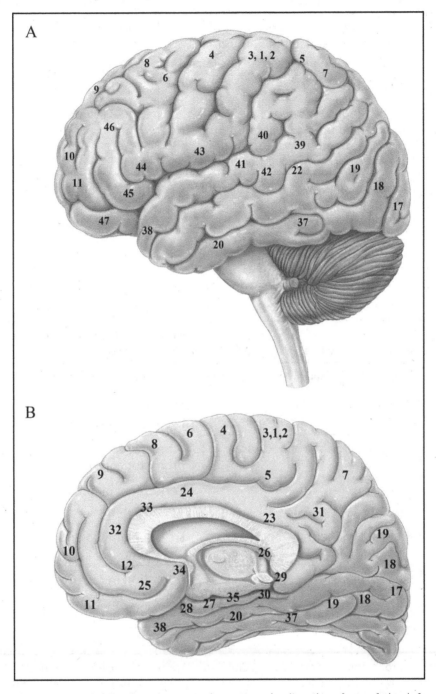

Figure 1–2. A. Brodmann areas shown on the literal surface of the left hemisphere. **B.** Brodmann areas shown on the medial surface of the right hemisphere. (From *Clinical neuroscience for communication disorders: Neuroanatomy and* neurophysiology, by M. Lehman Blake and J. K. Hoepner, 2023, p. 8, Figure 1–8. ©Plural Publishing.)

Table 1–1. Impacted Subnetworks and Structures and Corresponding Behavioral Consequences

Network	Structures Involved	Significant Correlations
Subnetwork 1	Left inferior and superior frontal gyrus, left superior and middle temporal gyrus, and left posterior–central gyrus.	Low performance on oromotor skills Low DDK rate Poor expressive grammar Poor lexical production
Subnetwork 2	Right supplementary motor area, left middle and inferior frontal gyrus, left precuneus and cuneus, right superior occipital gyrus, and right cerebellum	Low DDK rate
Subnetwork 3	Right angular gyrus, right superior temporal gyrus and right inferior occipital gyrus	No correlation found

Table 1–2. Neural Structures and Their Behavioral Correlates Impacted in Research Participants With CAS

Subnetwork	Neural Structures Involved	Proposed Functions of the Neural Structure
1	Middle and superior temporal gyri	Phonemic discrimination
1	Inferior frontal gyrus	Phonological and syntactic processing Feedback-based articulatory control
1	Temporal-frontal connectivity disruption	Mismatch between auditory feedback and oromotor control
2	Precuneus	Conceptual planning during lexical search Action initiation
2	Right supplementary motor area (SMA)	Speech planning and motor and cognitive triggering
2	Cerebellum Cerebellum + SMA	Alteration in feed-forward mechanisms of speech control Altered motor planning
3	Angular gyrus	Semantic representation

Note. Data from "Neuroanatomical Correlates of Childhood Apraxia of Speech: A Connectomic Approach," by S. Fiori, A. Guzzetta, J. Mitra, K. Pannek, R. Pasquariello, P. Cipriani, M. Tosetti, G. Cioni, S. Rose, and A. Chilosi, 2016, *NeuroImage: Clinical, 12*, pp. 894–901. https://doi.org/10.1016/j.nicl.2016.11.003

Treatment studies have provided additional information on neurological differences of the brain in children with CAS. In 2014, Kadis and colleagues found differences in cortical thickness in the *left posterior supramarginal gyrus* when using *vertex-based thickness analysis with high-resolution MRIs*. Prior to treatment, children with idiopathic CAS had thicker left posterior supramarginal gyri than controls. Eight weeks post PROMPT (*PROMPTS for Restructuring Oral*

Muscular Phonetic Targets) treatment, eight of the nine children with CAS showed thinning of this area, suggesting increased neural plasticity of the brain with the pruning of unnecessary neurons for more efficient motor speech planning. Fiori et al. (2021) examined the behavioral and neurological impact of PROMPT compared to a language, nonspeech oral motor training (LNSOM) approach. Results indicated both groups had a favorable change in the *corticobulbar pathways* for speech motor control, with greater changes in the PROMPT group. More specifically, the use of fractional anisotropy indicated an increase in the *left dorsal* and *ventral corticobulbar tracts*. When interpreting results of studies that use fractional anisotropy, it helps to understand the basic premise. "Reduction of *fractional anisotropy* and related increase of mean diffusivity are reported to be associated with impaired connectivity, whereas processes connected with learning can determine neuroplastic effects and have been associated with fractional anisotropy increase and mean diffusivity decrease" (Fiori et al., 2021, p. 965). Although a correlational analysis between severity of motor speech control and measures of diffusivity were unable to be performed, positive changes were seen in both areas. In addition to studies giving us insight into the compromised neural networks for children with CAS, they also show how appropriate therapy can strengthen these pathways. It is exciting to know that, with appropriate therapy implementation, SLPs have the tools to change the brain.

To summarize, the neuroanatomical and physiological differences found thus far in children with CAS include the following areas: left posterior central gyrus (1, 2, 3); primary motor cortex (4); left premotor cortex (6); left precuneus (7); left cuneus (17); right superior occipital gyrus (19); left middle temporal gyrus (21); left caudate nucleus (23); left cingulate cortex (32); left and right superior temporal gyrus (41); Broca area (44, 45); and left ventral prefrontal cortex (46); in addition to the basal ganglia and cerebellum. See Figure 1–2 for a reference to the Brodmann areas and Figure 1–3 for the basal ganglia and cerebellum.

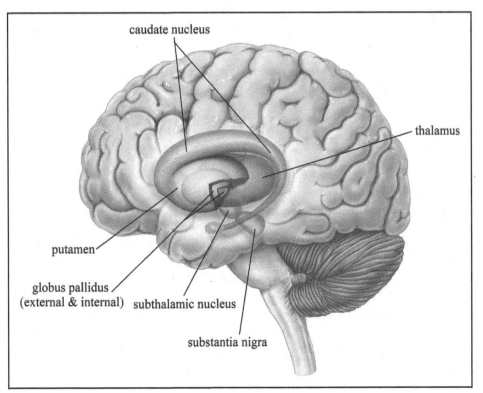

Figure 1–3. Structures of the basal ganglia, thalamus, and cerebellum from the lateral view of the left hemisphere. (From *Clinical neuroscience for communication disorders: Neuroanatomy and neurophysiology*, by M. Lehman Blake and J. K. Hoepner, 2023, p. 27, Figure 1–30. ©Plural Publishing.)

What Is Meant by Precision and Consistency of Movements?

As an SLP, you understand this. As a layperson, unfamiliar with how difficult acquisition of speech is for some children, the planning and executing of articulatory movement is a skill that is often taken for granted. Speech is a complex motor task requiring numerous muscles of the four speech subsystems (respiration, resonance, phonation, articulation) to work together efficiently in a coordinated manner. The coordination of these movements needs to be precise and consistent, yet flexible. To illustrate the motoric complexity of speech, think of all the steps that go into saying the word, "can" as in, "Can I go too?" It is a simple CVC, but let's break it down.

1. Cognitively, we need to have communicative intent to make this request.

2. Linguistically, we need to have the word in our lexicon, retrieve the word, and have a representation of it. For the full phrase, we need to have the sentence structure and know where to put stress.

3. Immediately prior to producing the sequence of phonemes (motor execution), we need to plan and program the movement parameters. For the word "can," we need to prepare to do the following:

    a. Take a quick inhalation to be ready to speak on exhalation.

    b. Raise the velum and constrict the pharyngeal walls to close off the velopharyngeal port so no air escapes out the nose while building pressure for /k/.

    c. Raise the back of the tongue to contact the soft palate while thinking ahead for where the /æ/ will be. (Note that placement for /k/ before /æ/ is different than for /u/.)

    d. Abduct the vocal folds for the /k/ so it is not voiced.

    e. Release pressure in ~50 ms to produce the /k/ sound.

    f. Get ready for /æ/ by opening the jaw slightly and dropping the tongue to the mid- front position and getting ready to phonate.

    g. Adduct and vibrate vocal folds while the tongue is in the front-low position for /æ/ with onset of voice occurring approximately 50 ms following initial onset of /k/.

    h. Start to open the velopharyngeal (VP) port to get ready for /n/ while still phonating /æ/.

    i. Continue phonation while fully opening the VP port and move tongue tip to the alveolar ridge to produce /n/.

    j. Drop the tongue tip and lower the jaw as you get ready for "I."

Wow, that was a lot of movement to plan for, and there are still several more words in the sentence to get through. When we appreciate the precision and speed of movement necessary for speech, it is amazing any of us can talk. That was just the precision part. Now think about the consistency. Speech is a motor skill, and some would add that it is a sensory-motor (or sensorimotor) skill, as you use your sensory feedback on how speech sounds and feels to know where to place the articulators. Early skill acquisition heavily relies primarily on a feedback strategy in which children observe the outcome of their action and make adjustments during future trials. With maturity, experience, and practice, children transition from reliance on feedback and begin to incorporate more feed-forward strategies, such as anticipating the required force, distance, and direction of movement prior to the execution of an action (Potter et al., 2009). This is why when learning a new motor skill, we tend to be inconsistent. It takes a lot of trial and error to get it right and hence a lot of practice.

What Is This About the Absence of Neuromuscular Deficits?

When this statement was initially written, many SLPs thought this meant that dysarthria had to be ruled out to diagnose a child with CAS. We now recognize that a child can have both CAS and dysarthria, among other challenges that impact communication. Of the 32 children Murray and colleagues (2015) studied with idiopathic CAS, four also had dysarthria. Hence, this is not an either/or situation. The SLP needs to tease out which aspects of the child's speech sound disorder are due to difficulty with *motor planning* and *programming* versus other underlying factors. A child with dysarthria will have imprecise movement due to difficulties with the execution portion of speech production, but the errors tend to be consistent, while the child with CAS will have inconsistent errors. This is addressed more in Chapter 2.

> *CAS may occur as a result of known neurological impairment, in association with* **complex neurobehavioral disorders** *of* **known** *or* **unknown origin,** *or as an* **idiopathic** *neurogenic speech sound disorder.*

What Is Known About Complex Neurobehavioral Disorders Associated With CAS?

Recent studies by Shriberg, Strand, Jakielski, and Mabie (2019) examined the prevalence of motor speech disorders in children with *complex neurodevelopmental disorders* (CNDs). In a companion study, Shriberg, Kwiatkowski, and Mabie (2019) calculated the prevalence of motor speech disorders in children with *idiopathic* speech delay (SD). Speech samples of 346 children with one of eight types of CNDs, with an average age of 13.3 years, were studied to determine prevalence of speech sound disorder classifications for this population. In the companion study, there were 415 participants with idiopathic speech delay, and most participants were preschool age or in early primary grades (M = 5.5 years of age; SD = 1.4). See Figures 1–4 and 1–5 for the percentage of children in each group diagnosed as not having a motor speech disorder (no MSD), speech motor delay (SMD), childhood dysarthria (CD), CAS, and childhood apraxia of speech with childhood dysarthria (CAS + CD).

 When interpreting these graphs, it is important to note that SSDs can evolve over time and that the speech samples used for this research captured only a moment in time. The children with idiopathic CAS were an average age of 5.5 years and had no co-occurring CD, whereas the children with complex neurodevelopmental disorder (CND) were an average age of 13.3 years, and 5% had both CAS and CD. It has been our experience, as SLPs who work primarily with children with motor speech disorders from early childhood through adolescence, that for some children a dysarthric component becomes more apparent as the motor sequencing improves. In other words, the child's sequence of articulatory movement becomes more accurate, but some of the phonemes are still weak and imprecise.

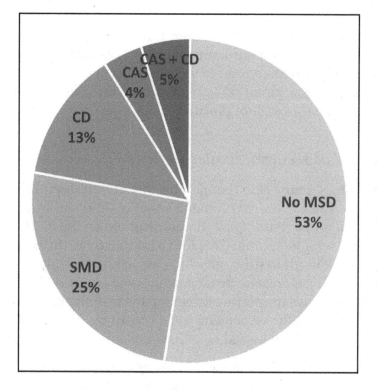

Figure 1–4. Estimates of prevalence of motor speech disorders in children with complex neurodevelopmental disorders. Adapted from Shriberg, L. D., Strand, E., Jakielski, K. J., & Mabie, H. L. (2019). Estimates of the prevalence of speech and motor speech disorders in persons with complex neurodevelopmental disorders. *Clinical Linguistics & Phonetics, 33*(8), 707–736. https://doi.org/10.1080/02699206.2019.1595732

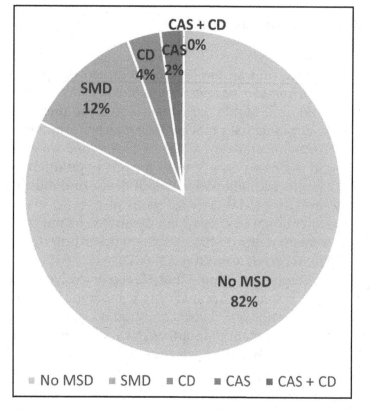

Figure 1–5. Estimates of prevalence of motor speech disorders in children with idiopathic speech delay. Adapted from Shriberg, L. D., Kwiatkowski, J., & Mabie, H. L. (2019). Estimates of the prevalence of motor speech disorders in children with idiopathic speech delay. *Clinical Linguistics & Phonetics, 33*(8), 679–706. https://doi.org/10.1080/02699206.2019.1595731

The relatively new classification of *speech motor delay* (SMD) may also be why our clinical perceptions are not consistent with the research. Speech motor delay used to be referred to as motor speech delay not otherwise specified (MSD-NOS). SMD is characterized by imprecise and unstable speech, prosody, and voice that does not meet criteria for either CD or CAS (Shriberg, Kwiatkowski, & Mabie, 2019; Shriberg, Strand, et al., 2019). It is considered a disorder of execution instead of motor planning and programming, as in CAS. It is "a delay in the development of neuromotor precision-stability of speech motor control" (Namasivayam et al., 2020, p. 16). Assessment methods used in the research by Shriberg, Kwiatkowski, and Mabie, (2019), Shriberg, Strand, et al., (2019), and Namasivayam et al. (2020) allow for more precise classification, which can provide insight for the SLP. However, the time it takes to do the detailed speech and kinematic analysis for the classification of SMD versus CAS versus CD versus CAS + CD is not typically feasible for the practicing SLP currently. Hence, Chapter 2 focuses on what is practical and helps guide the clinician to make an appropriate treatment plan.

What Have Studies Revealed About Genetic Variants Implicated in CAS?

Most cases of CAS are currently considered *idiopathic*, meaning we do not know what the cause is. However, with the rapid gains being made in genetics research, we are learning more about the gene mutations that play a role in neurodevelopment. SLPs involved in the research of genetics of CAS and other speech and language disorders (e.g., Graham & Fisher, 2015; Laffin et al., 2012; Lewis et al., 2011; Morgan, 2020; Peter et al., 2012; Vargha-Khadem et al., 2005; Velleman & Mervis, 2011) have helped our field tremendously in better understanding the link between gene variants and the behavioral characteristics related to speech, language, literacy, and cognition. It is currently estimated that 32% to 44% of children with CAS have an associated genetic variation (Eising et al., 2019; Hildebrand et al., 2020). Some of the variants are inherited, passed from the parent to the child, and many are new variants (de novo) (Hildebrand et al., 2020). The availability of new cost-efficient genetic technologies and the hard work of many researchers have brought us to a place of great discovery. If a parent had asked their SLP if genetic testing was worth the expense and effort prior to 2015, the answer probably would have been no. However, methods like whole genome sequencing have become more affordable at approximately one thousand dollars per individual in 2022. Children who present with neurodevelopmental conditions (e.g., attention deficit hyperactivity disorder [ADHD], epilepsy, autism spectrum disorder [ASD], motor impairments) in addition to CAS should be referred for genetic testing, as it can assist with a clearer diagnosis and prognosis (Dodd, 2021; Morgan et al., 2021; Peter et al., 2012). In addition, the diagnosis will guide intervention, may qualify a child for earlier intervention or increased insurance coverage, and potentially offer the family more support, as some genetic diagnoses have a related support group (e.g., *SETBP1* haploinsufficiency disorder, 22q11.2 deletion, and galactosemia). Genetic variations related to CAS can be divided into three categories: (a) single gene variants, where there is an alteration in the gene; (b) copy number variants (CNVs), where there can be small or large deletions, duplications, or rearrangements of sections of a chromosome; and (c) other genetic syndromes, where CAS sometimes occurs. Examples of single gene variants and CNVs are presented in Table 1–3. Some of the genetic syndromes and disorders that may or may not have a CAS component include Noonan syndrome, Down syndrome, fragile X syndrome, Klinefelter syndrome, and classic galactosemia (Potter et al., 2013).

These single gene variants, CNVs, and other genetic syndromes can be associated with a wide range of behavioral and physical characteristics. As with any genetic condition or

Table 1–3. Examples of Single Gene Variants and Copy Number Variations Associated With CAS

Single Gene Variants				Copy Number Variations
CDK13[a]	GNAO1[a]	MKL2	UPF2[a]	5q14.3q21.1[a]
CHD3	GNB1[a]	POGZ[a]	WDR5	7q11.23 duplication syndrome
DDX3X[a]	GRIN2A	SETBP1[a]	ZFHX4	16p11.2 deletion
EBF3[a]	KAT6A	SETD1A	ZNF142	17q21.31 microdeletion (Koolen de Vries syndrome)
FOXP2	MEIS2	TNRC6B		22q11.2 deletion syndrome

[a]These are de novo variations (i.e., not passed down from either parent).

Notes. 2018 Information from "A Set of Regulatory Genes Co-expressed in Embryonic Human Brain Is Implicated in Disrupted Speech Development," by E. Eising, A. Carrion-Castillo, A. Vino, E. Strand, K. Jakielski, T. Scerri, . . . S. Fisher, 2019, *Molecular Psychiatry*, *24*(7), 1065–1078, https://doi.org/10.1038/s41380-018-0020-x; "A Highly Penetrant Form of Childhood Apraxia of Speech Due to Deletion of 16p11.2," E. Fedorenko, A. Morgan, E. Murray, A. Cardinaux, C. Mei, H. Tager-Flusberg, . . . N. Kanwisher, 2016, *European Journal of Human Genetics*, *24*, 302–306, https://doi.org/10.1038/ejhg.2015.149; "Severe Childhood Speech Disorder: Gene Discovery Highlights Transcriptional Dysregulation," M. S. Hildebrand, V. E. Jackson, T. S. Scerri, O. Van Reyk, M. Coleman, R. Braden, . . . A. Morgan, 2020, *Neurology*, *94*(20), e2148–e2167, https://doi.org/10.1212/wnl.0000000000009441; "Novel Candidate Genes and Regions for Childhood Apraxia of Speech Identified by Array Comparative Genomic Hybridization," by J. J. Laffin, G. Raca, C. A. Jackson, E. A. Strand, K. J. Jakielski, and L. D. Shriberg, 2012, *Genetics in Medicine*, *14* (11), 928–936, https://doi.org/10.1038/gim.2012.72; "Deep Phenotyping of Speech and Language Skills in Individuals With 16p11.2 Deletion," by C. Mei, E. Fedorenko, D. Amir, A. Boys, C. Hoeflin, P. Carew, T. Burgess, S. Fisher, and A. Morgan, 2018, *European Journal of Human Genetics*, *26*, 676–686, https://doi.org/10.1038/s41431-018-0102-x

syndrome, no two children with the same diagnosis will present exactly alike. For example, where one child with 22q11.2 deletion may have velopharyngeal insufficiency, CAS, cardiac issues, and a language disorder, another might not have the CAS component but have ADHD and an intellectual disability. Regardless, if there is a known genetic diagnosis, it alerts the child's parents and primary health care provider to be on watch for the symptoms the child is at high risk for, which can lead to better precision medicine and access to the appropriate health care providers (Morgan & Webster, 2018) (information about current clinical trials can be found at https://www.geneticsofspeech.org.au/research/ or https://clinicaltrials.gov/).

*The **core impairment in planning and/or programming** spatiotemporal parameters of movement sequences results in errors in speech sound production and prosody.*

What Are the Underlying Deficits That Result in the Core Impairment of Planning and Programming of Movement Sequences?

Children diagnosed with CAS have various levels of challenge with planning and programming for speech, described eloquently by van der Merwe (2019). In the motor planning phase of speech, specifications are made related to placement and manner for articulatory movements, as well as the timing of specific movements for each sound. For example, to produce the word *bee,* the lips need to close but also to spread slightly in anticipation of the vowel "ee" to follow. For *boo,* the lips close but also round as an anticipatory response to the upcoming vowel "oo." At the same time, the brain is also specifying the raising of the velum and vibration of the vocal folds at just the right time, for if the vocal fold vibration begins too late, the result would be "pea" and "poo," rather than "bee" and "boo."

In the motor programming phase, the specifications of muscle movements related to muscle tone, velocity of movement, amount of force applied to the articulators, range of motion, and so on, are made. Both planning and programming these specifications of articulatory control occur prior to actual execution of the movement. When we consider the speed with which the brain needs to organize all this information, it becomes clearer how a breakdown in the planning and programming can have such a significant impact on speech in children with CAS.

Although it is well accepted that the core impairment of CAS is because of faulty sensory and motor planning and programming (ASHA Technical Report, 2007b; Overby et al., 2019; Rosenbek & Wertz, 1972, several other theories have been proposed as well. When reading through the literature, it can sometimes feel like a "Which came first, the chicken or the egg?" question. For example, do infants later diagnosed with CAS have decreased speech-like vocalizations because they are unable to motor plan or program the movement, or did the ability to plan and program movement fail to develop normally because there was a lack of sensorimotor feedback? During this time, an infant's brain is undergoing a mapping process, coupling articulator movements with sound production and sensory feedback. This phase is followed by a phonological stage where imitation and practice begin to solidify the mapping of articulatory movement to the specific goal (Overby et al., 2020).

To account for the findings of disordered prosody, Shriberg and colleagues (1997b) suggested that for at least a subtype of CAS, there is a "stress deficit at the level of representational planning processes rather than the motor-speech programming processes" (Shriberg et al., 1997b, p. 324). Stress assignment is thought to occur at the linguistic level, which would occur prior to motor speech programming. It is represented in the instructions sent for prearticulatory processing by the programmer. Although disordered prosody was listed as a characteristic of CAS, Shriberg and colleagues brought observations of disordered prosody more to the forefront for differential diagnosis.

Alternatively, Velleman and Strand (1994) posited that "children with CAS could be seen as impaired in their ability to generate and utilize frames, which would otherwise provide the mechanisms for analyzing, organizing, and utilizing information from their motor, sensory and linguistic systems for the production of spoken language" (pp. 119–120). Through this lens, we see the importance of paying attention to syllable shapes and syntax, areas in which the child with CAS is challenged. The focus of therapy is often on systematically increasing the complexity of the syllable shapes, while being mindful of the phonemes within those syllable shapes. Theoretically, this will allow the work on one set of phrases to generalize to a different set of phrases of similar syllable shape, length, and complexity.

Through the investigation of auditory perception, discrimination, syllable identification, and rhyming tasks, other linguistic theories emerged. Marquardt and colleagues (2002) found that children with CAS had difficulty perceiving syllableness and comparing syllable representations. Built on previous findings of children with CAS not being able to recognize or produce rhymes (Marion et al., 1993), they concluded that speech motor programming deficits alone could not explain their findings. Rhyming tasks necessitate internal representation of the phoneme. Hence, difficulty with identifying and producing rhymes indicates poor phonemic representations that allow rhyming to occur. Children with CAS also had difficulty performing syllable tasks that included awareness of syllables, identifying the location of phonetic differences, and constructing syllable shapes (Marquardt et al., 2002). Based on these findings, they hypothesized that the disorder is due to an impoverished phonological representation system, where the linguistic integrity of the underlying phonological structures is compromised. Because the neural substrates representing the phonological framework of the child's speech motor programming performance are disordered, the speech motor output is severely handicapped as the phonological targets driving articulation could be totally missing or marginal. This could account for the difficulty children with CAS have producing complex syllable shapes and multisyllabic words, in addition to spelling and decoding. In another body of research from the Netherlands, Groenen and colleagues (1996) found that children with CAS had poor discrimination of consonants with subtle acoustic differences and vowels, which leads to difficulty with speech.

There have also been discussions about CAS being linked to implicit motor learning difficulties, which interferes with procedural memory and learning, making it difficult for the child to automatize the sequence of sounds into words and words into phrases (Hildebrand et al., 2020; Iuzzini-Seigel, 2021; Vhaga-Khadem et al., 2005).

From careful review of the kinematic studies, Namasivayam and colleagues (2020) proposed that "speech variability issues in CAS may arise at the level of articulatory synergies (intra-gestural coordination)" (p. 15). For example, Grigos and colleagues (2015) found that children with CAS demonstrate higher lip-jaw spatiotemporal variability with increasing utterance complexity and greater lip aperture variability. Terband et al. (2011) saw that children with CAS had less stable tongue tip-jaw synergy and greater contribution of the lower lip for bilabial closure (Namasivayam et al., 2020).

Which one of these underlying deficit theories is correct? It could be all or any of them. As we discover the neuroanatomical and genetic differences, we have learned that there are many potential causes that impact neurodevelopment; thus, these children could have a variety of underlying deficits, leading to the wide range of CAS profiles.

What Do We Mean by Spatiotemporal Parameters of Movement Sequences, and How Does This Impact Speech Accuracy and Prosody?

First, let's break up the term *spatiotemporal*. This refers to "space" and "timing"—in other words, the exact movement of the tongue, jaw, lips, and soft palate with the correct timing of each movement. Watching a video of the vocal tract movement during speech or singing using MRIs and *electropalatography* allows us to appreciate more greatly what this entails. Studies using *electropalatography* have shown that children with CAS do not develop the more finely tuned speech movements with the specificity and precision that typically developing children do (Gibbon, 1999).

Core Characteristics of CAS

The ASHA 2007 technical report was the first publication to provide a list of core deficits to differentiate CAS from other SSDs. These core features include the following:

1. Inconsistent errors on consonants and vowels in repeated productions of syllables or words

2. Disordered prosody lengthened and disrupted coarticulatory transitions between sounds and syllables

3. Inappropriate prosody, especially in the realization of lexical stress

Although these characteristics are indicative of the underlying deficit of impaired motor planning and programming, the report provided a note of caution stating, "these features are not proposed to be the necessary and sufficient signs of CAS" (ASHA CAS Technical Report, 2007, Section Definitions of CAS). These signs will vary depending on the age of the child, comorbid diagnoses, severity of the disorder, and the task given. For example, a young child with severe CAS may only have a few sounds in their phonetic repertoire, making it unlikely they will be able to demonstrate any of these characteristics.

Since this report was written, researchers continue their efforts to better define and specify criteria for a diagnosis of CAS (Iuzzini-Seigel, 2021; Iuzzini-Seigel et al., 2015, 2017; Murray et al., 2015; Strand, 2020). The diagnostic checklists are similar to each other, while the exact criteria may vary. For example, while a diagnosis of CAS with Strand's 10-point checklist required any combination of at least four of the 10 features listed, Iuzzini-Seigel (2021) uses a list of 11 characteristics and recommends that a child needs to present with five or more of the features, in addition to inconsistent errors, three times each in three different contexts. Iuzzini-Seigel et al. (2015) assist the reader by operationally defining each of the characteristics. It can also be helpful to separate the characteristics into *segmental* characteristics and *suprasegmental* characteristics, as many SLPs have better training in listening for segmental (speech sound errors) than for suprasegmental errors (related to lexical stress and smooth coarticulation). For this reason, it is strongly encouraged to video-record the child's assessment, as it can be difficult to accurately judge all the characteristics in real time. See Table 1–4 for a list of widely accepted characteristics of CAS.

Inconsistency of errors (i.e., inconsistent errors on consonants and vowels in repeated productions of syllables or words) is listed as the top core characteristic for differential diagnosing of CAS but was not included in the table, as it requires a longer explanation. Inconsistency of errors refers to the variability in speech production, and it can be measured several different ways (Betz & Stoel-Gammon, 2005; Iuzzini & Forrest, 2010; Iuzzini-Seigel et al., 2017; Terband et al., 2019). For example, inconsistency can be measured based on multiple productions of the same whole word or phrase, as in the case of token-to-token inconsistency, or it can be calculated by measuring how inconsistent the speech sounds are from productions of different words and phrases. More details on how to obtain inconsistency measures will be provided in Chapter 2.

When relying on inconsistent errors as a measure for differential diagnosis, it is important to note that the developmental stage of the child's motor speech system will be a factor; thus,

Table 1–4. Diagnostic Criteria Frequently Used for CAS With Operational Definitions and Examples Divided Into Segmental and Suprasegmental Characteristics

Characteristic	Definition	Examples (including diacritical markers[a] as appropriate)
Segmental Characteristics		
1. Vowel errors	Vowel substitutions or distortions that are not due to dialect. The vowel does not sound like a prototypical production and may sound like it is in between two vowels.	Substitution errors: /bɑt/ for /bæt/ "bat" /bɑk/ for /baɪk/ "bike" Distortion errors: Shortened vowels as in /dădĭ/ for /dædi/ "Daddy"
2. Consonant distortion	A consonant that is recognizable but not produced accurately.	Lateralized /s/ and /z/ as in /drɛlsəɫz/ for "dresses"
3. Intrusive schwa	A schwa (epenthesis) that is added between consonants or at the end of a word	Addition of schwa in a cluster: /bəlu/ for "blue" Schwa between syllables: /bækəpæk/ for "backpack" Schwa at the end of a word: /maɪjə/ for "my" /mænə/ for "man"
4. Voicing errors	A sound is produced as its voiced cognate. This could also include productions that appear to be in between voicing categories, when it is not expected, as in an intervocalic stop, as in "little."	Substitution: /bɪk/ for "pick" Partially voiced: /t̬ɑp/ for "top"
5. Difficulty achieving initial articulatory configurations or transitional movement gestures	Initiations of words and sounds are difficult for the child to produce and may sound lengthened or uncoordinated. The child may also produce lengthened or disrupted coarticulatory gestures when transitioning from one sound or syllable to the next.	A delay in timing as the back of the tongue is raised with a lengthened release for /k/, as in /...kːæn..aɪ/ for "Can I?"
6. Groping	There are visible trial-and-error movements of the articulators prior to speaking.	Child's lips protrude, retract, and then open prior to saying "out."

Table 1–4. *continued*

Characteristic	Definition	Examples (including diacritical markers[a] as appropriate)
7. Increased difficulty with multisyllabic words	There are disproportionately more errors as the number of syllables increase as compared to words with fewer syllables.	Child can say "axe" and "dent" but says /æ.skɪ.dən/ for "accident."
8. Resonance or nasality disturbance	Nasal sounds are hyponasal or denasal /ˀ/ (not acoustic energy from the nose) and/or oral sounds are hypernasal /˜/ (too much acoustic energy from the nose). *Nasal resonance errors tend to be inconsistent for children with CAS if there is no coexisting dysarthria or velopharyngeal insufficiency.	Child is hyponasal on /m/ and /n/ but hypernasal on /b/ and /d/—in this example, /m̃aɪ.b̃rʌ.θɚz..ñeɪm.ɪz.d̃æn/ for "My brother's name is Dan."
Suprasegmental Characteristics		
9. Syllable segregation	Brief or lengthy pause between syllables that are not linguistically appropriate.	/fæn..tæs..tɪk/ for "fantastic"
10. Slow rate and/or slow DDK rates	Speech rate is not typical. *Decreased rate of speech is more noticeable when the child is attempting the correct articulatory configurations, or when asked to repeat a novel sound sequence like "pataka."	/kːæːnː..aːɪːhːæːvːwːʌːn/ for "Can I have one?" DDK rates are slower than age-matched norms.
11. Stress errors	When stress is placed on the wrong syllable or when all syllables receive equal stress. *Weak syllable deletion may also be included in this category (Strand & McCauley, 2019)	Equal stress on each syllable: /ˈbeɪˈbi/ for /ˈbeɪˌbi/ "baby" /ˈbjuˈtiˈful/ for /ˈbjuˌɾɪfəl/ "beautiful" For "beautiful," note that the vowels may be altered due to stressing the unstressed syllables. Misplaced stress: /ˈpoˌlis/ for /ˌpəˈlis/ "police" Weak syllable deletion: /næ.nə/ for "banana"

Note. Adapted from "Reliance on Auditory Feedback in Children With Childhood Apraxia of Speech," by J. Iuzzini-Seigel, T. P. Hogan, A. J. Guarino, and J. Green, 2015, *Journal of Communication Disorders, 54*, 32–42, https://doi.org/10.1016/j.jcomdis.2015.01.002

[a]See Appendix 2–G for common diacritics used for disordered speech.

the stimuli will need to be appropriate for the child's age and ability. For example, young typically developing children will have greater variability in their speech productions as they are rapidly acquiring speech. Conversely, a young child with CAS may show little variation because of having a restricted phonemic repertoire. As the typically developing child matures, their system becomes more stable and less variable, but as the child with CAS obtains more sounds and syllable shapes, their speech becomes more variable.

Part of the challenge of diagnosing CAS is the lack of a gold standard assessment or a single *pathognomonic* characteristic that is indicative of CAS. Many of the characteristics listed in Table 1–4 may be present in other SSDs but not to the same extent as they are in CAS. In addition, researchers vary on how many of these characteristics need to be observed, which characteristics need to be observed, and in how many conditions they need to be observed to make a diagnosis of CAS. For this reason, it is helpful to summarize how likely it is to see the characteristics frequently listed as core features of CAS in comparison to other SSDs. Table 1–5 provides a summary of the literature reviewed by Iuzzini-Seigel and Murray (2017) as it pertains to the occurrence of frequently listed characteristics of CAS compared to other SSDs.

Murray and colleagues (2015) employed a discriminant function analysis model to determine which combination of characteristics was the most indicative of CAS. Combined measures from syllable segregation (noticeable gaps between syllables), lexical stress matches, percentage phonemes correct (PPC) from a polysyllabic picture naming task, and articulatory accuracy on the sequential movement repetition task /pʌtʌkʌ/ reached 91% diagnostic accuracy when compared to expert diagnosis differentiating CAS from dysarthria and other SSDs. Given that salient characteristics can change over time, it is important to note that the participants in their study ranged in age from 4 to 12 years, and the mean age was 5.8. Syllable segregation, low PPC, and poor lexical stress matches were also observed in one child with ataxic dysarthria. Of all the different types of dysarthria, ataxic dysarthria can be the most difficult one to differentiate from CAS due to some of the overlapping characteristics. However, children with ataxic dysarthria will have more noticeable motor control challenges of the physiological speech subsystems (e.g., respiration, phonation, resonance, and articulation) (Allison & Hustad, 2018).

Benway and Preston (2020) compared multisyllabic word production in children with CAS to children with other types of SSDs between 7 and 17 years of age. The resulting features that differentiated the two groups were slightly different from what Murray and colleagues (2015) found. For example, percentage of consonants correct on multisyllabic words did not differentiate children with CAS from children with other SSDs. Characteristics that were statistically different included voicing change errors (e.g., prevocalic voicing errors), percentage of structurally correct words (i.e., correct syllable shapes), percentage stress correct, and percentage of full syllable deletion. Authors noted that their results may have differed from earlier research on multisyllabic word repetition error types that help distinguish CAS from other SSDs due to the age of their participants among other reasons. Varied results from different studies highlight several factors one should be aware of when reading the research. First, children with CAS compose a heterogenous group; second, salient characteristics change over time; and third, methods used for elicitation and data analysis and participant criteria vary greatly. Each study builds on information from the last, which allows us to learn more about this multifaceted disorder.

Table 1–5. A Research Summary of Core Characteristics Observed in CAS Compared to Other SSDs

Characteristic	CAS	Other Speech Sound Disorders (artic/phono/dysarthria)
Vowel errors	100% of children with CAS presented at least one vowel error on the GFTA-3.[b] 100% of preschoolers with CAS and 90% of school-age children had vowel errors.[c]	10% of children with speech delay had vowel errors on the GFTA-3.[b] 8% of preschoolers with isolated speech sound disorders and language disorders (SL) and 0% of school-age children with SL had vowel errors.[c]
Consonant distortions	*Consonant distortions are not a pathognomonic characteristic.[a]	Children and adults may have consonant distortions due to structural differences, dysarthria, and other SSDs.[a]
Intrusive schwa	75% of school-age children with CAS evidenced schwa insertion during a standardized articulation test.[b]	30% of school-age children with speech delay evidenced schwa insertion during a standardized articulation test.[b]
Voice onset time (VOT)/voicing	85% of school-age children with CAS had voicing errors.[b]	40% with SD had voicing errors.[b]
Groping	54% of preschool-age children had articulatory groping, and 29% had nonspeech oral groping.[d] *This behavior is not seen in all children with CAS and is not necessary for a diagnosis of CAS.[a]	0% of children with other SSDs showed evidence of groping.[d]
Resonance	50% of children with CAS had disturbance in resonance.[b]	10% of children with speech delay had disturbance in resonance.[b] *Disordered resonance can also occur in dysarthria and velopharyngeal insufficiency.
Syllable segregation	75% of children with CAS had syllable segregation.[b]	30% of children with phonological disorder had syllable segregation.[b]
Decreased rate	50% of school-age children with CAS had decreased rate.[b]	20% of children with speech delay had a decreased rate.[b] *Slow rate is also indicative of dysarthria.
DDK	Children with CAS only averaged 48% accuracy over two trials of /pʌtʌkʌ/, and children with CAS + dysarthria averaged 24% accuracy.[d]	Children with other SSDs averaged 76% over two trials.[d]
Stress errors	52% of children with CAS had inappropriate sentential stress.[a] 10% had accurate lexical stress matches on polysyllabic words.[d]	10% of children with SD had inappropriate sentential stress.[a] 67% of children with other SSDs (submucous cleft, phono disorder and dysarthria) had accurate lexical stress matches on polysyllabic words.[d]

continues

Table 1–5. *continued*

Characteristic	CAS	Other Speech Sound Disorders (artic/phono/dysarthria)
Inconsistency	Children with CAS produced inconsistent errors when repeating "Buy bobby a Puppy" repeated five times.[b] Children with CAS had a consonant substitute inconsistency percentage (CSIP) of over 24%.[e]	Children with other speech delays were consistent in their productions.[b] Children with phonological or articulatory disorders had a CSIP score of below 21%.[e]

[a]Data from "Speech Assessment in Children With Childhood Apraxia of Speech," by J. Iuzzini-Seigel and E. Murray, 2017, *Perspectives of the ASHA Special Interest Groups, 2*(2), 47–60, https://doi.org/10.1044/persp2.SIG2.47

[b]Data from "Speech Inconsistency in Children With Childhood Apraxia of Speech, Language Impairment, and Speech Delay: Depends on the Stimuli," by J. Iuzzini-Seigel, T. Hogan, and J. Green, 2017, *Journal of Speech, Language, and Hearing Research, 60,* 1194–1210, https://doi.org/10.1044/2016_JSLHR-S-15-0184

[c]Data from "School-Age Follow-Up of Children With Childhood Apraxia of Speech," by B. Lewis, L. A. Freebairn, A. J. Hansen, S. K. Iyengar, and H. G. Taylor, 2004, *Language, Speech, and Hearing Services in Schools, 35*(2), 122–140, https://doi.org/10.1044/0161-1461(2004/014)

[d]Data from "Differential Diagnosis of Children With Suspected Childhood Apraxia of Speech," by E. Murray, P. McCabe, R. Heard, and K. J. Ballard, 2015, *Journal of Speech, Language, and Hearing Research, 58*(1), 43–60, https://doi.org/10.1044/2014_JSLHR-S-12-0358

[e]Data from "A Comparison of Oral Motor and Production Training for Children With Speech Sound Disorders," by K. Forrest and J. Iuzzini-Seigel, 2008, *Seminars in Speech and Language, 29*(4), 304–311, https://doi.org/10.1055/s-0028-1103394

Suspected CAS in Children Before the Age of Three Years

Infants and toddlers who are not reaching the expected communication milestones in a timely manner may be suspected of having CAS and are unlikely to present with many of the characteristics listed earlier due to lack of vocalizations. For years, what was known about early communication skills in children later diagnosed with CAS was obtained by anecdotal reports (Highman et al., 2008). These children were often described as less vocal, having a limited sound repertoire, decreased babbling, simple syllable shapes, and limited suprasegmental patterns, with a later emergence of first words. In addition, it was reported they may experience a loss of words or phonemes, have difficulty with feeding, and have delayed fine and gross motor skills (Davis & Velleman, 2000; Highman et al., 2008). Highman et al. (2008) did a retrospective study comparing parent reports of children in three groups: (1) typically developing (TD), (2) suspected CAS (sCAS), and (3) specific language impairment (SLI). There were 20 children in each group, and they ranged from 3 to 5 years of age when their parents filled out the questionnaire. Their results supported previously reported observations, but there was some overlap of characteristics between children with CAS and children with SLI. Results are summarized in Table 1–6. Although it is helpful to know the red flags for CAS in the child's developmental history, it is important to be aware of the similarities and differences for the purpose of making a correct diagnosis.

In addition, 45% of children with SLI and sCAS were reported to have feeding problems compared to 15% of TD children. However, only 20% of children with SLI and 10% of TD

Table 1–6. Verbal and Motor Milestones of Typically Developing (TD) Children, Children With Specific Language Impairment (SLI), and Suspected CAS (sCAS)

Milestone	Typically Developing	SLI	sCAS
Verbal Milestones			
Vowel noises	4.9 months	8.2 months	8.2 months
Reduplicated babble	7.2 months	10.1 months	11.0 months
Variegated babble	9.2 months	12.2 months	Did not occur
First word	9.2 months	13.0 months	14.0 months
Two-word combinations	14.6 months	27.0 months	33.3 months
Nonverbal/Motor Milestones			
Smiled	6.9 weeks	16.8 weeks	8.6 weeks
Crawling	9.1 months	9.1 months	7.5 months
First steps unaided	11.7 months	12.5 months	13.6 months

Note. Adapted from "Retrospective Parent Report of Early Vocal Behaviours in Children With Suspected Childhood Apraxia of Speech (sCAS)," by C. Highman, N. Hennessey, M. Sherwood, and S. Leitao, 2008, *Child Language Teaching & Therapy*, *24*(3), 285–306, https://doi.org/10.1177%2F0265659008096294

children were reported to have dribbling issues compared to 45% of the children with CAS. When asked if their children babbled as *much as, more than,* or *less than* other children, 80% of parents of children with CAS and 70% of parents of children with SLI reported their children babbled less than other children, compared to only 5% of TD children (Highman et al., 2008).

Overby et al. (2019) analyzed home videos of infants and toddlers (birth to age 2 years) later diagnosed with CAS (LCAS) (*n* = 7), children with speech sound disorders (LSSD) (*n* = 5), and TD children (*n* = 5) to compare *volubility*, consonant emergence, and syllabic structure from birth to 2 years of age. Volubility refers to the amount of vocalization produced regardless of type. Early vocalizations were coded as *nonresonant vocalizations* (sounds that cannot be transcribed with the International Phonetic Alphabet, such as vegetative sounds) and *resonant vocalizations* (speechlike, including vowels and consonants, babbling, and words). Although children with LSSD had less volubility than TD children, children in the LCAS group had significantly less volubility of resonant utterances and consonants and higher volubility of nonresonant utterances than the children in the LSSD and TD groups. Examination of the diversity of resonant consonants and features of consonants revealed a similar trend, where children with LCAS had significantly less diversity of consonants and diversity of place and manner features than the other two groups. A summary of potential red flags for a later diagnosis of CAS from the findings of Overby et al. (2019) and Overby and Caspari (2015) are listed in Box 1–1.

When we consider the long-range implications of decreased variegated babble; reduced phonetic repertoire of sound, place, manner and voicing contrasts; and reduced syllable sequences, one can theorize that delays in these areas will not bode well for the child. If

■ **Box 1–1.** Early Vocal Characteristics Observed in Infants and Toddlers Later Diagnosed With CAS

1. Limited vocalization during the child's first 2 years

2. Lack of a resonant consonant by 12 months

3. Acquisition of three or fewer resonant consonants between 8 and 16 months old

4. Acquisition of five or fewer resonant consonants between 17 and 24 months of age

5. Dependency on bilabials, alveolars, stops, and nasals with a paucity of velars or posterior sounds before age 2 years

6. Productions of stops and nasals over a more diverse manner repertoire (e.g., fricatives and affricates)

7. Use of mostly vowels at 13–18 months with little use of simple consonant vowel sequences or more complex syllable structures

8. Lack of voiceless consonants between birth and 24 months of age

experience is the chief architect of the brain, the lack of vocalizations will negatively impact the cognitive-linguistic and motor aspects of phonology. This, in turn, will lead to less accurate phonological representations that affect language and literacy development (Miller et al., 2019; Overby et al., 2020; Velleman, 2011), which brings us to our next section.

Language and Literacy

The interaction of motor speech development, language, and literacy is fascinating and complex and will continue to keep researchers actively engaged for years to come. As we learn more about genetic variants that impact neurodevelopment and neural substrates and pathways implicated in CAS, one can see why a child with CAS is likely to be challenged in more than one area of motor and linguistic development. Hence, it is not surprising that as the child with CAS becomes more intelligible, we often begin to notice the co-occurrence of an expressive language disorder. Children with CAS frequently present with syntactic errors (e.g., word sequencing errors, omission of function words, and reduced mean length of utterance) and morphological errors (e.g., omission of plural "s" or past tense "ed" markers) (Crary, 1993; Ekelman & Aram, 1983; Murray et al., 2019). One might be inclined to believe that the linguistic errors are solely due to the child's motor speech challenges, since children with CAS have difficulty with complex syllable shapes and produce more errors as the utterance length increases (e.g., adding "s" to denote plurality or possession could increase the syllable shape complexity). However, some linguistic errors are not related to motor speech (e.g., gender pronoun errors ["she" for he], incorrect auxiliary substitutions ["is" for are], and omission of verbs in sentences) and may persist in children with CAS beyond the age at which these features should have been attained (Ekelman & Aram, 1983; Murray et al., 2019).

Research has also shown that children with CAS are at higher risk for difficulties in areas related to literacy, such as rhyming, word attack, word identification, spelling, phonological perception, phonological discrimination, and phonological memory (ASHA, 2007a). When a child has CAS or a persistent SSD, in addition to a language impairment, they are at even higher risk for having difficulties with reading and writing (Cabbage et al., 2018; Lewis et al., 2004; Miller et al., 2019). Lewis and colleagues (2004) conducted a follow-up of preschoolers with CAS and found that even when the children improved in articulation, they continued to have difficulties with syllable sequencing, nonsense word repetition, language, reading, and writing. Miller and colleagues (2019) assessed school-age children and adolescents (7–18 years) with sCAS and SSDs without CAS and compared measures on performance IQ, oral language, phonological awareness, rapid automatic naming, diadochokinetic rates, single word articulation, and multisyllable and nonsense word repetition. Results indicated that children with sCAS with language and phonological awareness deficits had poorer reading outcomes. Motor speech deficits and speech sound production also had an impact on reading outcomes, but to a lesser degree (Miller et al., 2019). The studies cited in this section represent a fraction of the research done in this area. Results of numerous studies looking at the relationship of CAS and linguistic-based disorders highlight the need for a comprehensive assessment of motor speech skills, in addition to language, phonological awareness, and literacy skills, when CAS is suspected.

Related Areas of Concern

Additional areas of concern are observed in some children with CAS. Parents may report problems with early feeding, clumsiness, or behavior challenges. The SLP may be the first person to observe delays in gross and fine motor coordination and/or sensory processing. These areas of related concern are described in more detail next.

Early Feeding Difficulties

Some children with CAS exhibit motor planning challenges during eating and drinking (Highman et al., 2008). They may have trouble coordinating their chewing and swallowing or their sucking and swallowing, causing them to eat slowly; stuff too much food in their mouths; hold the food for a long time before swallowing; or suck, suck, suck and then gulp their liquid, rather than using a rhythmic suck/swallow/breathe pattern. Management of mixed textures also may be challenging for some children with CAS. Feeding difficulties often are resolved by the time a child with suspected CAS is brought to the SLP for an initial screening or evaluation. Information about the child's prior feeding challenges can be obtained from a thorough case history. If feeding difficulties currently exist, it is important to determine if the underlying nature of feeding challenges in children with CAS is related to planning the coordinated oral movements for feeding tasks or to the child's muscular strength.

Gross and Fine Motor

Children with CAS often present with fine and gross motor delays (ASHA, 2007a), and many researchers have noted a relationship between *developmental coordination disorder* (DCD) and CAS (Duchow et al., 2019; Hodge, 1998; Iuzzini-Seigel, 2019).

DCD is a neurodevelopmental disorder in which a child's motor coordination difficulties significantly interfere with activities of daily living or academic achievement. These children typically have difficulty with fine and/or gross motor skills, with motor performance that is usually slower, less accurate, and more variable than that of their peers. (Zwicker et al., 2012, p. 573)

It is estimated that 5% to 6% of school-age children have DCD (Zwicker et al., 2012). When Duchow et al. (2019) examined results of standardized DCD parent questionnaires of 35 children with sCAS, they found that 49% of the children had possible DCD (pDCD). This supported their hypothesis of there being a significantly higher number of children with CAS having pDCD than the general population.

Iuzzini-Seigel (2019) examined fine and gross motor performance among 10 children with CAS, 16 children with SSD, and 14 TD children. The movement components assessed included manual dexterity, aiming and catching, and balance. When comparing the three groups, TD performed the best, followed by children with SSD, and then children with CAS. Eight of the 10 children with CAS obtained a standard score (SS) of 5 or lower, where the mean SS is 10, which indicates significant movement difficulty. When the children were compared based on the presence of a co-occurring language impairment (LI; CAS only = 3, CAS + LI = 7, SSD only = 10, SSD + LI = 6, and 14 TD children), children with CAS + LI had the poorest performance in all three areas. All seven of the children with CAS + LI received a SS of 5 or below, whereas only one of the three children with CAS performed this poorly. Although the sample size in this study was relatively small, the results highlight the importance of the additive risk factors that come with a diagnosis of CAS and LI, versus CAS alone. Research on concomitant fine and gross motor disorders also points to the importance of a team evaluation that includes occupational therapists and physical therapists.

Sensory Processing

It is also not uncommon for children with CAS to have some challenges with sensory processing (Newmeyer et al., 2009). This can include the ability to appropriately respond to and integrate auditory, vestibular, tactile, gustatory (taste), olfactory, visual, and/or proprioceptive input. Although parents and health care providers frequently see evidence of these issues in children with neurodevelopmental disorders such as ADHD, ASD, and CAS, the terms used to include it in a diagnosis vary and are not without controversy (Arky, n.d.; Newmeyer et al., 2009). For example, the diagnosis of Sensory Processing Disorder (SPD), often used by occupational therapists (OTs), may be listed on a child's report, but it is not in the *Diagnostic and Statistical Manual of Mental Disorders* (5th ed.; *DSM-5*; American Psychiatric Association, 2013) because it is not recognized as a distinct medical diagnosis. However, "sensory problems" is included as one of the criteria for the ASD diagnosis (Arky, n.d.). Hence, it is more prudent to describe the sensory issues a child exhibits than to use the term *SPD*. Keeping that in mind, it can certainly be helpful to obtain a sensory profile for children who appear to struggle in multiple areas, such as attention, behavior, and communication, since how they perceive their environment can influence how they respond in therapy. SLPs are wise to integrate activities that promote focus and motivation by considering the client's sensory preferences and aversions. Incorporating OT input on how to adapt activities to meet the sensory needs of the child, while working on the child's speech and language skills can be quite beneficial. Assessments and sensory profile checklists, which are further discussed in Chapter 2, can be helpful in identifying the areas in which a child exhibits difficulty.

Newmeyer and colleagues (2009) examined 38 children ages 3 to 10 years with sCAS using the *Sensory Profile* (Dunn, 1999). The *Sensory Profile* uses a parent/caregiver questionnaire and Likert scale to look at the areas of (a) sensory processing, (b) modulation, and (c) behavior and emotional responses, which are further broken down into other areas. Results indicated that the children with sCAS had significant differences in area (a) auditory, visual, touch, and multisensory processing; area (b) modulation of movement affecting activity level and sensory input affecting emotional responses; and area (c) behavioral outcomes of sensory processing. Factor cluster scores also revealed a significant difference in the areas of sensory seeking, emotionally reactive, oral sensory sensitivity, and inattention/distractibility.

Social-Emotional Considerations

Although research has looked at the social-emotional impact of speech and language disorders on children and adults in general, only a few studies have delved more into this concern for children, adolescents, and adults with CAS (Cassar et al., 2022; Lewis et al., 2021; Rusiewicz et al., 2018; Tarshis et al., 2020). In addition, Farinelli Allen and Babin (2013) and Rusiewicz et al. (2018) examined the social-emotional impact on the parent or caregiver of a child with CAS, as well. Tarshis and colleagues (2020) explore how communication challenges in CAS might impact social competencies in young children, as these young children are more apt to miss out on early opportunities to grow socially. Many parents of children with CAS fear that their children will not make friends when they go to school due to the isolation that comes with not being understood. This article takes a proactive approach to suggesting ways of implementing therapy to address both speech and social goals, which are discussed in Chapters 8 and 9.

Rusiewicz et al. (2018) examined the functional implications of CAS from the parent perspective. Forty parents of children ages 3 to 16 years with CAS were given two Likert-scale questionnaires and four open-ended questions about their personal experiences of living with a child with CAS. The majority of the parents (92%) reported a personal emotional reaction to their child being difficult to understand with feelings that ranged from frustration and sadness to heartbreak. Parents also reported that their children commented on feeling sad (33%), commented on feeling frustrated (22%), wished to be understood (22%), were asked why they had difficulty with speech production (11%), and expressed anger (11%). In addition, parents believed their child's speech impairment had a negative effect on peer interactions (42%), caused avoidance of situations (32.5%), affected play and play dates (27.5%), and decreased their participation in school and church activities (20%). Clinical recommendations to address these issues included creating online or face-to-face support networks for families impacted by CAS, empathizing with parents' stressors and anxiety related to their role as caregiver, and providing resources for professional support when possible.

As part of an ongoing longitudinal study, Lewis and colleagues (2021) examined the psychosocial outcomes of adolescents with a history of CAS and compared them to peers with histories of SSD only and SSD with language impairment. The psychosocial assessment battery included self-report and parent-report measures that looked at a wide range of mental health conditions, such as externalizing problems (e.g., aggression and destructive behavior), internalizing problems (e.g., anxiety, depression, withdrawal, somatic symptoms), ADHD, inattention, social problems, and thought problems (e.g., obsessive thoughts, self-harm, hallucinations, nervous twitching, strange behavior, or ideas). The most common areas in the borderline/

clinical range noted by the parents included social problems (41%), inattention (35%), and hyperactivity (24%), where children with histories of CAS self-reported social problems (29%), thought problems (29%), and internalizing problems (29%). Authors concluded that "adolescents with histories of CAS may experience more social problems, hyperactivity, and thought problems than adolescents with histories of milder SSD" (Lewis et al., 2021, p. 2578). Working with adolescents can be challenging regardless of there being a communication disorder or not. This study is a good reminder to monitor the client's mental health and realize that behavioral issues are often signs of needing additional help.

Cassar and colleagues (2022) examined the long-term consequences of CAS in adulthood. They looked at self-reported measures of speech, language, and literacy and the psychosocial impacts using the *Brief Fear of Negative Evaluation Scale-Revised (BFNE-R)* and the *State-Trait Anxiety Inventory (STAI)*. In addition, they obtained speech samples from 25% of the participants. On average, participants reported elevated levels of state anxiety (i.e., anxiety triggered by a stressful situation) and trait anxiety (i.e., anxiety due to a person's predisposition to react anxiously to a situation) when compared to normative data. In addition, 75% of respondents reported limited social interactions, 69% reported teasing or bullying, and 50% reported they avoided social functions because of their CAS. From the speech samples and self-reported measures, authors gleaned that many of the adults had ongoing segmental and suprasegmental errors. They concluded that both psychosocial effects and speech errors appeared to persist for adults with CAS. Consistent with prior research (Lewis et al., 2021; Rusiewicz et al., 2018; Tarshis et al., 2020), these findings stress the need for SLPs to be monitoring the mental health of their clients and be proactive in locating the psychosocial supports needed for optimal adjustment to the client's communication disorder. This is addressed further in Chapter 9.

Using the International Classification of Functioning, Disability and Health for Children and Youth (ICF-CY) to Guide Assessment and Treatment of Children With CAS

When choosing assessment tools, treatment goals, and ways of measuring progress, it is important to keep in mind the ICF-CY framework. This framework reminds the practitioner that it is imperative to have functional outcome measures that will ensure improved participation in all aspects of the child's life.

The ICF-CY offers a conceptual framework and a common language and terminology for recording problems manifested in infancy, childhood, and adolescence involving functions and structures of the body, activity limitations and participation restrictions, and environmental factors important for children and youth (WHO, 2007, p. xii).

The ICF-CY (WHO, 2007) is derived from the International Classification of Functioning, Disability and Health (ICF) (WHO, 2001). It was designed to be compatible with the ICF and provide more detailed information relevant to youth below the age of 18 years. It allows the person working with the child to focus on the interaction of how the health condition impacts the function of the body and how that, in turn, limits the child's participation in the environment they are in. Table 1–7 provides examples of the main areas under each category.

Consider how these areas interact with one another. Children with similarly severe CAS may have different levels of participation based on their environmental and personal factors.

Table 1–7. ICF-CY Components, Descriptions of Each Component, and Examples

ICF-CY Component	Description*	Examples
Health Condition/ Health Status	Disorder or Disease	1. CAS 2. Expressive language disorder 3. ASD
Functioning & Disability		
Body Functions & Structures	Physical, physiological, and cognitive processes that underlie a function. Deficits at any of these levels are impairments.	Impaired • Speech motor planning and programming • Language • Social communication
Activity	The integrated functional activity for which the body structures and mind are used. Deficits at this level are limitations.	Decreased • Intelligibility • Communication skills • Pragmatic skills
Participation	The integrated functional activity to accomplish tasks in daily life and participate in society. Deficits at this level are restrictions.	Restricted • Interaction with peers and turn-taking during games • Ability to answer questions appropriately in class • Interpersonal interactions and social relationships
Contextual Factors		
Environmental Factors	Attitudes and beliefs of the settings the child is in, such as school, home, clubs, and faith community.	• School provides appropriate services and there is a culture that does not tolerate bullying. • Supportive family, but financially struggling • Club members are not educated or understanding of neurodiversity.
Personal Factors	Attitude, beliefs, coping skills of the individual	• Low self–esteem • Easily frustrated • Able to laugh at their mistakes and works hard to overcome obstacles

*Descriptions of ICF–CY components were adapted from "Predicting Intelligibility: An Investigation of Speech Sound Accuracy in Childhood Apraxia of Speech," by K. Skoog and E. Maas, 2020, *CommonHealth*, 1, 44–56, https://doi.org/10.15367/ch.v1i2.397

Conversely, children with different diagnoses and levels of severity may have similar levels of participation based on their own environmental and personal factors. The beauty of the ICF-CY is that although we may not be able to remove the health condition, we can improve the child's activity and participation by making accommodations (e.g., providing augmentative and alternative communication, paraprofessionals, and increased time to respond) and decreasing the level of impairment (e.g., increasing speech intelligibility, language skills, and joint attention). We can also improve participation by addressing the contextual factors such as increasing understanding and inclusiveness of the people in the child's environment (e.g., school, home, community centers) and building resilience, persistence, and coping skills, in the child, themself.

References

Allison, K., & Hustad, K. (2018). Data-driven classification of dysarthria profiles in children with cerebral palsy. *Journal of Speech, Language, and Hearing Research, 61*, 2837–2853. https://doi.org/10.1044/2018_JSLHR-S-17-0356

American Psychiatric Association. (2013). *Diagnostic and statistical manual of mental disorders* (5th ed.). https://doi.org/10.1176/appi.books.9780890425596

American Speech-Language-Hearing Association. (n.d.). *Speech sound disorders: Articulation and phonology* [Practice portal]. https://www.asha.org/Practice-Portal/Clinical-Topics/Articulation-and-Phonology/

American Speech-Language-Hearing Association. (2007a). *Childhood apraxia of speech* [Position statement]. https://www.asha.org/policy/PS2007-00277/

American Speech-Language-Hearing Association. (2007b). *Childhood apraxia of speech* [Technical report]. http://static.crowdwisdomhq.com/asha/4735%20Technical%20Report.pdf

Arky, B. (n.d.). The debate over sensory processing: A look at the dispute over whether sensory symptoms constitute a disorder, and whether treatment works. *Child Mind Institute.* https://childmind.org/article/the-debate-over-sensory-processing/

Benway, N. R., & Preston, J. L. (2020). Differences between school-age children with apraxia of speech and other speech sound disorders on multisyllabic repetition. *Perspectives of the ASHA Special Interest Groups 2, 5*, 794–808. https://doi.org/10.1044/2020_PERSP-19-00086

Cabbage, K., Farquharson, K., Iuzzini-Seigel, J., Zuk, J., & Hogan, T. (2018). Exploring the overlap between dyslexia and speech sound production deficits. *Language, Speech, and Hearing Services in Schools, 49*, 774–786. https://doi.org/10.1044/2018_LSHSS-DYSLC-18-0008

Cassar, C., McCabe, P., & Cumming, S. (2022). "I still have issues with pronunciation of words": A mixed methods investigation of the psychosocial and speech effects of childhood apraxia of speech in adults.

International Journal of Speech-Language Pathology. https://doi.org/10.1080/17549507.2021.2018496

Chilosi, A. M., Lorenzini, I., Fiori, S., Graziosi, V., Rossi, G., Pasquariello, R., Cipriani, P., & Cioni, G. (2015). Behavioral and neurobiological correlates of childhood apraxia of speech in Italian children. *Brain and Language, 150*, 177–185. https://doi.org/10.1016/j.bandl.2015.10.002

Crary, M. A. (1993). *Developmental motor speech disorders.* Singular.

Davis, B. L., & Velleman, S. L. (2000). Differential diagnosis and treatment of developmental apraxia of speech in infants and toddlers. *Infant-Toddler Intervention, 10*(3), 177–192.

Dodd, B. (2021). Re-evaluating evidence for best practice in paediatric speech-language pathology. *Folia Phoniatrica et Logopaedica, 73*, 63–74. https://doi.org/10.1159/000505265

Duchow, H., Lindsay, A., Roth, K., Schell, S., Allen, D., & Boliek, C. (2019). The co-occurrence of possible developmental coordination disorder and suspected childhood apraxia of speech. *Canadian Journal of Speech-Language Pathology and Audiology, 43*(2), 81–93.

Dunn, W. (1999). *Sensory Profile.* Pearson.

Eising, E., Carrion-Castillo, A., Vino, A., Strand, E., Jakielski, K., Scerri, T., . . . Fisher, S. (2019). A set of regulatory genes co-expressed in embryonic human brain is implicated in disrupted speech development. *Molecular Psychiatry, 24*(7), 1065–1078. https://doi.org/10.1038/s41380-018-0020-x

Ekelman, B. L., & Aram, D. M. (1983). Syntactic findings in developmental verbal apraxia. *Journal of Communication Disorders, 16*(4), 237–250. https://doi.org/10.1016/0021-9924(83)90008-4

Farinelli Allen, L., & Babin, E. A. (2013). Associations between caregiving, social support, and well-being among parents of children with childhood apraxia of speech. *Health Communication, 28*(6), 568–576. https://doi.org/10.1080/10410236.2012.703120

Fiori, S., Guzzetta, A., Mitra, J., Pannek, K., Pasquari-ello, R., Cipriani, P., . . . Chilosi, A. (2016). Neuroana-tomical correlates of childhood apraxia of speech: A connectomic approach. *NeuroImage: Clinical, 12*, 894–901. https://doi.org/10.1016/j.nicl.2016.11.003

Fiori, S., Pannek, K., Podda, I., Cipriani, P., Lorenzoni, V., Franchi, B., . . . Chilosi, A. (2021). Neural changes induced by a speech motor treatment in childhood apraxia of speech: A case series. *Journal of Child Neurology, 36*(11). 958–067. https://doi.org/10.1177%2F08830738211015800

Fisher, S., Vargha-Khadem, F., Watkins, K., Monaco, A., & Pembrey, M. E. (1998). Localisation of a gene implicated in a severe speech and language disor-der. *Nature Genetics, 18*, 168–170. https://doi.org/10.1038/ng0298-168

Forrest, K., & Iuzzini-Seigel, J. (2008). A comparison of oral motor and production training for children with speech sound disorders. *Seminars in Speech and Language, 29*(4), 304–311. https://doi.org/10.1055/s-0028-1103394

Fowler, K. (2017). "An extended family with a domi-nantly inherited speech disorder" (1990), by Jane A. Hurst et al. *Embryo Project Encyclopedia* (2017, March 23). http://embryo.asu.edu/handle/10776/11455

Gibbon, F. E. (1999). Undifferentiated lingual ges-tures in children with articulation/phonological disorders. *Journal of Speech, Language, and Hearing Research, 42*(2), 382–397. https://doi.org/10.1044/jslhr.4202.382

Graham, S. A., & Fisher, S. E. (2015). Understanding language from a genomic perspective. *Annual Review of Genetics, 49*, 131–160. https://doi.org/10.1146/annurev-genet-120213-092236

Grigos, M. I., Moss, A., & Ying, L. (2015). Oral articula-tory control in childhood apraxia of speech. *Journal of Speech, Language, and Hearing Research, 58*(4), 1103–1118. https://doi.org/10.1044/2015_JSLHR-S-13-0221

Groenen, P., Maassen, B., Crul, T., & Thoonen, G. (1996). The specific relation between perception and production errors for place of articulation in devel-opmental apraxia of speech. *Journal of Speech, Lan-guage, and Hearing Research, 39*(3), 468–482. https://doi.org/10.1044/jshr.3903.468

Highman, C., Hennessey, N., Sherwood, M., & Leitao, S. (2008). Retrospective parent report of early vocal behaviours in children with suspected Childhood Apraxia of Speech (sCAS). *Child Language Teach-ing and Therapy, 24*(3), 285–306. https://doi.org/10.1177%2F0265659008096294

Hildebrand, M. S., Jackson, V. E., Scerri, T. S., Van Reyk, O., Coleman, M., Braden, R. O., . . . Morgan, A. (2020). Severe childhood speech disorder: Gene discovery highlights transcriptional dysregulation. *Neurology, 94*(20), e2148–e2167. https://doi.org/10.1212/wnl.0000000000009441

Hodge, M. M. (1998). Developmental coordination disorder: A diagnosis with theoretical and clinical implications for developmental apraxia of speech. *Language Learning and Education, 5*, 8–11. https://doi.org/10.1044/lle5.2.8

Hurst, J., Baraitser, M., Auger, E., Graham, F., & Norell, S. (1990). An extended family with a dominantly inherited speech disorder. *Developmental Medicine & Child Neurology, 32*, 347–355. https://doi.org/10.1111/j.1469-8749.1990.tb16948.x

Iuzzini, J., & Forrest, K. (2010). Evaluation of a com-bined treatment approach for childhood apraxia of speech. *Clinical Linguistics & Phonetics, 24*, 335–345. https://doi.org/10.3109/02699200903581083

Iuzzini-Seigel, J. (2019). Motor performance in children with childhood apraxia of speech and speech sound disorders. *Journal of Speech, Language, and Hearing Research, 62*, 3220–3233. https://doi.org/10.1044/2019_JSLHR-S-18-0380

Iuzzini-Seigel, J. (2021). Procedural learning, grammar, and motor skills in children with childhood apraxia of speech, speech sound disorder, and typically developing speech. *Journal of Speech, Language, and Hearing Research, 64*, 1081–1103. https://doi.org/10.1044/2020_JSLHR-20-00581

Iuzzini-Seigel, J., Hogan, T., & Green, J. (2017). Speech inconsistency in children with childhood apraxia of speech, language impairment, and speech delay: Depends on the stimuli. *Journal of Speech, Language, and Hearing Research, 60*, 1194–1210. https://doi.org/10.1044/2016_JSLHR-S-15-0184

Iuzzini-Seigel, J., Hogan, T. P., Guarino, A. J., & Green, J. (2015). Reliance on auditory feedback in chil-dren with childhood apraxia of speech, *Journal of Communication Disorders, 54*, 32–42. https://doi.org/10.1016/j.jcomdis.2015.01.002

Iuzzini-Seigel, J., & Murray, E. (2017). Speech assess-ment in children with childhood apraxia of speech. *Perspectives of the ASHA Special Interest Groups, 2*(2), 47–60. https://doi.org/10.1044/persp2.SIG2.47

Kadis, D., Goshulak, D., Namasivayam, A., Pukonen, M., Kroll, R., DeNil, L., . . . Lerch, J. (2014). Cortical thickness in children receiving intensive therapy for idiopathic apraxia of speech. *Brain Topography, 27*, 240–247. https://doi.org/10.1007/s10548-013-0308-8

Laffin, J. J., Raca, G., Jackson, C. A., Strand, E. A., Jak-ielski, K. J., & Shriberg, L. D. (2012). Novel candidate genes and regions for childhood apraxia of speech identified by array comparative genomic hybridiza-tion. *Genetics in Medicine, 14*(11), 928–936. https://doi.org/10.1038/gim.2012.72

Lehman Blake, M., & Hoepner, J. K. (2023). *Clinical neuroscience for communication disorders: Neuroanatomy and neurophysiology*. Plural Publishing

Lewis, B., Avrich, A., Freebairn, L., Hansen, A., Sucheston, L., Kuo, I., . . . Stein, C. (2011). Literacy outcomes of children with early childhood speech sound disorders: Impact of endophytes. *Journal of Speech, Language, and Hearing Research, 54*(6), 1628–1643. https://doi.org/10.1044/1092-4388(2011/10-0124)

Lewis, B., Benches, P., Tag, J., Miller, G., Freebairn, L., Taylor, G., Iyengar, S., & Stein, C. (2021). Psychosocial comorbidities in adolescents with histories of childhood apraxia of speech. *American Journal of Speech-Language Pathology, 30*, 2572–2588. https://doi.org/10.1044/2021_AJSLP-21-00035

Lewis, B. A., Freebairn, L. A., Hansen, A. J., Iyengar, S. K., & Taylor, H. G. (2004). School-age follow up of children with childhood apraxia of speech. *Language, Speech, and Hearing Services in Schools, 35*(2), 122–140. https://doi.org/10.1044/0161-1461(2004/014)

Liégeois, F., Morgan, A. T., Connelly, A., & Vargha-Khadem, F. (2011). Endophenotypes of *FOXP2*: Dysfunction within the human articulatory network. *Official Journal of the European Paediatric Neurology Society, 15*, 283–288. https://doi.org/10.1016/j.ejpn.2011.04.006

Marion, M., Sussman, H., & Marquardt, T. (1993). The perception and production of rhyme in normal and developmentally apraxic children. *Journal of Communication Disorders, 26*(3), 129–160. https://doi.org/10.1016/0021-9924(93)90005-U

Marquardt, T., Sussman, H., Snow, T., & Jacks, A. (2002). The integrity of the syllable in developmental apraxia of speech. *Journal of Communication Disorders, 35*(1), 31–49. https://doi.org/10.1016/S0021-9924(01)00068-5

Miller, G., Lewis, B., Benches, P., Freebairn, L., Tag, J., Budge, K., . . . Stein, C. (2019). Reading outcomes for individuals with histories of suspected childhood apraxia of speech. *American Journal of Speech-Language Pathology, 28*, 1432–1447. https://doi.org/10.1044/2019_AJSLP-18-0132

Morgan, A. T. (2020). Severe childhood speech disorder: Gene discovery highlights transcriptional dysregulation. *Neurology, 94*(20), e2148–e2167. https://doi.org/10.1212/WNL.0000000000009441

Morgan, A., Lauretta, M., & Feldman, H. (2021). CAS and genetics: Causes and testing, *Apraxia-Kids*. https://www.apraxia-kids.org/wp-content/uploads/2021/08/CAS-and-Genetics-Article.pdf

Morgan, A., & Webster, R. (2018). Aetiology of childhood apraxia of speech: A clinical practice update for paediatricians. *Journal of Paediatrics and Child Health, 54*(10), 1090–1095. https://doi.org/10.1111/jpc.14150

Morley, M., Court, D., & Miller, H. (1954). Developmental dysarthria. *British Medical Journal, 1*, 8. https://doi.org/10.1136/bmj.1.4852.8

Murray, E., McCabe, P., Heard, R., & Ballard, K. J. (2015). Differential diagnosis of children with suspected childhood apraxia of speech. *Journal of Speech, Language, and Hearing Research, 58*(1), 43–60. https://doi.org/10.1044/2014_JSLHR-S-12-0358

Murray, E., Thomas, D., & McKechnie, J. (2019). Comorbid morphological disorder apparent in some children aged 4–5 years with childhood apraxia of speech: Findings from standardized testing. *Clinical Linguistics & Phonetics, 33*(1–2), 42–59. https://doi.org/10.1080/02699206.2018.1513565

Namasivayam, A., Coleman, D., O'Dwyer, A., & van Lieshout, P. (2020). Speech sound disorders in children: An articulatory phonology perspective. *Frontiers in Psychology, 10*, 1–16. https://doi.org/10.3389/fpsyg.2019.02998

Newmeyer, A., Aylward, C., Akers, R., Ishikaway, K., Grether, S., deGrauw, T. . . . White, J. (2009). Results of the sensory profile in children with suspected childhood apraxia of speech. *Physical & Occupational Therapy in Pediatrics, 29*(2), 203–218. https://doi.org/10.1080/01942630902805202

Overby, M., Belardi, K., & Schreiber, J. (2020). A retrospective video analysis of canonical babbling and volubility in infants later diagnosed with childhood apraxia of speech. *Clinical Linguistics & Phonetics, 34*(7), 634–651. https://doi.org/10.1080/02699206.2019.1683231

Overby, M., & Caspari, S. S. (2015). Volubility, consonant, and syllable characteristics in infants and toddlers later diagnosed with childhood apraxia of speech: A pilot study. *Journal of Communication Disorders, 55*, 44–62. https://doi.org/10.1016/j.jcomdis.2015.04.001

Overby, M. S., Caspari, S. S., & Schreiber, J. (2019). Volubility, consonant emergence, and syllabic structure in infants and toddlers later diagnosed with childhood apraxia of speech, speech sound disorder, and typical development: A retrospective video analysis. *Journal of Speech, Language, and Hearing Research, 62*, 1657–1675. https://doi.org/10.1044/2019_JSLHR-S-18-0046

Peter, B., Matsushita, M., & Raskind, W. (2012). Motor sequencing deficit as an endophenotype of speech sound disorder: A genome-wide linkage analysis in a multigenerational family. *Psychiatric Genetics, 22*(5), 226–234. https://doi.org/10.1097/YPG.0b013e328353ae92

Potter, N. L., Kent, R. D., & Lazarus, J. A. C. (2009). Oral and manual force control in preschool-aged children: Is there evidence for common control? *Jour-

nal of Motor Behavior, 41(1), 66–82. https://doi.org/10.1080/00222895.2009.10125919

Potter, N., Nievergelt, Y., & Shriberg, L. (2013). Motor and speech disorders in classic galactosemia. *Journal of Inherited Metabolic Disorders Reports, 11*, 31–41. https://doi.org/10.1007/8904_2013_219

Rosenbek, J., & Wertz, R. (1972). A review of fifty cases of developmental apraxia of speech. *Language, Speech, and Hearing Services in Schools, 1*, 23–33 https://doi.org/10.1044/0161-1461.0301.23

Rusiewicz, H., Maize, K., & Ptakowski, T. (2018). Parental experiences and perceptions related to childhood apraxia of speech: Focus on functional implications. *International Journal of Speech-Language Pathology, 20*, 569–580. https://doi.org/10.1080/17549507.2017.1359333

Shriberg, L. D., Aram, D., & Kwiatkowski, J. (1997a). Developmental apraxia of speech: I. Descriptive and theoretical perspectives. *Journal of Speech, Language, and Hearing Research, 40*, 273–285. https://doi.org/10.1044/jslhr.4002.273

Shriberg, L. D., Aram, D. M., & Kwiatkowski, J. (1997b). Developmental apraxia of speech II. Toward a diagnostic marker. *Journal of Speech, Language, and Hearing Research, 40*(2), 286–312. https://doi.org/10.1044/jslhr.4002.286

Shriberg, L. D., Kwiatkowski, J., & Mabie, H. L. (2019). Estimates of the prevalence of motor speech disorders in children with idiopathic speech delay. *Clinical Linguistics & Phonetics, 33*(8), 679–706. https://doi.org/10.1080/02699206.2019.1595731

Shriberg, L. D., Strand, E., Jakielski, K. J., & Mabie, H. L. (2019). Estimates of the prevalence of speech and motor speech disorders in persons with complex neurodevelopmental disorders. *Clinical Linguistics and Phonetics, 33*(8), 707–736. https://doi.org/10.1080/02699206.2019.1595732

Skoog, K., & Maas, E. (2020). Predicting intelligibility: An investigation of speech sound accuracy in childhood apraxia of speech. *CommonHealth, 1*(2), 44–56. https://doi.org/10.15367/ch.v1i2.397

Strand, E. A. (2020). Dynamic temporal and tactile cueing: A treatment strategy for childhood apraxia of speech. *American Journal of Speech-Language Pathology, 29*(1), 30–48. https://doi.org/10.1044/2019_AJSLP-19-0005

Strand, E. A., & McCauley, R. J. (2019). *Dynamic Evaluation of Motor Speech Skill (DEMSS) manual.* Brookes.

Tarshis, N., Garcia Winner, M., & Crooks, P. (2020). What does it mean to be social? Defining the social landscape for children with childhood apraxia of speech. *Perspectives of the ASHA Special Interest Groups, 5*(4), 843–852. https://doi.org/10.1044/2020_PERSP-19-00116

Terband, H., Maassen, B., van Lieshout, P., & Nijland, L. (2011). Stability and composition of functional synergies for speech movements in children with developmental speech disorders. *Journal of Communication Disorders, 44*(1), 59–74. https://doi.org/10.1016/j.jcomdis.2010.07.003

Terband, H., Namasivayam, A., Maas, E., van Brenk, F., Mailed, M., Diepeveen, S., . . . Maassen, B. (2019). Assessment of childhood apraxia of speech: A review/tutorial of objective measurement techniques. *Journal of Speech, Language, and Hearing Research, 62*, 2999–3032. https://doi.org/10.1044/2019_JSLHR-S-CSMC7-19-0214

Vargha-Khadem, F., Gadian, D., Copp, A., & Mishkin, M. (2005). *FOXP2* and the neuroanatomy of speech and language. *Nature Reviews of Neuroscience, 6*, 131–138. https://doi.org/10.1038/nrn1605

Vargha-Khadem, F., Watkins, K. E., Price, C. J., Ashburner, J., Alcock, K. J., Connelly, A., . . . Passingham, R. E. (1998). Neural basis of an inherited speech and language disorder. *Neurobiology, 95*(21), 12695–12700. https://doi.org/10.1073/pnas.95.21.12695

Velleman, S. L. (2011). Lexical and phonological development in children with childhood apraxia of speech—A commentary on Stoel-Gammon's "relationships between lexical and phonological development in young children." *Journal of Child Language, 38*(1), 82–86. https://doi.org/10.1017/s0305000910000498

Velleman, S., & Mervis, C. (2011). Children with 7q11.23 duplication syndrome: Speech, language, cognitive, and behavioral characteristics and their implications for intervention. *Perspectives on Language Learning and Education, 18*(3), 108–116. https://doi.org/10.1044/lle18.3.108

Velleman, S., & Strand, K. (1994). Developmental verbal dyspraxia. In J. E. Bernthal & N. W. Bankson (Eds.), *Child phonology: Characteristics, assessment, and intervention with special populations* (pp. 110–139). Thieme Medical Publishers.

World Health Organization. (2001). *International classification of functioning, disability and health (ICF).* https://www.who.int/classifications/international-classification-of-functioning-disability-and-health

World Health Organization. (2007). *International classification of functioning, disability and health: Children and youth version (ICF-CY).* https://apps.who.int/iris/handle/10665/43737

Zwicker, J., Missions, C., Harris, S., & Boyd, L. (2012). Developmental coordination disorder: A review and update. *European Journal of Paediatric Neurology, 16*, 573–581. https://doi.org/10.1016/j.ejpn.2012.05.005

Assessment and Differential Diagnosis of Childhood Apraxia of Speech

As discussed in Chapter 1, children with childhood apraxia of speech (CAS) often have difficulties with expressive language, phonological awareness, speech perception, and literacy (Iuzzini-Seigel, 2019; Lewis et al., 2004; Murray et al., 2021; Zuk et al., 2018). In addition, they may exhibit dysarthria (Murray et al., 2015; Shriberg et al., 2019) and developmental coordination disorder (Duchow et al., 2019; Iuzzini-Seigel, 2019). Given the complexity of CAS, the overlapping characteristics with other speech sound disorders, and the likelihood of co-occurring disorders, differential diagnosis often requires a battery of assessments. Recent research on genetics and brain imaging further illustrates that CAS is often just one part of the puzzle to tease out in the midst of other potential challenges. The purpose of this chapter is to guide the reader with the most up-to-date assessments that can be used in the clinic, while accounting for the child's stage of development and potential co-occurring disorders. Our goal is to be as informed as possible regarding the nature of the sensorimotor planning deficit (in relation to any other deficits, such as cognitive, linguistic, and motor execution) (Strand, 2017).

Who Diagnoses CAS?

The American Speech-Language-Hearing Association (ASHA) Ad Hoc Committee on Apraxia of Speech in Children (ASHA, 2007) suggests that "A *well-trained speech-language pathologist with specific experience in pediatric speech sound disorders, including motor speech disorders* [emphasis added], is the appropriate professional to assess and diagnosis CAS" (ASHA Childhood Apraxia of Speech Technical Report, p. 53). Although other professionals working with a pediatric population—such as pediatricians, pediatric neurologists, or psychologists—may suspect apraxia, the speech-language pathologist (SLP) with training in sensorimotor speech disorders is specifically qualified to make a differential diagnosis and determine a course of action for treatment.

Conceptualizing Assessment

When a child is referred for an assessment for a speech delay or disorder, it is helpful to first conceptualize the basic elements of what is necessary for speech production. This is important for caregivers to understand as well. Few people fully appreciate the multiple processes that need to be intact to utter an intelligible meaningful utterance. Figure 2–1 may be useful when explaining the assessment outcomes to the parent, especially when there are cognitive and linguistic components involved.

A child can have decreased verbal output for a multitude of reasons. Hence, there is a lot to factor in during the assessment process for the SLP to determine which deficits are impacting the child the most and what strengths are available to build communicative success. Table 2–1 provides an overview of the key areas of assessment and why it is pertinent for a child suspected to have CAS. Each area is discussed in greater detail throughout the course of the chapter.

A Developmental Lens

How one assesses CAS is dependent on the child's age, other diagnoses, and the child's ability to imitate. ASHA's Childhood Apraxia of Speech Practice Portal (n.d.) suggests that making a definitive diagnosis of CAS prior to age 3 years is difficult due to the challenge of obtaining a sufficient speech sample. Hence, if characteristics of difficulty with sensorimotor planning and programming for speech are observed prior to age 3 years, ASHA recommends using the phrases "CAS cannot be ruled out," "signs are consistent with problems in planning the movements required for speech," or "suspected to have CAS." Additionally, diagnosing CAS before age 3 years can be problematic because the core characteristics of CAS do not easily differentiate children with CAS from other children. In other words, prior to age 3 years, even a typically developing child may present with inconsistent errors, vowel errors, and lexical stress errors (e.g., weak syllable deletion) (Iuzzini-Seigel & Murray, 2017; Kent & Rountrey, 2020; Masso et al., 2018). The child may also not be able or willing to attempt imitation. There is research, however, to guide the SLP to look for early signs of CAS (Overby & Caspari, 2015; Overby et al., 2019, 2020).

Assessment Recommendations for Children Under Age Three Years

Case History

Obtaining a case history and observing the child's vocalizations and communicative behaviors will assist in obtaining a good clinical picture of the toddler with delayed speech development. Given that CAS tends to be overdiagnosed (Shriberg et al., 2017), it is helpful to know which etiologies, vocal characteristics, and communicative behaviors are consistent with CAS versus other disorders. Clark and Baas (2021) remind the SLP to be mindful of the prevalence of CAS versus other speech sound disorders, as to not overdiagnose CAS. When children are younger, there are more overlapping characteristics between CAS and other causes for reduced verbal communication. It is helpful to remember that CAS accounts for less than 3% of speech sound

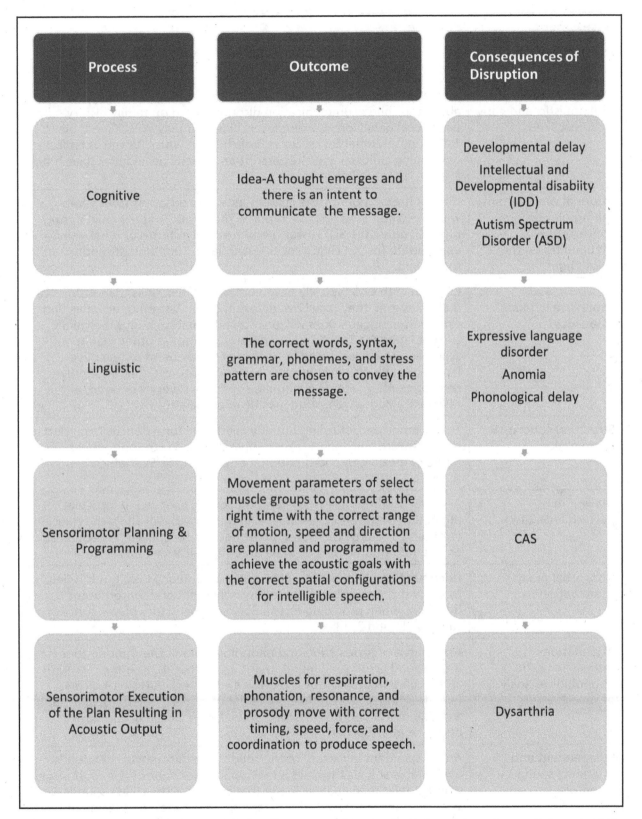

Figure 2–1. Basic conceptualization of what is necessary for speech. (Adapted from Caruso & Strand, 1999; Strand, 2020.)

Table 2–1. Key Areas of Assessment for Determining Relative Contribution of CAS to the Communication Disorder

Assessment	Purpose
Hearing evaluation	Make sure hearing acuity is optimal for speech development and that middle ear health is monitored.
History of feeding, prelinguistic, and early linguistic skills	A careful case history can yield information that leads to a hypothesis about the child's communication disorder based on family history, early vocal behaviors, sensorimotor skills, and play skills. (See Table 1–6 for developmental milestones of children with CAS versus typically developing children and the description of early developing speech that follows for reference.)
Informal observations during play or conversation (depending on the child's age)	It is not uncommon for the child to look very different from what was expected based on prior reports. Thus, watching the child during play will guide the SLP's assessment protocol in terms of what will be appropriate for the child's speech, language, cognition, attention, and social skills.
Receptive and expressive language assessment	Children with CAS typically have higher receptive skills than expressive skills; however, they may have delays in both. Assessing receptive and expressive language skills will provide information about the child's current language functions and determine if areas other than speech skills need to be addressed in treatment. Assessment of receptive language skills also may provide a window into the child's cognitive development. If receptive language skills are severely delayed, a referral for cognitive testing may be appropriate.
Structural-functional examination	This is important for ruling out any overt structural deficits (e.g., cleft palate, severe ankyloglossia) as well as deficits in strength, speed, range of motion, or coordination (i.e., dysarthria). See Tables 2–4 through 2–10.
Maximum performance tasks	Assessment of the five subsystems for speech production (articulation, phonation, respiration, resonance, and prosody) will allow the clinician to observe the physiological support needed for speech. Weakness and/or incoordination in any of these areas is indicative of dysarthria.
Nonverbal praxis examination	Nonverbal oral apraxia may or may not accompany CAS, but it is helpful to know if the child is able to follow nonverbal oral sensorimotor directions when providing instruction for articulatory placement. See Tables 2–11 and 2–12.
Articulation assessment with phonological analysis of speech errors	Assessment of articulation and phonology allows the clinician to see if the sound errors are limited to just a few sounds, as is the case with an articulation disorder or if there is a consistent pattern of errors (e.g., fronting, cluster reduction, initial consonant deletion), indicating a phonological delay or disorder. *A child with CAS may also have a phonological disorder.*
Independent and relational sound inventory	An independent inventory of the child's speech refers to the sounds and syllable shapes the child is making independent of the adult target, where a relational analysis is one that compares the child's sounds and syllable shapes to the adult target to see what they are missing or have in error. *For children with CAS, their independent inventory typically has more sounds than their relational inventory.*

Table 2–1. *continued*

Assessment	Purpose
Vowel assessment	Unlike children with phonological error patterns only (i.e., phonological delays/disorders), children with CAS often present with vowel errors in addition to errors on consonants. Special attention needs to be paid to the production of vowels during the articulation assessment and other speech samples, as these errors could easily go missed since vowel production is given less consideration in most standardized articulation tests. In addition, assessment of vowel errors is often overlooked in the training of SLPs. See Chapter 5 for additional information on assessment of vowels.
Prosody	Informal probes of the child's lexical and sentential stress patterns, use of pitch and loudness variation to signal linguistic differences, and observations of linguistically inappropriate pauses between sounds and syllables are all elements of prosody that can be impacted in CAS. (See Chapter 5 for additional information on assessment of prosody.)
Assessment of sensorimotor speech skills	A sensorimotor speech evaluation is designed to assess the child's ability to plan and program sequences of sounds by systematically increasing phonetic complexity, syllable shape, syllable length, and phrase length. The goal is to see where the child breaks down and if the child improves with cueing, such as saying the target word simultaneously while watching the clinician and responding to tactile cues. This element of the examination is crucial for choosing appropriate targets for treatment.
Phonological awareness and literacy skills	Children with CAS often have difficulty with phonological awareness, reading, and writing. Even after their sensorimotor speech skills have improved, there may still be delays in literacy. Assessment of phonological awareness and literacy skills will help determine if these skills need to be addressed in addition to or in the context of speech and language therapy.
Speech perception	Children with CAS and a co-occurring language impairment can have weak acoustic-phonetic representation, which can impact the ability to produce target phonemes.

disorders in preschool children, while developmental articulation and phonological disorders account for over 80% of speech sound disorders (Shriberg et al., 2019). In addition, it is not uncommon to see children with autism spectrum disorder (ASD) given a diagnosis of CAS, as they both present with reduced communication during the early stages of development. The prevalence of ASD is currently 1 in 44 (Maenner et al., 2021), much higher than CAS, which only occurs in 1 to 2 children per 1,000 (Shriberg et al., 2019). Since pediatricians are encouraged to screen for ASD at age 18 and 24 months (Lipkin & Macias, 2020) it would be appropriate for the SLP to inquire if the child had received the ASD screening during their well-child visit, especially if ASD is suspected. If the child did not receive a screening and ASD is suspected, an ASD checklist, such as the *Autism Parent Screen for Infants* (APSI; Sacrey et al., 2018), for children ages 6 to 24 months could be useful for determining if a referral for further testing is warranted. In addition, *Autism Navigator* (https://autismnavigator.com/) provides the *16 by 16 online screener for ASD*. If the parent notices eight or more of these 16 early signs by age 16 months, it is recommended they ask their doctor for a full diagnostic evaluation. Examples of these early signs include the child rarely sharing enjoyment or interests with the parent, not responding to their name, and little or no imitation of others or pretending. (See Table 2–25 for the URL.)

Although there are no standardized screening tools or assessment protocols for infants and toddlers that can provide a definitive diagnosis of CAS, there is research that supports observations that lead one to suspect CAS, such as reduced speech-like vocalizations, limited phonetic inventory of consonants and vowels, late emergence of first consonants and first words, and predominant use of simple syllable shapes (Davis & Velleman, 2000; Overby & Caspari, 2015; Overby et al., 2019). The case history questions in Appendix 2–A and the observation checklist in Appendix 2–B will guide and support the SLP's evaluation of the toddler. To get a better sense of the child's functioning in their home environment, it helps to ask the parent to walk you through a typical day with their child. This can bring to light information that we do not always get from the standard questionnaire. For example, the parent may share how difficult it is to get the child fed and dressed due to sensory issues or how their child does not vocalize as much as the other children in their play group. Providing a way for the parent to share their story in this manner can also help facilitate a stronger sense of connection and gives the SLP a chance to validate the feelings the parent may have. In addition to looking for early signs of CAS, the case history should address age of attainment of motor milestones and any concerns about ASD, auditory comprehension, dysarthria, feeding and swallowing, sensory issues, and behavioral concerns (e.g., difficulty getting joint attention, dislikes change in routine, frequent temper tantrums, aggressive behavior, etc.).

Considerations for Internationally Adopted Children

One population that is often overlooked when taking a case history are internationally adopted children (IAC). The vast majority of IAC are adopted after age 1 year, and thus the parent may feel there is not much to offer the SLP for diagnostic information on the traditional case history form. However, there are several variables that have been shown to impact the speech, language, social-emotional, cognitive, gross, and fine motor development of IAC that the parent can provide information about.

The SLP should inquire about the type of attention the child received prior to adoption. Each country has different standards of care, which can impact the child's development. Orphanage care varies greatly by region. Some children receive excellent care and services, while others are strained for resources, and children get minimal attention. A general rule of thumb is for every 3 months in an institution, expect 1 month of delay (Jenista, 1997). Some countries have foster care as an option to orphanages or large institutions. Children raised in foster care typically get more attention and language stimulation resulting in reaching developmental milestones at the appropriate times. Some children live in an orphanage prior to being placed in a foster home. It is also possible that the IAC were raised by their biological family and had to be adopted due to the loss of their parents. Although these children often fare better with attachment and development because of the attention they received in early development, the trauma of losing their birth family and being brought to another country needs to be considered.

The examiner will also want to know if there were any medical diagnoses that the child arrived with. These diagnoses are not always consistent with what is observed at the assessment but can be a good place to start. Some countries over diagnose disorders to make it easier for the country to relinquish the child, while other countries may downplay issues to make the child more likely to be adopted. If there are any medical records that came with the child, it helps to know there are international adoption clinics around the country that specialize in reviewing the adoptees' records. This is beneficial, as different countries use different terminology, and the international adoption clinic is able to discern the information that the records provide as they know what to expect from each country.

In regard to speech and language development, IAC often have delays in their first language due to environmental deprivation (Glennen, 2014). In addition, IAC will go through a quiet period as they transition to their new language. Unless the adopted family speaks the child's first language, they lose their first language and are usually caught up in their adopted family's language in 1 to 2 years. Studies done on age of adoption have shown that the younger the age of adoption, the faster the child should be acquiring their new language. Glennen's (2014) results on age of adoption and time needed exposed to the new language to achieve age-appropriate language skills is provided in Box 2–1. Box 2–2 provides additional resources for internationally adopted children.

Table 2–2 gives the SLP an alternative or supplemental developmental history questionnaire that will be more relevant to an adoptive parent than the traditional history forms.

■ Box 2–1. Amount of Time Exposed to New Language Needed for Acquisition

Age at adoption	Time to achieve expected language skills
1–2 years	15 months
3 years	2 years
4 years	3 years

■ Box 2–2. Additional Resources for Internationally Adopted Children

Resources

Working with Internationally Adopted Children
https://www.asha.org/practice/multicultural/intadopt/

Phonemic Inventories and Cultural and Linguistic Information Across Languages
https://www.asha.org/practice/multicultural/phono/

International Adoption Clinics
https://www.barkeradoptionfoundation.org/sites/default/files/International%20Adoption%20Medical%20Resources.pdf

Table 2–2. Questionnaire for Parents of Internationally Adopted Children (IAC)

1. How old was your child at the time of adoption?

2. Where was your child adopted from?

3. Was your child raised in an orphanage, foster care, or both?

4. Did the child have any time with their birth family prior to adoption?

5. What was the ratio of caregiver to child where your child was raised?

6. What medical diagnoses were you made aware of from the adoption agency?

7. Has your child or their records been reviewed by an international adoption clinic? If so, do you have that report to share?

8. What information did you receive about your child's speech and language development?

9. Describe the child's speech and language skill development since joining your family.

Speech and Language Assessment for Children Under Age Three Years

A child referred to an SLP at an early age for their lack of speech development is not apt to be at the point where they can participate in a formal articulation assessment. Hence, information from the case history and observations while building rapport during the play portion of the assessment will aid the SLP in checking for signs consistent with characteristics in children who later have a CAS diagnosis. The SLP will want to observe the child interacting with whomever they are most verbal to obtain the child's sound inventory and syllable shape inventory. Infants and toddlers do not always perform on command, so it may also be helpful to ask the caregiver to bring videos of the child from home. In addition to observing vocalizations and sounds, the SLP will want to note which communicative intents (e.g., request for help, items, activities, and attention, refusing or rejecting items and activities, labeling, describing, commenting, and expressing feelings) and what communication modalities they are using (e.g., gestures, sign, verbal approximations). Appendix 2–B provides a form to record this information and a checklist of the characteristics frequently observed in children later diagnosed with CAS.

It is important to note that these observations do not provide a definitive diagnosis. They do, however, indicate the child should receive early intervention. Sometimes families are told to take a "wait and see" approach. If this is the case, the family and/or physician may need additional evidence, encouragement, and support to obtain the appropriate services for their child in a timely manner.

Standardized expressive language assessments that require verbal responses will not be reliable measures of nonverbal or minimally verbal children for obvious reasons. In addition to it being too motorically difficult for the child to verbally respond, the parent may try to interpret what the child is saying, which can skew results. When assessing expressive language with a minimally verbal child, the informal observations listed earlier and in Appendixes 2–A and 2–B may reveal more than a test. However, receptive language assessments are especially useful for obtaining a more accurate diagnostic profile of the child's communication skills.

Parents often report that their child understands everything and that they just cannot talk. Sometimes this is accurate, but these observations are not necessarily valid and reliable, as the child can give the impression they understand more than they do by following the visual cues and routines that occur in the home rather than actually comprehending the sentences and vocabulary used in the directions. Appropriate language assessments and screenings for the birth to age 3 years population include the following:

- *Communication and Symbolic Behavior Scales (CSBS)* (Prizant & Wetherby, 2003) for ages 8 to 24 months (or up to 72 months if developmental delays are present)
- *Bayley Scales of Infant and Toddler Development Screening Test (Bayley-4 Screening Test)* (Bayley & Aylward, 2019) for ages 16 days to 42 months
- *Receptive-Expressive Emergent Language Test, Third Edition (REEL-3)* (Bzoch et al., 2003) for up to age 3.
- *MacArthur-Bates Communicative Development Inventories (MB-CDIs)* (Fenson et al., 2007)
  - *MB-CDI Words and Features* is designed for 8- to 18-month-old children.
  - *MB-CDI Words and Sentences* is designed for 16- to 30-month-old children.

The case history provided in Appendix 2–A will alert you to other areas that should be screened (e.g., ASD and cognition, sensory and motor deficits) to assist with making the appropriate referrals. ASD screenings were discussed earlier. Following are examples of screenings for other areas of development:

- *Hawaii Early Learning Profile (HELP: 0–3)* (Parks Warshaw, 2013) assesses cognitive, language, gross motor, fine motor, social-emotional, and self-help in children birth to age 3 years.
- *Westby's Symbolic Play Scale* (Westby, 1980) for children ages 17 months to 5 years (URL is provided in Table 2–25.)

Screening of hearing is also important, but an audiologist will be needed for children too young to respond to play audiometry.

Structural-Functional Exam for Children Under Age Three Years

Children under age 3 years may not be able or willing to follow instructions to participate in a formal structural-functional exam, as outlined in Tables 2–5 through 2–12. However, observing the child's face at rest is feasible and essential for checking to see if there is any dysmorphology that could impact function and/or be associated with a syndrome. It will also be vital to observe if the child is able to breathe at rest with a closed-mouth posture. An open-mouth posture can be indicative of a restricted upper airway (e.g., enlarged adenoid tissue, *choanal atresia*, deviated septum) and can negatively impact the development of the upper jaw, palate, dental occlusion, and muscles of the tongue. Function of the articulatory structures can be observed during eating, drinking, swallowing, laughing, and giving their parent a kiss. If the child happens to yell and/or cry during the evaluation, this will give you additional information on phonatory and respiratory support. Of course, we do not encourage eliciting these behaviors, but if it happens you can note voice quality, duration of phonation, and ability to vary loudness. Last, to determine function of the velopharyngeal mechanism, elicit oral and nasal consonants in syllables (e.g., "pa" or "pop" when popping bubbles and "mama" to get the mother's attention). Note if there is any nasal emission or nasalizing of oral sounds and if these errors are consistent or inconsistent to discern if the disordered resonance is due to structure, dysarthria, or CAS.

Assessment Report Summary for Children Under Age Three Years

The report should provide the SLP's diagnostic impressions of all areas of development observed and assessed during the evaluation. As previously stated, ASHA recommends using terms like *suspected CAS (sCAS)* if the child is under age 3 years, has characteristics consistent with CAS but does not have enough. It is not uncommon for parents to want a definitive diagnosis. This is understandable, as it gives them a place to look for help, such as other parents support groups, books, and online resources. At this point of the journey, parents need to be assured that their child is being treated in a manner that addresses all areas of concern to ensure the best outcomes for optimal communication. These little ones are dynamic beings who can change quickly in a period of months. In addition, it can take several therapy sessions to build trust and rapport to see what the child is truly capable of. In addition, there will be more time for dynamic assessment that will allow the SLP and parents to see the techniques the child responds to best. For example, a child with expressive language delay may not need the therapist to hold the toy up to their mouth to see the movement of the articulators to attempt imitation, where the child with a sensorimotor speech disorder will. Explaining these nuances to the parents may help them understand that a more definitive diagnosis will become easier over time.

Assessment for Children Over Age Three Years

When children are more capable of imitative tasks and following directions, which typically happens after age 3 years, there are more assessment tools available for the SLP. The next part of this chapter goes through the assessments that can be used for children in preschool through early school age. However, if the child has a developmental delay, is resistant or unable to do some of these tasks, it may be more appropriate to use the tools listed in the previous section. The areas of assessment listed do not have to be completed in any particular order. It is recommended to start in an area in which the child will be successful, such as pointing to pictures for a receptive vocabulary test versus labeling pictures for an articulation test. In addition, not all assessments will be appropriate for all children. For example, if the child is unable to attempt most of the words on a standardized articulation test, move on to the dynamic sensorimotor speech exam with simple syllable shapes and maximal cuing. Last, it can be helpful to set up a visual schedule of the assessments you hope to get through and make a game out of it. One trick is to put the pictures representing the tasks on a treasure map and when they get to the end of the map, they get to pick a prize out of the prize box. Between tasks, the examiner and child can play a mind-reading game where the child gets to put a different colored sticker on each pictured task once it is completed. The examiner is not allowed to look and has to guess which color the child chose. If the examiner gets it wrong, the child gets a point; if the examiner gets it right, the examiner gets a point. Needless to say, the child wins in this scenario, giving the child something to feel good about. Dr. Nancy Potter, who came up with this motivator, has managed to assess thousands of children with this little game, so it comes highly recommended.

Case History

The case history form provided in Appendix 2–C is appropriate for young children in general; however, as the child enters kindergarten, other questions related to language and early literacy are essential. As mentioned before, it is helpful to ask the parent to walk you through a typical day with their child. This will provide additional insight into how this child's communication and coping skills are impacting them in their activities of daily living. An example case history form for children preschool age through second grade can be found in Appendix 2–C. For children grades 3 and up, it will be important to ask about the child's family history of communication and/or learning challenges, therapy history, academic history, how the child copes with having a communication disorder, and what the child enjoys and has strengths in. In regard to their therapy history, we want to know the services they have received (e.g., occupational therapy, physical therapy, speech-language therapy, etc.), when they started receiving services, how often they received services, what were their goals, what therapy techniques they did and did not respond well to, how much progress they made, and what were the results of past assessment reports. For academic history, ask about services the child received and currently receives from the school and for past and present Individualized Education Programs (IEPs).

Hearing Screening

All children should receive a hearing screening. Refer to ASHA guidelines on Pure-Tone Screening Procedures provided in the link in Table 2–25. Play audiometry may be needed for conditioning children between 3 and 5 years of age to respond appropriately. Table 2–3 provides basic instructions and an example of a hearing screening form.

Structural-Functional Assessment (SFA)

It is not uncommon for SLPs to overlook doing a structural-functional assessment. A study by Murray and colleagues (2015) found that of the 47 participants in their study on differential diagnosis of CAS, three had undiagnosed submucous cleft, and six had dysarthria. This is consistent with a recent study, where the majority (60%) of SLPs surveyed had low or no confidence

Table 2–3. Basic Hearing Screening Protocol

Pure-tone hearing screening in quiet room: Administer 2+ conditioning trials @ 40 dB HL prior to hearing screen. Limited to four presentations/pure tone.				
	500 Hz @ 25 dB HL	1000 Hz @ 20 dB HL	2000 Hz @ 20 dB HL	4000 Hz @ 20 dB HL
Right				
Left				

in diagnosing dysarthria and 40% reported they don't make the diagnosis (Iuzzini-Seigel et al., in press). A cursory SFA should be done on all children with a speech sound disorder, and a more thorough SFA will be necessary for children with suspected neurological deficits and/or craniofacial anomalies. The full structure-function praxis exam is in Appendix 2–D, as well as in the online materials, and can be copied for your use. For the purpose of this chapter, each part is broken down. Table 2–4 illustrates the portion of the exam that provides observation of the structures at rest and a place to comment on relevant history. The examiner is just being

Table 2–4. Assessment of Structures

Name: _____ Date: _____ Age: _____

History regarding chewing, drooling, swallowing, oral aversion, sensory issues, TMJ issues, etc.

Structure & Tone (observe at rest)

Structure (STR)	Comments	Within Functional Limits (WFL)	Deviant
Cranial/facial symmetry			
Eyes			
Ears			
Lips			
Mandible			
Dentition			
Occlusion			
Tongue (symmetry at rest)			
Length of lingual frenulum			
Hard palate			
Velum			
Observations Relating to Tone		**Absent**	**Present**
Drooling			
Open mouth posture			

asked to judge if structures and muscle tone appear within functional limits (WFL) or deviant. If a structure is marked as deviant, a description should be provided in the comments section. When observing structures at rest, note any involuntary movements in addition to structural differences. Although not directly related to speech production, eyes and ears are included in the list to guide the examiner to look for features that often accompany a syndrome. As discussed in Chapter 1, there are several syndromes in which CAS may occur. For example, children with Noonan syndrome, who sometimes present with CAS, often have wide-set eyes and low-set ears. Sometimes these features are subtle at birth and become more apparent as the child grows; hence, they could have been missed by other practitioners. If a child presents with noticeable dysmorphology, they should be referred to a geneticist for further testing.

The next portion of this assessment involves the functions of the structures for articulation and resonance and the cranial nerves that innervate them (Table 2–5). This part of the exam allows the SLP to see if there is any evidence of dysarthria. Characteristics of dysarthria include decreased *strength*, speed, range of motion, and coordination of the muscles needed for speech. There may also be increased or decreased *tone*. Tone is related to strength, but it is not the same thing. Tone refers to the tension of the muscle at rest. Strength refers to the child's ability to recruit the muscles during contraction (i.e., not at rest) and is observed during purposeful movement. A child may have low tone, but strength is WFL for speech, which can be seen in children with CAS. If tone is too low (hypotonia) or too high (hypertonia), the muscles will not

Table 2–5. Oral Motor Function (OMF) Section of the Structural Functional Assessment

Structure	Performance		
Tongue-CN XII	WFL	Mild–Moderately Impaired	Severely Impaired
Protrusion *"Stick out your tongue."* Look for deviation to left or right and range of motion (ROM).			
Elevation *"Can you touch your tongue to your nose?"* (Or place a tongue depressor over the upper lip and say, *"Touch the stick with your tongue."*) Tongue tip should elevate to the upper lip without lower lip/jaw assistance.			
Tongue wag *"Can you move your tongue like mine?"* Model tongue movement from corner to corner for three complete back-and-forth sequences. Observe child's attempt for speed, coordination, and ROM.			
Lateral tongue strength *"I'm going to try to push your tongue. Don't let me."* With jaw approximately half open, have the child push against tongue depressor on each side. Note resistance.			

continues

Table 2–5. *continued*

Structure	Performance		
Lips-CN VII	**WFL**	**Mild–Moderately Impaired**	**Severely Impaired**
Pucker *"Say (oo)"* Look for symmetry and ROM.			
Retraction *"Say (ee)"* Look for symmetry and ROM.			
Pucker to retraction *"Say (oo-ee x 3)"* Look for symmetry, ROM, and speed.			
Strength of lips pressed together *"Bite your teeth together. Now press your lips together. I'm going to try to pull your lips apart, but don't let me."* Apply upward pressure against upper two quadrants and downward pressure against lower two quadrants to check for resistance with a tongue depressor or gloved finger. If any weakness is observed, note which quadrant—upper right (UR), upper left (UL), lower right (LR), lower left (LL).			
Jaw-CN V			
Symmetry, ROM, and stability during jaw opening and closing *"Open and close your jaw x 2."* Look for smooth movement, symmetry, appropriate excursion, and evidence of jaw sliding.			
Velum-CN IX and X			
Velar elevation during sustained "ah" *"Say ah for 5 seconds. I'll tell you when to start and stop."* Look for timing of movement, ROM, symmetry, and endurance.			
Velar elevation during staccato production of "ha" *"Say ha-ha-ha."* Look for timing of movement, symmetry, and ROM.			

be able to respond to resistance as well. For example, when the child is told to resist having their tongue pushed to the side with the tongue depressor, a tongue that seems soft and mushy would indicate hypotonia. When assessing these structures, it can be helpful to have a reference of the cranial nerves on hand, as in Figure 2–2.

A summary of findings from the structural-functional exam should include observations of symmetry and tone of structures at rest, dysmorphology, and observations of range of motion, symmetry, speed, strength, and coordination during movement tasks. If all structures and function of structures appear WFL, this will be important to note as it decreases the possibility of the speech sound disorder being due to dysarthria or structural differences, such as cleft or a severe malocclusion. Conversely, list anything that appears not to be WFL and how these differences may or may not impact the child's speech production.

Assessing the Subsystems

The next section of the structural-functional exam assesses the subsystems of speech (i.e., respiration, phonation, articulation, resonance, prosody) and how they work together. This is particularly important when differentiating dysarthria from childhood apraxia of speech when a motor speech disorder is suspected (Iuzzini-Seigel et al., in press; Levy et al., 2021). Levy and colleagues (2021) diagnose dysarthria as present when characteristics are observed in at least two of the speech subsystems.

Resonance

Table 2–6 provides oral and nasal speech tasks to assess the resonance. SLPs are good at judging if resonance is disordered or not but have difficulty perceiving if the child sounds hypernasal versus hyponasal. To assist with judgment of resonance, use a listening tube or straw going from under one of the client's nostrils to the listener's ear, or place a small mirror under the nostrils while the client repeats the following stimuli. If the child is hypernasal, /b/ will sound more like /m/, which the listening tube will make more noticeable. If they have nasal emission, it will be felt through the tube or seen on the mirror as fog. If the child is hyponasal, /m/ will sound more like /b/, and there will be very little acoustic energy coming through the listening tube. Try listening to the differences using this technique on yourself before using it with a child and experiment with being hyponasal, hypernasal, and producing nasal emission to become acquainted with the differences. If the phrases are too difficult, have the child repeat the syllables instead. If resonance is consistently hypernasal or hypernasal with nasal emissions, the child may have dysarthria (velopharyngeal impairment) or insufficient tissue, as in the case of submucous cleft, unrepaired cleft, or a repaired cleft that needs a secondary repair for better closure. If the child is consistently hyponasal, there is most likely an obstruction keeping them from having good airflow through the nose. If it is inconsistent, it is more apt to be due to sensorimotor planning and indicative of CAS. If the child uses glottal stops /ʔ/ in place of /b/, /p/, and /s/ on the stimuli that follow, you will not be able to judge velopharyngeal (VP) function, as the child is bypassing the need to close the VP port. Children with velopharyngeal insufficiency often use this substitution to avoid nasal air escape on oral consonants. However, children with CAS may also use a glottal stop substitution as part of their reduced phonetic repertoire.

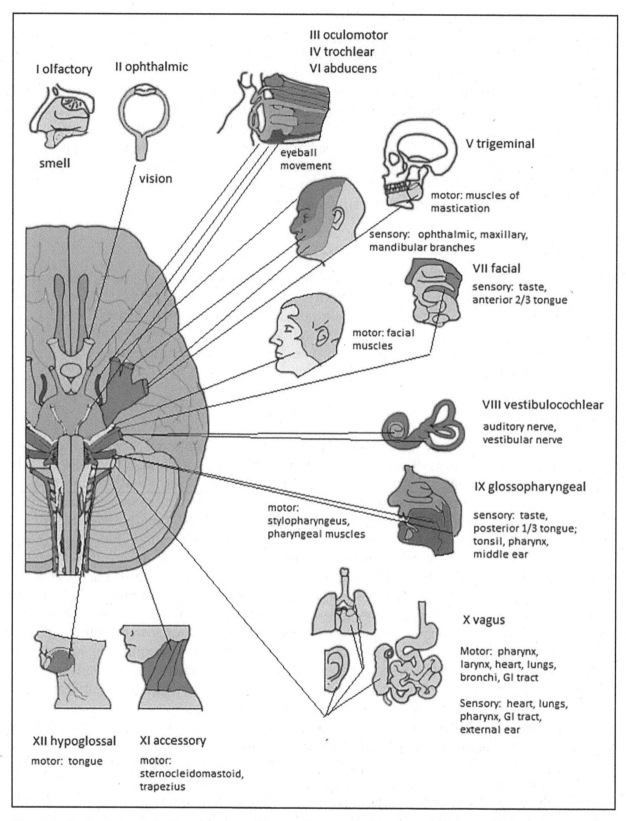

Figure 2–2. Cranial nerves. (From *Neuroanatomy and neurophysiology for speech and hearing sciences*, by A. Seikel, K. Konstantopoulos, and D. Drumright, 2020, p. 219, Figure 7–1A. "Source: After view of Carpenter," 1991. Copyright 2020 by Plural Publishing.)

Table 2–6. Resonance

	Normal	Hypernasal	Nasal Emissions	Hyponasal
Buy Bobby a puppy* **Pa pa pa**				
Seesaw, Seesaw, Seesaw **Sa sa sa**				
Mama made lemonade **Ma ma ma**				
Conversational speech				

*"Buy Bobby a puppy" will also be used later in the assessment to look at inconsistency.

Maximum Performance Tasks for Respiration, Phonation, and Articulation

Maximum performance tasks (MPTs) are also part of the structural-functional examination and are useful in determining the relative involvement of dysarthria versus CAS. They are used to "determine the upper limits of the speech-motor capacities of respiration, phonation, and articulation" (Thoonen et al., 1999, p. 5). Assessment of maximum duration of phonation and exhalation allows the clinician to judge the respiratory and phonatory subsystems, while the multiple syllable rate tasks provide a measure to assess articulatory movement speed, coordination, sequencing, and accuracy. Thoonen et al. (1999) were able to differentiate children with *spastic dysarthria* from children with CAS, children with other speech sound disorders (e.g., articulation and phonological delay/disorder), and children without speech sound disorders based on diadochokinetic (DDK) rates, articulatory accuracy of trisyllabic sequences, and length of maximum phonation duration.

Table 2–7 provides the respiration and phonation portions of the exam. The child should be given multiple attempts and models to obtain their maximum performance, especially if they appear reticent about the task. For the maximum exhalation duration (MED) task, instruct the child to take a deep breath, then blow steadily for as long as they can through a standard elbow straw submerged in 5 cm of water in a cup. Tell them to avoid splashing water when they blow bubbles to get a steady airstream. Sometimes children just give it all they have in one or two seconds, which does not give the examiner a true sense of how long they can sustain controlled exhalation. For the maximum phonation duration (MPD), instruct the child to take a deep breath then say /ah/ with a normal volume for as long as they can. These tasks are not standardized, so providing coaching and motivators is encouraged. For example, it could be turned into a contest among the examiner, the parent, and the child, being sure to allow the child to win. Showing your stopwatch or using visual feedback of a real-time waveform on Audacity can help the child see how long they are holding the sound out for, while providing the clinician the time. For younger kids, the Bla Bla Bla app might be fun (Bravo, 2017). The Bla Bla Bla app is free on iPads and iPhones and has a cast of black-and-white drawn characters to choose from. The louder the child is, the larger the character's mouth gets. The child could be instructed to keep the character's mouth open as long as possible.

Table 2–7. Assessment of Respiration and Phonation

Phonation-Respiration Duration	Trial 1	Trial 2	Trial 3	Longest of Three Trials
Maximum exhalation duration (MED) Have a cup of water with a straw positioned so the low end is 5 cm below the surface of the water. You may need to plug the child's nose to avoid air escape. *"Blow through the straw and make bubbles for as long as you can in one breath. I'll go first."*				
Maximum phonation duration (MPD) *"Say /ah/ for as long as possible. I'll go first."*				
If the child is able to produce multisyllable utterances, note the number of syllables the child can say in one breath group and if the child appears to be running out of breath by the end of the sentence or taking a breath in linguistically inappropriate places. _____ _____				

Phonation-CNX

Observations of Phonatory Quality and Control	Normal	Abnormally High or Low Pitch	Reduced Pitch Range	Strained/ Strangled	Breathy	Rough	Tremor/ Flutter/ Pitch Instability
Sustained Phonation* *"Say /ah/ steadily for as long as you can. I'll go first."*							
Pitch Range *"Sing ah, then go as low as you can. Sing ah again and then go as high as you can. I'll go first."*							
Spontaneous Speech Observe the child's pitch range and voice quality during a connected speech sample.							

*You can note your observations of sustained phonation from the last task, rather than having the child sustain phonation again.

When interpreting results from the maximum phonation duration and exhalation duration tasks, compare them to normative data. Table 2–8 provides norms for children ages 3 to 12 years based on 160 typically developing children (Potter, unpublished data). Reduced exhalation and phonation duration can be indicative of dysarthria, especially when a strained or breathy voice quality is present and DDK rates are reduced. The ability to vary pitch may be reduced for children with CAS, as well as dysarthria; however, it will be more difficult for the child with dysarthria when phonation and respiration are involved. Using an app like Voice Analyst that provides real-time feedback for pitch may help in eliciting a wider pitch range for children with CAS, as it provides a visual target.

Articulation-DDK Task

The last portion of the structural-functional exam is the DDK task, the maximum performance task for articulation. DDK rates are calculated for two different types of tasks: (a) the alternate movement rate (AMR) task, where the client repeats the same syllable multiple times, as in /pʌpʌpʌpʌpʌ/; and (b) the sequential movement rate (SMR) task, as in /pʌtʌkʌ/. DDK rates are calculated using a time-by-count measurement (Fletcher, 1972), where you calculate syllables per second by dividing the number of repetitions produced by the number of seconds it took to produce them. The child may be instructed to say as many repetitions of the stimuli as fast as they can for 5 seconds. If they produced 20 syllables in that time, they would have a DDK rate of four syllables per second. Conversely, you could determine the amount of time used to produce a set number of repetitions. For example, the child is timed on how long it takes to produce seven repetitions. The calculation is the same in terms of dividing the number of repetitions by the amount of time it took. For a more representative rate, remove the first production and last production of the repetitions. For example, if the child produced seven repetitions in an SMR task, calculate syllables per second on the middle five productions. If they produced five repetitions in an AMR task, remove the first and last /pʌtʌkʌ/ (Potter, 2004).

Table 2–8. Normative Data on Maximum Phonation Duration (MPD) and Maximum Exhalation Duration (MED) Based on 20 Males and 20 Females Per Age Group

Ages in Years	MPD Mean (SD) in Seconds	MED Mean (SD) in Seconds
3–4	3.45 (1.23)	6.08 (2.61)
5–7	11.65 (4.09)	11.13 (6.00)
8–9	14.23 (4.96)	13.72 (6.18)
10–12	15.77 (6.02)	17.55 (7.75)

Note. Adapted from "Developmental Outcomes in Duarte Galactosemia," by G. S. Carlock, T. Fischer, M. E. Lynch, N. L. Potter, C. D. Coles, M. P. Epstein, . . . J. L. Fridovich-Keil, 2019, *Pediatrics, 143*(1), p. e20182516; *Oral/ speech and manual motor development in preschool children* (Publication No. 3155158), by N. L. Potter, 2004 [Doctoral dissertation, University of Wisconsin–Madison], ProQuest Dissertations and Theses Global.

To prepare for the DDK task, you will need a stopwatch and an audio recorder. Alternatively, you can do the recording on any free sound editing software, like Audacity. This is efficient and provides more accurate results. Figure 2–3 provides example waveforms of typical speech and disordered speech during repetitions of /pʌtʌkʌ/. Each burst represents a syllable, and the time is visible on the *x*-axis above the waveform. In example A (typical speaker's production), there are 32 syllables produced over 5 seconds, yielding a DDK of 6.4 syllables a second. Note that the waveform is fairly rhythmic. In example B, the speaker has a reduced

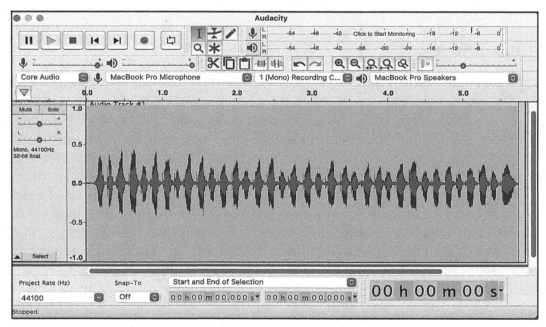

A

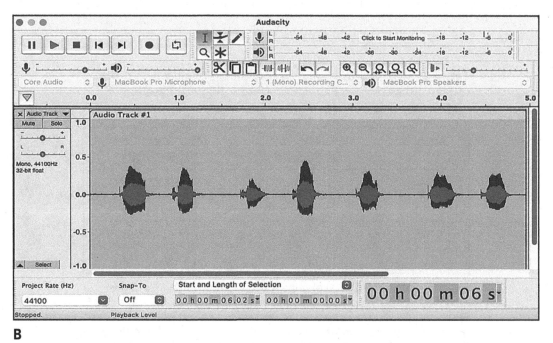

B

Figure 2–3. A. Waveforms representing /pʌtʌkʌ/ being repeated multiple times over 5 seconds by a speaker with typically developing speech. **B.** A speaker with CAS + dysarthria.

rate of 1.4 syllables a second, and the production is dysrhythmic. This is more indicative of a child with a sensorimotor speech disorder. Table 2–9 provides an example of the recording form for calculating the DDK rates.

Table 2–10 provides comparative data from a compilation of multiple studies for children without speech disorders (Kent et al., 2021). The ranges represent the lowest mean DDK rate to the highest DDK rate reported in these studies, with outliers removed from averages and ranges.

Table 2–9. Diadochokinetic (DDK) Calculation Form

DDK	Trial 1	Trial 2	Trial 3	Highest DDK Rate of the Three Trials
/pʌ/	_____ syllables/ _____ seconds = _____ syll/sec	_____ syllables/ _____ seconds = _____ syll/sec	_____ syllables/ _____ seconds = _____ syll/sec	= _____ syll/sec
/tʌ/	_____ syllables/ _____ seconds = _____ syll/sec	_____ syllables/ _____ seconds = _____ syll/sec	_____ syllables/ _____ seconds = _____ syll/sec	= _____ syll/sec
/kʌ/	_____ syllables/ _____ seconds = _____ syll/sec	_____ syllables/ _____ seconds = _____ syll/sec	_____ syllables/ _____ seconds = _____ syll/sec	= _____ syll/sec
/pʌtʌkʌ/	_____ syllables/ _____ seconds = _____ syll/sec	_____ syllables/ _____ seconds = _____ syll/sec	_____ syllables/ _____ seconds = _____ syll/sec	= _____ syll/sec

Table 2–10. Diadochokinetic (DDK) Comparative Data in Syllables/Second for Ages 2–15 Years

Ages in Years	/pʌ/ Mean (range)	/tʌ/ Mean (range)	/kʌ/ Mean (range)	/pʌtʌkʌ/ Mean (range)
2–3[a]	3.86 (3.46–4.74)	3.83 (3.38–4.56)	3.56 (3.36–3.75)	3.41 (2.82–4.23)
4–5	4.21 (3.62–4.92)	4.35 (3.54–4.82)	3.89 (3.00–4.76)	3.70 (2.86–4.47)
6–7	4.45 (3.93–5.56)	4.46 (3.42–5.88)	4.04 (3.33–4.74)	3.86 (2.91–4.74)
8–9	4.78 (4.54–5.88)	4.7 (4.30–5.88)	4.26 (4.12–4.49)	4.32 (3.85–5.19)
10–11	5.1 (4.63–5.56)	5.03 (4.66–5.56)	4.62 (4.50–5.00)	4.92 (4.22–5.46)
12–15	5.9 (4.76–6.06)	5.25 (4.46–6.06)	4.91 (4.39–5.40)	5.55 (4.35–6.66)

[a]Although data are available for 2- to 3-year-old children, it is not always possible to elicit the productions in a reliable and valid manner.

Note. Adapted from "Oral and Laryngeal Diadochokinesis Across the Life Span: A Scoping Review of Methods, Reference Data, and Clinical Applications," by R. D. Kent, Y. Kim, and L. Chen, 2021, *Journal of Speech, Language, and Hearing Research*, 1–50 (https://doi.org/10.1044/2021_JSLHR-21-00396).

In addition to comparing the child's DDK rates to the norms, note observations on rhythmicity, articulatory accuracy, voicing errors, sequencing errors, addition of a segment, deletion of a segment, consistency of errors, and ability to complete task. You can also compare the effort observed in producing AMRs to the SMR task. By the end of the structural-functional examination, you will be able to provide a summary that provides evidence of indicators for apraxia, dysarthria, a combination of the two, or neither.

Another helpful part of the exam is the nonverbal oral motor apraxia (NVOA) exam. Children who have difficulty with sensorimotor planning of sequences of movement for speech may also have difficulty sequencing oral movement for nonspeech tasks. However, a child does not have to have NVOA to be diagnosed with CAS, nor does a child necessarily have CAS if they have NVOA. Table 2–11 provides a brief examination of NVOA.

To provide scores for comparison on this NVOA task, data were retrieved from a study where children with galactosemia were compared to a control group (Carlock et al., 2019). The data provided in Table 2–12 are from 261 children ages 6 to 12 years without a speech sound disorder, as judged by having a *GFTA-3* standard score of 76 or higher. These scores indicate

Table 2–11. Examination for Nonverbal Oral Apraxia (NVOA)

Single Nonspeech Oral Movements

Give verbal directions, then model if necessary.

0 = imitates immediately
1 = mild groping; or delayed but successful
2 = groping or sequential efforts (up to four tries), then success
3 = could not achieve imitation even though there is purposeful effort
4 = Child does not/cannot attempt to do the task

	Blow out a candle	Smile	Puff out your cheeks	Smack your lips together	Clear your throat	Bite your lower lip
Score						

Sum Single Nonspeech Oral Movements Score _____ (0–24 possible)

Nonspeech Movement Sequencing (NSMS)

Give verbal directions, then model if necessary (same scoring as above).

	Smile, Blow, Smile	Smack your lips together, then clear your throat	Sip through a straw, then bite your lower lip	Open your mouth wide, then lick the back of your top teeth	Smile, Blow, Smile	Smack your lips together, then clear your throat
Score						

Sum NSMS Score _____ (0–16 possible)

Sum PRAXIS Score _____ (0–40 possible)

Table 2–12. Nonverbal Oral Apraxia Average Scores With Standard Deviations and Ranges of Children With Typical Speech Development (GFTA-3 Standard Score of Over 75)

	Boys	**Girls**
6- to 7-year-olds (boys n = 35; girls n = 30)	4.3 (3.6) Normal range 0–10	2.5 (1.96) Normal range 0–6
8- to 9-year-olds (boys n = 50; girls n = 36)	2.3 (2.5) Normal range 0–6	1.9 (2.5) Normal range 0–6
10- to 12-year-olds (boys n = 51; girls n = 59)	1 (1.3) Normal range 0–3	1 (1.3) Normal range 0–3

that even children without speech sound disorders may have some difficulty with these tasks, and performance varies according to age and gender.

As with all portions of the assessment, there should be a summary statement regarding the child's performance on the NVOA including if the child's performance fell within the normal range or not. For children below age 6 years, just descriptive results can be provided. The information provided by a NVOA assessment can guide how instructions are given during therapy. For example, if a child has NVOA and is having difficulty obtaining the articulatory configuration for /k/, the therapist would be better off providing tactile and visual cues than verbal instructions.

Standardized Articulation and Phonology Assessment

If a child is able to attempt word productions for the stimuli in a standardized articulation and phonology test, it can be helpful to do this prior to the sensorimotor speech exam, as it provides a way to sample all sounds in all word positions, enabling the examiner to obtain both an independent and relational sound inventory and a syllable shape inventory. Appendix 2–G provides diacritics typically used for disordered speech, exercises to practice identifying syllable shapes, and practice calculating percentage consonants correct (PCC) and percentage vowels correct (PVC). Table 2–13 provides a summary of commonly used standardized articulation and phonology tests and the ages they are normed for.

When the child speaks a language other than English, it will be important to assess them in their first language as well (McLeod & Verdon, 2014). Table 2–25 provides a link to published tests and word lists in other languages (McLeod et al, 2012a).

Getting More Out of Your Standardized Articulation/Phonology Exam

In addition to obtaining standardized articulation scores, the SLP can adapt how they administer the exam and use supplemental scoring methods to obtain information on inconsistency, vowel errors, segmentation errors, lexical stress matches, and response to dynamic cuing, as long as the standard score is based off the child's first production (unless directed otherwise in the instruction manual). For example, eliciting multiple repetitions for a set of words (*Diagnostic*

Table 2–13. Standardized Articulation and Phonology Examinations and the Components They Include

Test	Inconsistent Errors	Stimulability	Vowel Errors	Phonological Patterns	Sentence Level	Oral-Motor Screening
Goldman-Fristoe Test of Articulation 3 (GFTA-3; Goldman & Fristoe, 2015) (2;0–21;11)		X		*When used with the *Kahn–Lewis Phonological Analysis, Third Edition* (KLPA-3; Kahn & Lewis, 2015)	X	
Diagnostic Evaluation of Articulation and Phonology (DEAP; Dodd et al., 2002) (3:0–8:11)	X	X	X	X		X
Arizona Articulation and Phonology Scale, Fourth Edition (Arizona-4; Fudala & Stegall, 2017) (18 months–21;11)		X	X	X	X	
Hodson Assessment of Phonological Patterns, Third Edition (HAPP-3; Hodson, 2004) (3:0–8:0)			X	X		
Glaspey Dynamic Assessment of Phonology (Glaspey, 2021) (3;0–10;11)		*Includes 15-point cuing system that factors into the score			X	

Evaluation of Articulation and Phonology [*DEAP*] uses 25) can be used to obtain a token inconsistency score. Iuzzini-Seigel (2021) uses stimuli from the *GFTA-3* to calculate an inconsistency severity percentage (ISP) score, which you can learn more about from her online materials. Links are provided in Table 2–25. The SLP could use the child's productions to compare the target syllable structure of the stimuli to the child's production to obtain a percentage of articulatory accuracy for each syllable shape (e.g., CV, CVC, CCVC) at different syllable and word lengths. However, since most standardized articulation tests use primarily single syllable and bisyllabic words, additional stimuli will be needed to sample more complex syllable shapes and longer words, such as a picture description task. Patel and Connaghan (2014) published a free accessible picture description task of a Park Play scene with guidelines for analysis. Items in the scene include words with a variety of sounds, syllable shapes, and word lengths (e.g., *boy, glasses, gingerbread, caterpillar*). To access, go to the URL for the article provided in Table 2–25, and then go to the supplemental material link for the picture and analysis form.

Taxing the Sensorimotor Speech System

The sensorimotor speech evaluation (typically referred to as a motor speech evaluation) should sufficiently tax the child's sensorimotor planning system to precisely identify the levels at which breakdowns are occurring. Because the core impairment in CAS is the sensorimotor planning and/or programming of speech movement sequences, the evaluation for CAS should incorporate the production of movement sequences that vary in *syllable shape complexity, number of syllables, phonetic complexity,* and *linguistic complexity*. Children's production of increasingly complex syllable/word structures, as measured by *syllable shape complexity* and *number of syllables*, should be completed to determine whether the complexity of utterances impacts the child's production accuracy. The point at which the syllable structure of the words becomes too complex or the number of syllables in the word becomes too great for the child to produce accurately should be documented. Test items included in traditional articulation or phonology tests are not structured in a hierarchical format of syllable shape complexity. Many of the formal tests for CAS, which are included in Table 2–14, are structured in a format that moves from simple to more complex syllable shapes. For some children with CAS, the breakdown in accuracy may occur even at the level of the CV syllable. Other children may be able to maintain the integrity of the utterance until the utterance becomes longer (multiply/multiplication; fridge/refrigerator) or the syllable structure is more complex (CVC, as in "top," versus CCVCC, as in "stopped").

As the *phonetic complexity* of an utterance increases, the child also may demonstrate greater articulatory challenge. Words that contain consonant phonemes that require shifts in place, manner, and voicing—as well as vowels that require shifts in tongue backing and height, and lip shaping—likely will be more difficult for a child. Consider the following words: "cocoa," "cookie," and "cozy." Each has two syllables and four phonemes, but the phonetic complexity builds with each target. In "cocoa," the consonants and vowels are the same for each syllable; meanwhile in "cookie," the consonants remain the same, but the vowel shifts from a high, back, lip-rounded vowel /ʊ/ to a high, front, lip-retracted vowel /i/. The same vowel shifting occurs in "cozy," but there also is an additional change between the two consonants, with /k/ being a voiceless velar stop and /z/ being a voiced alveolar fricative. All of these articulatory changes can be taxing on the child's sensorimotor planning system.

The evaluation can uncover challenges when the *linguistic complexity* of utterances is increased as well. For children whose language is beyond the single-word level, it is essential to compare the child's single-word productions to phrase- and sentence-level productions and conversation. Inconsistencies may be more noticeable during conversational speech than during single-word productions, especially for older children with CAS who are more conversational. Note any deterioration in phonetic or phonotactic accuracy or prosody as the utterance length increases, as these findings may be reflective of a breakdown at the level of sensorimotor planning and indicative of CAS. Connected speech-level analysis also is very important because it allows the clinician to observe the functional impact of the child's speech disorder. Barrett and colleagues (2020) created a protocol for analyzing connected speech samples. The URL is provided in Table 2–25.

The confirmation of the diagnosis of CAS is the part of the assessment that warrants the most attention. In lieu of a single gold standard assessment, perceptual assessments of core features through a variety of tasks that tax the sensorimotor system are what is typically used to diagnose CAS (Iuzzini-Seigel & Murray, 2017). Several studies have used Strand's 10-point checklist (Shriberg et al., 2009), where the presence of CAS is confirmed if there is any combination of at least four of the 10 segmental and suprasegmental features listed, in addition to inconsistency (Murray et al., 2015). Iuzzini-Seigel (2021) proposes a 5-3-3 rule, where the child must demonstrate at least five of the core characteristics, three times each in three different contexts. Table 2–14 lists commonly used formal assessments and informal tasks that provide the examiner a variety of ways to measure and document the core characteristics and the age range for which they are appropriate.

Assessments and Tasks That Tax the Sensorimotor Speech System in Developmental Order

There are currently three published pediatric sensorimotor speech exams available for purchase. They are all designed to tax the sensorimotor speech system by increasing phonetic and syllable shape complexity and length of the word. The *Kaufman Speech Praxis Test for Children* (*KSPT*; Kaufman, 1995) is norm-referenced for children age 2 to 5;11 years. It assesses imitation of oral movements, simple and complex phoneme production, simple to increasingly complex word shapes, and overall speech intelligibility. It also provides analysis and descriptive elements of other core characteristics observed during speech production, such as groping, inconsistency, vowel distortions, and atypical phonological patterns. Treatment recommendations are based on the level of complexity the child breaks down at and uses progressive approximation to help the child go from a motorically simpler version of a word to the correct production of the word following the order of how a typically developing younger child would say the word at different stages of development. For example, if the child struggles with CV-CV and says "ah-ah" for "bubble," the child will work on the duplicated syllable, "buh-buh," and then "bu-bo," and then "bubble." The *Kaufman Speech to Language Protocol* (*K-SLP*) provides materials using this method and is discussed further in Chapter 4.

The *Dynamic Evaluation of Motor Speech Skill* (*DEMSS*; Strand & McCauley, 2019) is a criterion-referenced assessment to use with young children, ages 3 years and older with severe SSDs and reduced phoneme and syllable shape inventories. Stimuli include simple syllable shapes of increasing levels of complexity with early developing sounds. In addition, bisyllabic and trisyllabic words elicit both trochaic and iambic stress patterns. Words build in complexity in the following order: CV (e.g., go), VC (e.g., up), reduplicated syllables (e.g., **pa**pa), single sylla-

Table 2–14. Tasks for Identifying Core Features of CAS and Suggested Age Range

Characteristic	Test or Task						
	DEMSS (3;0 and older with severe SSDs)	Kaufman (2;0–5;11)	VMPAC-R (3;0–12;0)	DDK task (4;0 to adult)	Multisyllabic word repetition (4;0 to adult)	Phrase repetition (when able)	Connected speech sample (all ages)
Inconsistent errors	X		X	X	X	X	X
Vowel errors	X	X	X		X	X	X
Intrusive schwa	X	X	X		X	X	X
Consonant distortions/ distorted substitutions	X	X	X	X	X	X	X
Increased difficulty with increased phonetic complexity, syllable shape and syllable length	X	X	X	X	X	X	X
Difficulty with initial articulatory configurations or transitional movement gestures	X		X	X	X	X	X
Syllable segmentation	X		X	X	X	X	X
Slow rate	X		X	X	X	X	X
Equal or excess stress	X		X	X	X	X	X
Resonance or nasality disturbance		X	X	X	X	X	X
Groping	X	X	X	X	X	X	X

Notes. DDK, diadochokinetic; DEMSS, *Dynamic Evaluation of Motor Speech Skill;* SSD, speech sound disorder; VMPAC-R, *Verbal Motor Production Assessment for Children–Revised.*

bles with the same consonant (e.g., pop), with different consonants (e.g., home), bisyllabic words with one consonant and two vowels (e.g., **ba**by), bisyllabic words with varied sounds, syllable shapes, and stress patterns (e.g., **O**pen/to**day**), multisyllabic words (e.g., ba**na**na/ **pee**kaboo). The examiner scores vowel accuracy, articulatory accuracy after the first attempt, articulatory accuracy after cuing, and inconsistency after three repetitions of each word. Bisyllabic and trisyllabic words receive a score for prosodic accuracy.

Scoring on this exam is multidimensional. For example vowels are scored as correct (2), uncertain (1), or distorted (0). To account for how children perform with additional cuing or if their errors fall more into a phonological error pattern, the articulatory accuracy score is judged as correct on first attempt (4), consistent developmental substitution error (3), correct after self-correction with no intervening model (2), correct after first cued trial (2), correct after additional cued trials (1), and not correct on final noncued elicitation after all cued attempts (0). Consistency and prosody scores are binary, meaning either correct (1) or incorrect (0).

In addition to the scoring, the *DEMSS* provides a place for the examiner to tally the different types of prosodic errors they are hearing (e.g., segmented, equal stress, incorrect stress) and other characteristics consistent with CAS, such as inconsistent voicing errors, groping, intrusive schwa, slow rate, and awkward movement transitions. The examiner then calculates scores for vowels, articulatory accuracy, prosody (lexical stress accuracy), and consistency. Scores can fall in the range of "significant evidence for CAS," "some evidence for CAS," and "little or no evidence of CAS." The other core characteristics observed are tallied but do not factor into the score.

This provides a rich interpretation of the data, even if the child is unable to complete the assessment. The only characteristic not explicitly listed in the protocol is resonance. However, this could be included in the comments section. The *DEMSS* manual comes with a link to online resources that include fillable protocols and tutorials on how to score. The tutorials are very helpful, as it can take some practice to get reliable with the multidimensional scoring and scoring prosody and vowels accurately. SLPs often have a lot of training articulation errors when it comes to consonants. Many of us need additional practice with correctly judging vowels and prosody. Results from the *DEMSS* provide a natural segue into implementing the Dynamic Temporal Tactile Cuing (DTTC) approach. In DTTC, functional words and phrases are targeted that are within the *zone of proximal development* (ZPD) and can be achieved with maximal cuing. As the child's motor sequencing of articulatory movement improves, cuing is faded. See Chapter 4 for more information on DTTC.

The *Verbal Motor Production Assessment for Children–Revised* (*VMPAC-R*; Hayden & Namasivayam, 2021) has the same elements as the original *VMPAC* (Hayden & Square, 1999) but is now completely digital and is administered and scored on a computer. It is designed to assess the neuromotor integrity of the motor speech system for children ages 3 to 12 years with SSDs. The VMPAC-R tests motor complexity of speech and nonspeech movements in terms of coordinating planes of movement with increasing linguistic (e.g., phoneme, syllabic, word, and phrase level) and cognitive load (e. g., picture formulation/narration). Planes of movement including *vertical* movement of the jaw opening; *horizontal* movement of the lips in terms of rounding and retraction; and *anterior-posterior* movement of the tongue are aligned with the *Prompts for Restructuring Oral Muscular Phonetic Targets* (*PROMPT*) Motor Speech Hierarchy (MSH), which is explained further in Chapter 4.

This allows the clinician to systematically study the impact of higher cognitive load on the breakdown of sequencing ability in children. It also has a dynamic component, where the examiner can see which modalities (e.g., auditory, visual, tactile) help the child with their motor speech control. The five test components are as follows:

- *global motor control*, which includes head and trunk stability, respiratory and phonatory support, reflexes, and the vegetative functions of chewing and swallowing
- *focal oromotor control* of mandibular, labio-facial, and lingual structures during nonspeech and speech movements
- *sequencing* of nonspeech and speech movements
- *connected speech and language control*
- *Speech characteristics*, which comprise oromotor production in automatic verbal sequences and self-formulated speech to assess overall speech characteristics, such as voice quality, pitch, loudness, and prosody

The new digital administration format provides video instructions embedded into the exam and training materials, which help standardize the administration of the assessment and scoring, and interpretation of results are online. The scores from each section auto populate onto the results page and are presented as a graphic display of the child's percentage accuracy and percentile for each area. The results page also provides the examiner with the corresponding severity rating for each area. Results of this exam guide the therapist to start treatment where the child needs support (i.e., where their performance falls on the motor speech hierarchy using *PROMPT*). Targets for treatment are carefully constructed to systematically address physiological support and movement parameters for speech. You can preview the video tutorials and learn more about the *VMPAC-R* online. (See URL in Table 2–25.)

If formal assessments are not available, the SLP can construct their own stimuli to see where the child breaks down and provide cuing to see what supports the child needs to improve articulatory accuracy. Tables 2–15 through 2–17 provide examples.

Table 2–15. Build Upon Words (One, Two, Three Syllables)

Ann	anna	animal
bass	basket	basketball
me	meaty	medium
some	summer	summertime
won	wonder	wonderful

Table 2–16. Build Upon Syllables (One-Syllable Words)

soup	scoop/coops	scoops
cap	scam/camp	scamp
wish	swish/wished	swished
lamb	clam/lamp	clamp
well	dwell/welled	dwelled
rat	raft	draft
sad	sand	scanned
puck	punk	spunk
wet	sweat/wept	swept
gas	grass	grasp

Table 2–17. Phrases of Increasing Length

I want more.	I want more milk.	I want more milk please.
Can we go?	Can we go home?	Can we go home now?
Wanna play?	Wanna play house?	Wanna play house with me?
Let me.	Let me try.	Let me try one.

School Age

As the child becomes more able to sequence articulatory movement for single and bisyllabic words and basic sentences, the previously listed formal and informal sensorimotor speech assessments may no longer be adequate. Several studies have shown that children with CAS often struggle with multisyllabic words up through adolescence (e.g., Benway & Preston, 2020). "By 7;11 years, most children with typically developing speech and language will produce all consonants, vowels, syllable shapes, and stress patterns correctly" (Masso et al., 2018, p. 44). Carefully designed multisyllabic word repetition and/or picture naming tasks can tax the sensorimotor speech system at the next level and help differentiate children with CAS from other speech sound disorders (Benway & Preston, 2020; Murray et al., 2015). How the child performs on the multisyllabic word task can also guide the SLP in determining the next step of phonotactic complexity to address in therapy. Working on multisyllabic words for improved sensorimotor speech skills has the additional benefit of addressing tier II and tier III vocabulary and morphology, allowing the child to feel more confident when engaging with peers in and outside of the classroom. When choosing multisyllabic stimuli, the examiner will want to use or construct a word list that contains a variety of syllable shapes in words ranging from three to five syllables with different lexical stress patterns. Table 2–18 provides an abbreviated version of our *Dynamic Multisyllabic Word Probe* (DMWP) for the purpose of instruction. The full probe can be found in Appendix 2–E. This *DMWP* recording form was created based off of the characteristics often cited in the research, in addition to the authors' combined 70 years of clinical experience. Core characteristics observed in school-age children with CAS have included syllable segregation, decreased PCC, decreased lexical stress matches, more voicing errors, lower percentage of structurally correct words (i.e., syllable shape), and more syllable deletions compared to peers with other SSDs (Benway & Preston, 2020; Murray et al., 2015).

For this probe, use the child's first production to score articulatory accuracy, coarticulation, and lexical stress accuracy. The recording form provides a place to transcribe incorrect words or simply mark the sound the child omitted, distorted, or substituted on the word written in International Phonetic Alphabet. This will allow for a quick calculation of percentage phonemes correct (PPC), PCC, and PVC analysis, if desired. Table 2–18 provides an example of how to adapt the form for these calculations. Otherwise, the examiner can mark the word with a + if correct and transcribe if incorrect. The form provided in Appendix E does not include PPC, PCC, and PVC, but it could easily be written in. It is important to note that the IPA transcriptions provided on the form are not representative of all dialects; thus, the examiner needs to be mindful of what is acceptable in the child's dialect and score accordingly. Appendix 2–G provides instructions on how to calculate these scores. If only consonants are in error, it is not necessary to calculate PVC. In the following example, it shows how you could average these scores for words at each syllable length. This is helpful for seeing if accuracy decreases as syllable length increases.

Table 2–18. Dynamic Multisyllabic Word Probe

Target Word	Transcribe or mark sounds that were incorrect, added, or omitted, if incorrect	Smooth coarticulation + good smooth coarticulation – poor coarticulation – syllable segmentation	Lexical stress accuracy + correct – incorrect	If incorrect, is there improvement with backward chaining or other cuing methods? Y/N If so, note the method that was helpful.
Three-Syllable Words				
vacation /veˈkeɪ.ʃən/	___/7 P ___/4 C ___/3 V			
subtraction /səbˈtræk.ʃən/	___/10 P ___/7 C ___/3 V			
principal /ˈprɪn.sə.pəl/	___/9 P ___/6 C ___/3 V			
Total for three-syllable words	___/26 P ___/17 C ___/9 V			
Four-Syllable Words				
avocado /ɑ.və.ˈkɑ.doʊ/	___/7 P ___/3 C ___/4 V			
television /ˈte.lə.vɪ.ʒən/	___/9 P ___/5 C ___/4 V			
experiment /ɛk.ˈspɛ.rɪ.mənt/	___/11 P ___/7 C ___/4 V			
Total for four-syllable words	___/25 P ___/14 C ___/12 V			

continues

Table 2–18. *continued*

Target Word	Transcribe or mark sounds that were incorrect, added, or omitted, if incorrect	Smooth coarticulation + good smooth coarticulation – poor coarticulation – syllable segmentation	Lexical stress accuracy + correct – incorrect	If incorrect, is there improvement with backward chaining or other cuing methods? Y/N If so, note the method that was helpful.
Five-Syllable Words				
congratulations /kən͵græ.ˌt͡ʃə'leɪ.ʃənz/	___/14 p ___/9 c ___/5 v			
enthusiasm /ɛn.'θu.zɪ.jæ.zəm/	___/11 p ___/6 c ___/5 v			
evaporation /ɪ.væ.pə.'reɪ.ʃən/	___/10 p ___/5 c ___/5 v			
Total for five-syllable words	___/35 p ___/20 c ___/15 v			

Note. Adapted from "Dynamic Multisyllabic Word Probe," by A. Skinder-Meredith and M. Fish, 2022 [Unpublished].

The third column of the record form provides a place to mark if the word was said with smooth coarticulation or if it sounded segmented. The presence of linguistically inappropriate silent pauses is a strong indicator of CAS (Shriberg et al., 2017). However, the time it takes to do the acoustic analysis necessary to determine silent pause markers, as defined by Shriberg and colleagues (2017), is not clinically feasible. Noting if a word was produced with poor coarticulation and/or syllable segmentation is a perceptual task that is relatively quick and shown to be indicative of CAS as well. In the fourth column, the examiner notes if the lexical stress pattern was correct or not. If the child uses a different stress pattern and/or deletes any of the syllables, it is marked as incorrect.

In the last column, the examiner notes if backward chairing or any other cues helped improve accuracy. Backward chaining, also called backward build-ups, facilitates improved articulatory accuracy while maintaining the correct stress pattern versus saying one syllable at a time, which leads to segmented syllables and an equal stress pattern with longer duration on the last syllable. To demonstrate, let's use the word, "majestic." You would first have the child repeat the last syllable, "stic," and then the last two syllables "**ge**stic," and then put the word all together, "ma**ge**stic." Now try the traditional one syllable at a time method, "ma....je....stic." Do you hear the difference? Knowing that children with CAS struggle with prosody and coarticulation, the backward chaining method is preferable. For more on this technique, see Chapters 3 and 5. If the child is struggling on one syllable in particular, you can work on that syllable in isolation with additional cuing, such as simultaneous production and tactile cuing, and then put it back into the whole word. If the child said the word correctly the first time, you could write NA for not applicable. This will be helpful when planning treatment. You do not need to elicit all words on the *DMWP*, just enough to get a sense of where the child breaks down.

There are several multisyllabic word lists available online, such as the 10 Clinically Useful Words available on Caroline Bowen's website and the *Single Word Test of Polysyllables* (Gozzard et al., 2008) in addition to word lists that are provided in the research (Benway & Preston, 2020; Masso et al., 2018). URLs for the 10 Clinically Useful Words and the Single Word Test of Polysyllables (Gozzard et al., 2008) are presented in Table 2–25.

Considerations for Taxing the Sensorimotor Speech System in Children Who Speak Languages Other Than English

When working with children who speak a language other than English, the SLP can determine appropriate stimuli by using the same principles previously discussed. In other words, the SLP can find words and phrases from the child's language that build in phonetic complexity, syllable shape, word length, and phrase length. An example of stimuli for Spanish is in Box 2–3. In addition to building complexity, the SLP can use the dynamic cuing discussed on the *DEMSS* and note the level the child makes errors and where they improve with additional cuing. Also note observations of inconsistency, stress errors, and segmentation of sounds and syllables.

Determining the appropriate stimuli will require some homework on the part of the SLP. Fortunately, access to information on the phonology of different languages, order of sound acquisition, and first words spoken in most languages can be found by doing a literature search (McLeod & Crowe, 2018). The Charles Sturt University website on multilingual children's speech (http://www.csu.edu.au/research/multilingual-speech/home) and ASHA's Practice Management/Multicultural page (https://www.asha.org/practice/multicultural/phono/) provide links to multiple resources for finding this information.

Inconsistency Measurements

Inconsistency is the most commonly listed core characteristic of CAS. However, there are many ways to measure inconsistency, and sensitivity of the type of measure used can depend on the age of the child and the complexity of the task (Iuzzini-Seigel, 2021; Iuzzini-Seigel et al., 2017). *Token-to-token inconsistency* measures are used to calculate the inconsistency of words or phrases over multiple repetitions. For example, on the *DEAP*, a child repeats 25 words three times each, and if 12 of the words are produced differently in at least two of the three

■ Box 2–3. Example of Building Stimuli in Spanish

Isolated vowels: /i/, /e/, /a/, /o/, /u/

CV syllables: mí (my), no (no), yo (I), tú (you), sí (yes)

VC syllables: en (on), el (the)

$C_1V_1C_1V_1$: mamá, papá

CVC syllables: pan (bread), con (with), más (more), mal (bad), luz (light)

VCV: ojo (eye), oso (bear), hola (hello), año (year)

$C_1V_1C_1V_2$: dedo (finger)

$C_1V_1C_2V_1$: vaca (cow), cama (bed), taza (cup)

$C_1V_1C_2V_2$: pato (duck), gato (cat), queso (cheese)

Words with clusters: flan (custard), flauta (flute), plato (plate), gris (gray), blanco (white)

Multisyllabic words: tenedor (knife), juguete (toy), cuchara (spoon), comida (food), cumpleaños (birthdays)

Words of increasing length: es (is), está (is); pa (pa), pato (duck), zapato (shoe); gato (cat), gatito (little cat/kitten)

Phrases of increasing length: Quiero (I want), Quiero más (I want more), Quiero más leche (I want more milk), Quiero más leche por favor (I want more milk please)

Functional phrases: Hola mamá/papá (hi mom/dad), Me gusta (I like), No me gusta (I don't like), ayúdame (help me), Lo hago (I do it), ¿Quieres jugar? (Do you want to play?), No sé (I don't know), Yo también (Me too)

Elicit automatic speech tasks as well, such as counting to 10 ("Cuenta hasta diez") and saying the alphabet ("Dime el alfabeto").

---

repetitions, they would have a token-to-token inconsistency score of 48%. If the task was to repeat the same phrase five times and the child said it differently in two of the productions, they would receive an inconsistency score of 40%.

Phonemic-level inconsistency (i.e., segmental-level inconsistency, speech error variability, or type-token ratio [TTR]) measures inconsistency of a phoneme across multiple productions of the phoneme in the same words and phrases or different words and phrases. This allows for a more sensitive measure and has been found to differentiate typically developing children from children with CAS at younger ages (Iuzzini-Seigel & Murray, 2017). An inconsistency severity percentage (ISP) by dividing the total number of different error types, minus one for each phoneme, by the total number of target opportunities (Iuzzini & Forrest, 2010). Table 2–19 provides a comparison of a child with CAS and a child with phonological impairment when scoring inconsistency using ISP. For the purpose of demonstration, the example is only looking at the phoneme /s/. However, this can be done on more than one sound at a time, as is illustrated in Iuzzini-Seigel's tutorial on measures of inconsistency.

When distinguishing children with CAS from children with speech delay, Iuzzini-Seigel and colleagues (2017) found that token-to-token inconsistency of monosyllabic words and five repetitions of the phrase "*Buy Bobby a puppy*" were the most sensitive measures for differentiating between the two groups. For the phrase repetition, a *sentence inconsistency percentage* score is calculated by dividing the number of different ways the sentence was produced by the total number of trials and multiplying by 100. Table 2–20 provides an example of a child with CAS and a child with phonological impairment for scoring inconsistency using the sentence inconsistency percentage. Examples used in Tables 2–19 and 2–20 are based on theoretical cases consistent with the characteristics of the disorder to illustrate how the child with CAS is more apt to have higher inconsistency scores than children with phonological delay based on variability of consonant and vowel production.

Table 2–19. Productions of Five Words Targeting /s/ Produced by a Child With CAS and a Child With Phonological Delay With Inconsistency Severity Percentage Calculation

Target Production	Child With CAS	Child With Phonological Delay
messy	/mɛdɪ/	/mɛtɪ/
scissors	/dɪdɪ/	/tɪdɚz/
mass	/mæk/	/mæt/
house	/haʊʔ/	/haʊt/
swimming	/hwimɪŋ/	/twɪmɪŋ/
Inconsistency severity percentage	Four error types –1/ Five opportunities × 100 = 60%	One error type –1/ Five opportunities × 100 = 0%

Table 2–20. Five Repetitions of "*Buy Bobby a Puppy*" Produced by a Child With CAS and a Child With Phonological Delay

Repetition	Child With CAS	Child With Phonological Delay
First repetition	/ba.bɑpi.ʌ.pʌʔi/	/baɪ.babi.ʌ.bʌbi/
Second repetition	/ba.babi.ʌ.bʌʔi/	/baɪ.babi.ʌ.bʌbi/
Third repetition	/baɪ.babi.ʌ.bʌbi/	/baɪ.babi.ʌ.bʌbi/
Fourth repetition	/baɪ.babi.ʌ.bʌbi/	/baɪ.babi.ʌ.bʌbi/
Fifth repetition	/baɪ.baʔi.ʌ.ʌʔi/	/baɪ.babi.ʌ.bʌbi/
Sentence inconsistency percentage	Four different productions/ Five trials × 100 = 80%	Zero different productions/ Five trials × 100 = 0%

Prosody

Prosody refers to the *suprasegmental* aspects of speech and includes variation of pitch, loudness, duration, and articulatory effort. Assessing prosody can be done a number of ways. As already discussed, the *DEMSS* and multisyllabic word tasks provide a way of measuring lexical stress accuracy. In these tasks, we are listening for the stress to go on the correct syllable. A frequent observation of children with CAS is the characteristic of equal and excessive stress pattern. This means that the child does not unstress the unstressed syllable(s). For example, in the word "ba.**na**.na," only the second syllable should be stressed. The child with CAS may stress every syllable, so it is "**ba.na.na**," or delete the weak syllable(s) and only produce the stressed syllable, "**na**." We also vary our prosody in sentences by changing our intonation patterns for statements versus questions or changing which syllable receives the stress for emphasis. Just as we used multisyllabic words to see where the child correctly matched the lexical stress pattern, we can use sentences to see if they can match the sentential stress and intonation pattern. Appendix 2–F includes a list of 10 three- to four-word sentences with a variety of intonation contours to denote a question, an exclamation, and a statement. The sentences are scored for ability to match the intonation contour, stress the correct syllable, and include all of the syllables. Phrases are intentionally short and syllable shapes are simple as to not tax the child's memory or articulatory sequencing. It is also helpful to judge prosody in connected speech. Additional probes for assessing various features of prosody are discussed in Chapter 5, Table 5–7.

Speech Intelligibility and Comprehensibility

Now let us come back to what is essential as we think about the International Classification of Functioning, Disability and Health–Children and Youth (ICF-CY) framework. At the end of the day, we want the child to be able to participate fully in all of their environments (e.g., home, school, extracurricular activities, etc.) with a variety of communication partners (e.g., family, friends, community members, etc.). To do this, one needs to be understood. Hence, *speech intelligibility*, "the degree to which the acoustic signal is understood by a listener" (Yorkston, Strand, & Kennedy, 1996, p. 55), is an important measure that corresponds with the "activity" and "participation" portions of the ICF-CY. The lower the child's intelligibility, the more limited and restricted they are.

Intelligibility can be measured by calculating the percentage of words understood (i.e., a word identification task) or using a scaled rating system (e.g., a Likert scale ranging from unintelligible to intelligible). Each of these methods has their pros and cons. Where word identification approaches provide more specific measures for tracking progress, they are time consuming and not always feasible (Allison, 2020). Scaled rating approaches provide the option of giving an overall measure of severity and are more ecologically valid, especially when used with a variety of listeners (McLeod et al., 2012b). Although there are many variables to consider when determining intelligibility (e.g., length of sentence, knowledge of context, phonetic complexity and length of the words, speech elicitation method, etc.), strictly speaking, the measure is dependent on the acoustic signal alone. See Table 2–21 for a summary of intelligibility methods.

Table 2–21. Tasks and Procedures for Measuring Speech Intelligibility

Task	Procedure
Single-word identification, open set	The child is recorded saying a list of target words. The targets could be elicited using picture naming or imitation. An unfamiliar listener transcribes the words they heard. The percentage of words correctly identified is calculated.
Single-word identification, closed set	Elicitation is the same as above, but rather than transcribing the word, the listener is given a choice of phonetically similar words and circles the one they heard. The percentage of words correctly identified is calculated.
Word identification at the sentence level	The child produces a set of target utterances following a model, and the listener transcribes the sentences they heard. The percentage of words correctly transcribed is calculated. To track progress over time, the sentences should be similar in length and complexity, as illustrated in Table 2–22.
Intelligibility of words from a spontaneous speech sample	The listener transcribes the recording of what the child said and places an X for each word they did not understand. To compare scores over time, the SLP could elicit the connected speech from a picture description task, a narrative of a familiar story, or while playing with the same set of toys that were used in their prior speech sample.
Percent Consonants Correct (PCC)	PCC can be derived from transcriptions of articulation test productions or spontaneous speech. PCC has been shown to have moderate to strong positive correlations with intelligibility.

Comprehensibility is a broader term and goes beyond just the auditory signal. Comprehensibility refers to how well the listener understands the speaker when using all of the available cues, such as gestures, pictures, sign language, augmentative and alternative communication, body language, and knowing the context. For this reason, comprehensibility will be higher than intelligibility. Comprehensibility measures are more ecologically valid but do not directly reflect the accuracy of the speech signal (Allison, 2020). Goals can be written for improving both intelligibility and comprehensibility.

There are a number of options for calculating a percentage of speech intelligibility score and variables to consider when choosing the option that is the most appropriate for the child you are assessing. When using an intelligibility measure for the purpose of tracking progress, the procedure used needs to be consistent due to the many factors that can impact the score, such as predictability of the word or sentence, length of the stimuli (e.g., word vs. sentence), phonetic complexity of the words, and familiarity of the listener. This is especially important to consider when a child goes from one therapist to another. The new therapist will need to know how the previous therapist determined the intelligibility score for reliable tracking of progress.

Intelligibility assessments for children have been primarily used for research purposes, and the ones that have been published for clinical use are no longer in print (Allison, 2020).

Hence, the SLP is somewhat limited for options. The SLP can either make their own stimuli or use word and sentence lists published in the research (Ertmer, 2010). The URL addresses for a few of these measures are provided in Table 2–25.

When using an imitation task for words and phrases, the recording will need to be edited or paused each time the model says the utterance, so the listener is naïve to the target. Ideally, the listener should not be familiar with the speaker and only be allowed to listen to the child's productions twice (Allison, 2020). If the listener is familiar with the child's speech, this should be noted when providing the intelligibility score, since an increase in familiarity with the speaker can increase the intelligibility score.

Morris and colleagues (1995) created the *Preschool Speech Intelligibility Measure (PSIM)*, which was developed in a manner similar to the *Sentence Intelligibility Test (SIT)* (Yorkston, Beukelman, & Hakel, 1996) for adults. The *PSIM* provides 50 sets of 12 phonetically similar words and is an example of a single-word identification with a closed set. For example, in list one, the words are as follows: *warm, store, swarm, for, horn, corn, door, torn, born, floor, storm, form*. The child repeats the words the clinician has preselected from each list. The SLP records the list set number and asks the child to repeat a word from the set and then records the child's production only. There is approximately a 7-second pause between items, and then the SLP states the next item number, and the child repeats a word from that set. This continues until the child has been recorded saying one word from each of the 50 sets. The unfamiliar listener is then provided the recording and circles the word they heard using a multiple-choice format, which includes the 12 words for each set.

The *Beginner's Intelligibility Test (BIT*; Osberger et al., 1994) and the *Monsen-Indiana University Sentences (M-ISU*; Monsen, 1981) are examples of tasks used for word identification at the sentence level. The *BIT* consists of grammatically simple sentences that a young child who cannot read could easily repeat. In addition, the sentences are easy to demonstrate with objects and toys. For example, "The baby falls" would be modeled while having a baby doll fall. The *M-ISU* was developed for children in second grade or higher who can read, and the phrases range in phonetic complexity and length. Although both of these sentence intelligibility probes were developed for young children with hearing loss, they can be used with other pediatric populations as well. The URL for the article that contains the *BIT* and *M-ISU* stimuli is in Table 2–25.

The sentence lists in Table 2–22 were created to be consistent with the principles used for the *M–ISU*. The sentences in these lists are two to six words in length and include the following features: multiple phonetic contexts, with and without consonant clusters, including final bound morphemes, early and later developing phonemes, words of one to three syllables in length, familiar vocabulary, and declarative and interrogative forms. The child is recorded while either repeating or reading these utterances and the naïve listener transcribes the sentences exactly as they heard them. The percentage of correctly transcribed words is then calculated for the intelligibility score. For example, if the listener heard "Mom walk baby" for "Mom walks the baby" the score would be 50% of words intelligible for that item. Note that each list of phrases is similar in terms of length and complexity. This allows the examiner to use a different list of phrases each time the child is recorded for the purpose of tracking improvement in speech intelligibility at the sentence level.

Measures of PCC and percentage phonemes correct (PPC) have been found to correlate with intelligibility scores (Skoog & Maas, 2020). Some researchers and clinicians use the percentage of consonants correct–revised (PCC-R) score in single words and connected speech (Shriberg

Table 2–22. List of Phrases and Sentences to Produce for Word Intelligibility at the Sentence Level

Phrase and Sentence-Level Intelligibility Stimuli		
List 1	**List 2**	**List 3**
1. My toys	1. Go home.	1. Help me.
2. I see you.	2. I know Sue.	2. We saw two.
3. Where is daddy?	3. Why not, mommy?	3. Where is puppy?
4. Stop the car.	4. Stay right here.	4. She stayed home.
5. Mom walks the baby.	5. Dad takes the bus.	5. Bob bakes the cake.
6. It rained all day yesterday.	6. My friend touched the computer.	6. We laughed at the magician.
7. We can't go to the library.	7. She won't be at home tomorrow.	7. They don't like to exercise much.
8. I'm putting the trucks away.	8. She's dressing in fancy clothes.	8. Her plant needs more watering.
9. My special blanket is dirty.	9. I started planting seeds today.	9. Don't stand on the flowers.
10. Is Saturday your grandfather's birthday?	10. Can your grandmother make sandwiches?	10. Did the principal want lemonade?

et al., 1997). The PCC-R score can be useful for describing severity and can serve as a baseline for later comparisons. The following equation is used to calculate PCC-R:

$$\text{PCC-R} = \text{Number of correct consonants (excluding distortions)} \div \text{Total number of consonants} \times 100$$

Shriberg and Kwiatkowski (1982) used the following rating system for PCC scores:

- Mild: 85%–100%
- Mild-moderate: 65%–85%
- Moderate-severe: 50%–65%
- Severe: below 50

Obtaining a percentage of intelligibility from orthographic transcription, even when provided a closed set to choose from, can be a time-consuming task. With the advent of speech recognition software, more products are being developed that measure speech intelligibility. For example, Rose Medical Speech Therapy Software & Instrumentation, out of the United Kingdom sells Pronunciation Coach 3D software for home use and for the commercial user. As part of the package, the speaker can record their speech and compare it with the pronunciation model to obtain an intelligibility score. For more information, go to the URL provided in Table 2–25. This software was developed with the intended use of improving speech intelligibility of English-language learners and people with speech sound disorders. Although the developers have not determined validity and reliability measures with people with disordered speech and are not SLPs, they are open to feedback and are continually working on making their products more clinically useful.

Scaling scores for intelligibility are often used for rating spontaneous speech samples and can be used with a variety of listeners. McLeod and colleagues (2012) developed the *Intelligibility in Context Scale (ICS)* to measure functional intelligibility of young children with speech sound disorders and CAS. Given that the rater is provided contextual cues, the *ICS* and other rater scales are more of a comprehensibility measure than a strict intelligibility measure. The *ICS* is filled out by the caregiver and consists of seven questions relating to how well the child is understood by different communication partners (e.g., parents, friends, family, acquaintances, teachers, and strangers). It has a 5-point rating scale, ranging from 1, the child is never understood, to 5, they are always understood. This *ICS* can be found online and is available to download in 60 languages by going to the URL listed in Table 2–25. See Figure 2–4 for the English version.

Intelligibility in Context Scale (ICS)
(McLeod, Harrison, & McCormack, 2012)

Child's name:_____

Child's date of birth:_____Male/Female:_____

Language(s) spoken:_____

Current date: _____Child's age:_____

Person completing the ICS:_____

Relationship to child:_____

The following questions are about how much of your child's speech is understood by different people. Please think about your child's speech over the past month when answering each question. Circle one number for each question.

	Always	Usually	Sometimes	Rarely	Never
1. Do **you** understand your child[1]?	5	4	3	2	1
2. Do **immediate members of your family** understand your child?	5	4	3	2	1
3. Do **extended members of your family** understand your child?	5	4	3	2	1
4. Do your **child's friends** understand your child?	5	4	3	2	1
5. Do other **acquaintances** understand your child?	5	4	3	2	1
6. Do your **child's teachers** understand your child?	5	4	3	2	1
7. Do **strangers**[2] understand your child?	5	4	3	2	1
TOTAL SCORE =	/35				
AVERAGE TOTAL SCORE =	/5				

[1] This measure may be able to be adapted for adults' speech, by substituting *child* with *spouse*.
[2] The term *strangers* may be changed to *unfamiliar people*

Figure 2–4. Intelligibility in Context Scale. (*Intelligibility in Context Scale* by S. McLeod, L. J. Harrison, and J. McCormack, 2012, Charles Sturt University, http://www.csu.edu.au/research/multilingual-speech/ics. Used with permission of Sharyn McLeod.)

Although there are many scales available, the *ICS* is the only one that has been translated into 60 languages and has tested validity and reliability across 14 languages (McLeod, 2020). In a study by Soriano and colleagues (2021), ICS composite scores were compared to transcription intelligibility scores of 48 children with cerebral palsy (CP). The transcription intelligibility score was based off of the percentage of words transcribed correctly from 60 multiword utterances. Given the efficiency of filling out the ICS, it was encouraging to see that the ICS composite scores were moderately strong predictors of transcription intelligibility scores (Soriano et al., 2021). In this study, a composite score below 4 indicated the child had a speech motor impairment. This is a helpful cutoff score to be aware of when interpreting results of the *ICS*.

Comprehensibility

Some children with poor speech intelligibility have figured out ways to be understood by using a variety of strategies. When working to improve a child's comprehensibility, we can work on both increasing the child's articulatory and prosodic accuracy, while also giving them ways to compensate for their difficulties with motor planning and programming. Table 2–23 provides a comprehensibility strategies checklist for the parent to fill out. If working with a child in the school, this may also be appropriate for the teacher to fill out. The list is in developmental order of strategies we may expect to see a child use.

Table 2–23. Comprehensibility Strategies Checklist

Check the strategies your child uses to be understood	Yes	No	Unsure
Pantomimes and/or uses gestures			
Points to the object of a picture of what they are referring to			
Uses prosody and emphatic stress with word approximations (e.g., "I WA ta o O!" for "I want to go home.")			
Uses sign language and/or other forms of augmentative communication			
Decreases rate of speech			
Repeats the part of the message not understood			
Types or writes what is not understood			
Uses synonyms for what is not understood			
Provides context for what is not understood			
Pulls up an image or story on the Internet to show what they are referring to			
Other			

Differential Diagnosis and Relative Contribution

When Morley and colleagues (1954) first noted characteristics of apraxia in children, SLPs were only aware of pediatric dysarthria, and it took a long time for many to accept that CAS even existed (ASHA, 2007). However, as noted earlier, current studies indicate that SLPs are not as comfortable with diagnosing childhood dysarthria as they are with diagnosing CAS and may miss potential dysarthric components impacting the child's speech production (Murray et al, 2015; Iuzzini-Seigel et al., in press). In addition, it can be easy to overlook a phonological disorder when the focus is on CAS. We are now more aware that children with severe speech sound disorders may have CAS, dysarthria, a phonological disorder, or a combination of any of the three. Table 2–24 provides a comparison of the characteristics observed in CAS, dysarthria, and phonological disorder. To aid in differential diagnosis and determine the relative contribution of each underlying deficit to the child's speech disorder, the examiner can highlight the saliant characteristics listed in Table 2–24 to get a more comprehensive picture as to what may be going on for a particular child. This can then help guide the clinician's treatment plan to address the issues that are having the biggest impact on speech intelligibility.

The *Profile of Childhood Apraxia of Speech and Dysarthria* (ProCAD) is a new checklist that will be helpful in discerning CAS from childhood dysarthria (Iuzzini-Seigel et al., 2022). The ProCAD uses a binary scoring system (present or not present) for twenty speech features organized by subsystem, which are characteristic of dysarthria, CAS, or both. For example, short breath groups, which falls under respiration and phonation would be indicative of dysarthria; slow rate, which falls under prosody, could suggest both CAS or dysarthria; and intrusive schwa, under articulation, would be symptomatic of CAS. The examiner completes the feature checklist across three different speech tasks (e.g., articulation test, multisyllabic words, and connected speech). A diagnostic flowchart is then used to determine if dysarthria or CAS are present, should be further tested, or ruled out.

Table 2–24. Differentiating Characteristics of CAS, Dysarthria, and Severe Phonological Disorder

Speech Features	CAS	Dysarthria	Severe Phonological Disorder
Weakness	No weakness, incoordination, or paralysis of speech musculature *However, children with CAS may present with low tone.	Decreased strength and/or coordination of speech musculature that leads to deficits in respiratory support and/or coordination; voice impairment and imprecise speech production, slurring and distortions	No weakness, incoordination, or paralysis of speech musculature
Involuntary motor control	No difficulty with involuntary motor control for chewing, swallowing, etc.	Difficulty with involuntary motor control for chewing, swallowing, etc., due to muscle weakness and incoordination	No difficulty with involuntary motor control for chewing and swallowing

Table 2–24. *continued*

Speech Features	CAS	Dysarthria	Severe Phonological Disorder
Inconsistent speech errors	Inconsistencies in articulation performance—the same word may be produced several different ways	Articulation may be noticeably "different" due to imprecision, but errors generally consistent	Consistent errors that can usually be grouped into categories (fronting, stopping, etc.)
Types of sound errors	Sound errors may include vowel distortions, omission of initial consonants, and additions. Tendency to centralize vowels to a "schwa" or produce syllable final schwa	Errors are generally weak and imprecise distortions	Errors may include substitutions, omissions, distortions, etc. Omissions in final position more likely than initial position. Vowel distortions not as common.
Increased errors with increased word/phrase length	Number of errors increases as length of word/phrase increases	May be less precise in connected speech than in single words	Errors are generally consistent as length of words/phrases increases
Rate, rhythm, stress	Rate, rhythm, and stress of speech are disrupted, some groping for placement may be noted	Rate, rhythm, and stress are disrupted in ways specifically related to the type of dysarthria (spastic, flaccid, ataxic, etc.)	Typically, no disruption of rate, rhythm, or stress
Pitch and loudness	Generally good phonatory quality and normal volume, and physiological control of pitch and loudness is typically normal.	May have difficulty controlling pitch and loudness depending on the type of dysarthria	Good control of pitch and loudness, not limited in inflectional range for speaking
Speech prosody	Prosodic deficits often noted: equal stress, segmentation, lexical stress errors	Prosodic deficits common, varying with type of dysarthria	Typically, no prosodic deficits
Voice quality	Age-appropriate voice quality	Voice quality may be harsh, hypernasal, etc., depending on type of dysarthria	Age-appropriate voice quality
Nasal resonance	May be hypernasal due to mistiming but also look for structural deficits (e.g., submucosal cleft)	Often see hypernasality	Not typically associated with phonological impairment

Note. From Dave Hammer, MA, CCC-SLP, Ruth Stoeckel PhD, CCC-SLP, and Edythe Strand PhD, CCC-SLP, 2018. Updated 2021 by Margaret Fish, MS, CCC-SLP. Updated 2022 for Apraxia Kids website. Used with permission from Apraxia–Kids.

Other Areas of Assessment

Up to now, this chapter has focused on the components of the assessment battery that allow the examiner to determine if the underlying deficit of the child's speech sound disorder is structural, phonological, motor execution, sensorimotor planning and programming, or a combination of factors. As mentioned earlier, it will also be important to assess language, phonological awareness, and literacy skills, in addition to screening for fine motor and gross motor skills, and sensory processing, and monitoring social-emotional well-being.

Language Testing

- **Receptive language.** Describe the child's receptive language capacities in the following areas. When receptive language challenges co-occur with CAS, the child may exhibit difficulty understanding the instructions for the tasks presented. Adaptations may need to be made in the length and format of verbal instruction provided to the child during treatment.
  - Vocabulary and concept knowledge
  - Syntax and morphology
  - Question comprehension
  - Following directions of increased length and complexity
  - Language processing
  - Working memory

- **Expressive language.** A thorough examination of expressive language (vocabulary, syntax, morphology, narrative language) will help guide the treatment goals as well as the target vocabulary and utterances. More detailed information related to target selection and elicitation of phrases and sentences can be found in Chapters 6 and 8 of this book.
  - Syntax and morphology challenges may be a result of phonetic inventory limitations (e.g., child produces "cup" for cups because CVCC is not in the child's inventory). Even those errors not impacted by a child's phonetic inventory are a common finding in children with CAS (e.g., child produces "go" for goes even though the child's word shape inventory does include CVC). Other linguistic challenges may include reduced length and complexity of utterances, omission of function words, word sequencing errors, and incorrect pronoun usage.
  - Word retrieval concerns, if any, should be noted. Word retrieval challenges may be unrelated to the child's apraxia or may reflect difficulty with planning the phoneme sequences of the target utterances.
  - Narrative language in children who are conversational should be assessed and addressed if the child exhibits difficulties in the ability to share stories in a sequential, cohesive, and age-appropriate manner.

- **Social-pragmatic language.** Social language differences may result from a child's limited opportunities for early verbal interactions but also may be indicative of a co-occurring social language disorder. The following should be noted:

- **Conversational reciprocity with peers and adults.** For children who are conversational, note whether there are any difficulties in reciprocal conversational skills, and whether the child demonstrates a better ability to be reciprocal with adults than with peers.

- **Language functions.** Indicate whether the child demonstrates use of a limited variety of language functions, which may be an indication of concomitant social language challenges. Some examples of language functions include greeting, requesting objects, actions, or assistance, rejecting, protesting, sharing information, narrating events, expressing humor, getting attention, and commenting.

- **Level of engagement and interaction** (verbal and nonverbal). Indicate whether the child prefers to play alone or with others and whether the child engages in cooperative play with peers. If the child's play tends to be parallel or solitary beyond the age of 4 years, the age at which cooperative play would be expected, this should be noted and may need to be addressed in treatment.

Phonological Awareness and Literacy

As noted in Chapter 1, children with CAS often have difficulty with phonological awareness and literacy skills. There are many good screening tools and assessments for children age 4 years and up. There are also many online materials that can be used to assess phonological and phonemic awareness in the areas of alphabet knowledge, segmenting sounds and syllables of a word, blending sounds, rhyme awareness, and manipulation of phonemes (e.g., adding, substituting, and deleting sounds) to make new words. One such online screener is the *Phonological Awareness Screening Test* (*PAST*; Kilpatrick, 2019) for Pre-K through adult. The link is provided in Table 2–25. Following is a list of frequently used assessments for phonological awareness and literacy:

Standardized Assessments Phonological Awareness Tests and Literacy

- *Comprehensive Test of Phonological Processing, Second Edition* (*CTOPP-2*) (Wagner et al., 2013) (ages 4;0–24;11)
- *Lindamood Auditory Conceptualization Test, Third Edition* (*LAC-3*) (Lindamood & Lindamood, 2004) (ages 5;0–18;11)
- *Test of Phonological Awareness, Second Edition: PLUS* (*TOPA-2+*) (Torgensen & Bryant, 2004) (5 through 8 years)
- *Test of Integrated Language & Literacy Skills* (*TILLS*) (Nelson et al., 2016) (ages 6 through 18 years)

Speech Perception

Zuk et al. (2018) found that children with CAS and language delay did significantly worse than children with CAS without language delay in their ability to distinguish "da" from "ga." Given the comorbidity of CAS and language disorders and results from previous studies showing that children with CAS often have difficulty with speech perception (Groenen et al., 1996; Ingram et al., 2019; Maassen et al., 2003; Nijland, 2009), we suggest assessing discrimination of the sounds in error. For example, if they make prevocalic voicing errors, probe their ability to discriminate voiced and voiceless cognates. The authors' experience of working with children with CAS has shown them that voicing errors, especially prevocalic voicing, as in "big" for "pig" and vowel errors could be due to poor discrimination, in addition to sensorimotor planning and programming. Examples of assessments for speech perception are as follows:

- *Speech Assessment and Interacting Learning* (*SAILS*) (Rvachew & Brosseau-Lapré, 2021) has been updated from the original computer-based tool and is now available as an app for iPads. It is designed for younger children and provides graphics and auditory stimuli with a variety of voices (e.g., adult and children). The child hears the word with the target sound said correctly and incorrectly and makes a binary choice as to if the production is correct or incorrect.

- *The Locke Speech Perception-Speech Production Task* (Locke, 1980) examines the child's ability to perceive the errors they are making. For example, if the child says the initial sound in "ship" incorrectly, the examiner will then see if the child can perceive the correct production of this word by showing an image of a ship and then asking the child to judge if the examiner said the right word when providing incorrect and correct productions of the word (e.g., Is it a "fip"? Is it a "sip"?, Is it a "ship," etc.)? Three or more errors out of six opportunities indicates the child is having difficulty correctly perceiving the target phoneme. For the test protocol and further information on this task, go to Caroline Bowen's website (URL is provided in Table 2–25).

- *The Test of Language Development Primary, Fifth Edition* (*TOLD-P5*) (Newcomer & Hammill, 2019) Word Discrimination subtest measures the child's ability to recognize differences in speech sounds by having them respond if two words are similar or different. The child is presented pairs of words that are either the same or differ by one phoneme.

Gross and Fine Motor Skills

As noted in Chapter 1, studies have found children with CAS to be at high risk for co-occurring deficits in fine and gross motor skills. Because the SLP is often the first person to evaluate a child with suspected CAS, it is important to make some general observations of the coordination of the child's gate during walking and running and coordination of the hands while the child is handling toys, cutting with scissors, and drawing or writing to make appropriate referrals to a physical therapist (PT) and/or occupational therapist (OT) if warranted. It may also be helpful to provide the parent the *Developmental Coordination Disorder Questionnaire* (*DCDQ*; Wilson & Crawford, 2007) for ages 5 to 15 years for additional information to pass onto the PT and OT to see if they qualify for additional assessment. The *DCDQ* is free, and the URL addresses can be found in Table 2–25.

Sensory

There are several ways to check sensation, such as stimulus localization and two-point discrimination. However, noting whether the child demonstrates either hypersensitivity or reduced sensitivity (hyposensitivity) to sensory stimulation is often the most useful information for the clinician. A child with tactile hypersensitivity may resist tooth brushing or face washing or may express an unwillingness to accept certain food textures. These signs should be viewed with caution, as they may be normal reactions of young children without tactile sensitivity differences. A child who exhibits hyposensitivity to tactile input may not be aware of food in the mouth, around the lips, or on the chin, or may appear unaware of drooling. Hyposensitivity also may lead to greater difficulty developing the somatosensory awareness required to support online speech production accuracy. The *Sensory Profile-2* (Dunn, 2014) for birth to 14;11 is a tool that could be used to help us screen a child's sensory processing patterns in all of their environments. However, it is best to consult with an OT for interpretation of results and recommendations for therapy. A URL to an online sensory checklist can be found in Table 2–25.

Social-Emotional Well-Being

As discussed in Chapter 1, when a child has a severe communication disorder, it can impact their lives in many ways. It is well-documented that children with communication disorders are at higher risk for being bullied and feeling isolated (van den Bedem et al., 2018). When getting to know a child during the initial assessment, we may ask about their experiences with school, clubs, family, and friends to get a sense of how fully they are included in all of their communication circles. However, we may not get complete answers, as it takes time to establish trust to discuss these sensitive topics. Social-emotional well-being is an ongoing concern for many children, regardless of communication skills. Using good listening skills and creating a safe and brave space in our therapy session will allow us to stay connected and share concerns with parents and related professionals when they arise.

Interpretation of Evaluation Findings

When the formal and informal elements of the speech and language evaluation have been completed and the data and findings are analyzed, a diagnosis (or diagnoses) may be made, and an appropriate treatment plan developed. A child is rarely ever only apraxic, so this should not be the only diagnosis listed. When we write the report, we want to be mindful of the whole child, as depicted in Figure 2–5. In other words, what is getting in the way of their communicative success, and what can we (SLPs, teachers, other therapists, family members, community) do to improve upon this success.

When reporting the assessment findings, the following sequence is recommended:

1. Describe the purpose of the evaluation including who made the referral and why.

2. Summarize the case history in a manner that provides rationale for the evaluation and the areas that were assessed.

3. Describe the child's overall demeanor (e.g., shy, hesitant, clingy with the parent, easily engaged, slow to warm up). With a young child, describe the child's play, modes of communication, and responsiveness to attempts to interact.

4. Summarize results of the SFA in a way that provides evidence for the diagnosis or diagnoses you have determined from each part of your assessment. For example, did your findings from the SFA assessment reveal any signs of dysarthria, CAS, or NVOA? If so, what were they. If not, state "no signs of ____ were observed." From the formal articulation/phonology test, provide results indicating evidence for an

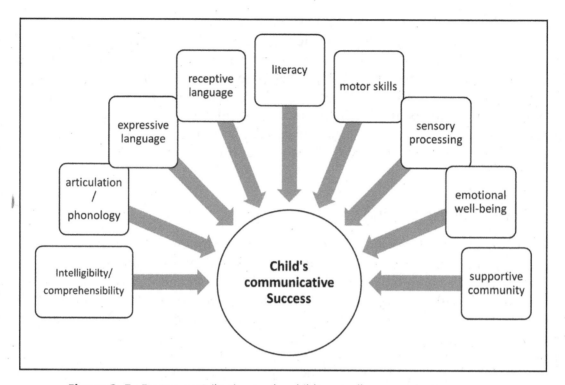

Figure 2–5. Factors contributing to the child's overall communicative success.

articulation or expressive phonological impairment and list the *active phonological processes*. If the child was unable to do a formal articulation test, provide the sound and syllable shape inventory gathered from informal assessment.

5. Assuming the child was referred for an assessment because of concern with CAS, results from the motor speech portion of the exam will be a key component of the report. Here you will want to provide the measures from the tasks that provided evidence of CAS, such as inconsistency of errors, disordered prosody, poor-coarticulation, segmented syllables, intrusive schwa, and so on. If there was no evidence of CAS, you will want to be clear to state that as well. If CAS was present, provide the level of phonetic and phonotactic complexity the child broke down at and include what cues helped the child improve. For example, "John was able to produce Vs, CVs, and VCs in two-syllable utterances with early developing sounds in direct imitation. He needed simultaneous and tactile cueing to correctly produce CVCs and three-syllable utterances." Knowing where the child was successful with cuing will guide your recommendations that address improving the child's sensory motor skills.

6. The next section should address all areas related to language and literacy. For young children, this may be based on informal observations, especially for the expressive language portion. Depending on the age of the child, results from phonological awareness and literacy measures should also be included. Since it is not always possible to assess all areas of concern in the diagnostic session, you could include a statement in your recommendations to assess the other areas you noted of concern at another time. Note additional concerns related to gross and fine motor, sensory issues/preferences, behavior, and social-emotional well-being.

7. Provide a list of recommendations that address all the areas of concern and referrals if warranted.

8. Last but not least, be sure to point out relative strengths of the child, as reading everything that is wrong with your child can be quite overwhelming. For example, was the child actively engaged and hardworking during the assessment? Did they demonstrate perseverance? Did they have a sense of humor? When writing attributes, look for the best possible way to describe them. For example, a child who was "hyperactive" could be referred to as enthusiastically energetic. Given that this is a lot to process, consider scheduling a follow-up call or visit to go through the assessment results after the parent has had time to absorb the information.

Case studies illustrating children with different communication profiles are available in the online materials.

A variety of online resources for assessment were referenced throughout this chapter. The URL or source for each of these assessment tools is listed in Table 2–25.

Table 2–25. Online Resources for Screening and Assessment Tools

Area of Assessment	Source and URL
ASD screener	Autism Navigator https://autismnavigator.learnercommunity.com/Files/Org/b7feabe6ed9e4713b02511fc0003214c/site/16-Early-Signs-of-Autism-Checklist.pdf
Symbolic play scale	*Revised Concise Symbolic Scale* (Westby, 2000) https://www.smartspeechtherapy.com/wp-content/uploads/2017/07/Revised-Concise-Symbolic-Play-Scale.pdf
ASHA's hearing screening guidelines	https://www.asha.org/practice-portal/professional-issues/childhood-hearing-screening/#collapse_1
Articulation assessments and word lists in other languages	https://www.csu.edu.au/research/multilingual-speech/speech-assessments
Measuring inconsistency	Jenya Iuzzini-Seigel, PhD, CCC-SLP provides great resources for explaining and measuring inconsistency, in addition to other CAS-related topics on her lab's Instagram account (@maquette_CML_lab); https://campsite.bio/marquette_cml_lab See links for "Buy Bobby a Puppy" and "Calculating ISP" Another link to Iuzzini's ISP tutorial: https://drive.google.com/file/d/12rQeWqCh9QqZAzHuEcJJuL3R0Nu5L7Kw/view
Picture description	Park Play: A picture description task for assessing childhood motor speech disorders (Patel & Connaghan, 2014) https://www.tandfonline.com/doi/full/10.3109/17549507.2014.894124?scroll=top&needAccess=true

continues

Table 2–25. *continued*

Area of Assessment	Source and URL
Connected speech analysis	Protocol for Connected Speech Transcription of Children with Speech Disorders (Barrett et al., 2020) https://www.ncbi.nlm.nih.gov/pmc/articles/PMC6940559/
Multisyllabic word lists	Ten clinically useful words from Caroline Bowen's website https://speech-language-therapy.com/index.php?option=com_content&view=article&id=46 Single-word test of polysyllables (Gozzard et al., 2006) https://www.academia.edu/22333231/Children_s_productions_of_polysyllables
Intelligibility	*The Preschool Speech Intelligibility Measure* (Morris, Wilcox, & Schooling, 1995), Appendix B https://doi.org/10.1044/1058-0360.0404.22 *Beginner's Intelligibility Test* and *Monsen-Indiana University Sentences* available in "Relationships between speech intelligibility and word articulation scores in children with hearing loss" (Ertmer, 2010), Appendixes A and B https://doi.org/10.1044/1092-4388(2010/09-0250)
Software for calculating intelligibility	Pronunciation Coach 3D software https://rose-medical.com//pronunciation-coach-3d.html
Intelligibility/ comprehensibility	*Intelligibility in Context Scale* available in 60 languages (McLeod et al., 2012b) http://www.csu.edu.au/research/multilingual-speech/ics
Phonological awareness	*The Phonological Awareness Screening Test* (Kilpatrick, 2019) https://www.thepasttest.com/
Speech perception	*The Locke Speech Perception-Speech Production Task* is available on Caroline Bowen's website. Directions for task: https://www.speech-language-therapy.com/index.php?option=com_content&view=article&id=46:speechax&catid=9:resources&Itemid=117 Protocol: https://www.speech-language-therapy.com/pdf/locketask.pdf
Gross motor	*Developmental Coordination Disorder Questionnaire (DCDQ)* https://www.dcdq.ca/uploads/pdf/DCDQAdmin-Scoring-02-20-2012.pdf
Sensory	Sensory checklist https://www.sensorysmarts.com/sensory-checklist.pdf
Hearing	Childhood Hearing Screening https://www.asha.org/practice-portal/professional-issues/childhood-hearing-screening/#collapse_1

References

Allison, K. (2020). Measuring speech intelligibility in children with motor speech disorders. *Perspectives of the ASHA Special Interest Groups 2, 5*(4), 809–820. https://doi.org/10.1044/2020_PERSP-19-00110

American Speech-Language-Hearing Association (n.d.). *Childhood apraxia of speech* [Practice portal]. http://www.asha.org/Practice-Portal/Clinical-Topics/Childhood-Apraxia-of-Speech/

American Speech-Language-Hearing Association. (2007). *Childhood apraxia of speech* [Technical report]. https://doi.org/10.1044/policy.TR2007-00278

Audacity [Computer Software]. (2021). https://www.audacityteam.org/

Barrett, C., McCabe, P., Masso, S., & Preston, J. (2020). Protocol for the connected speech transcription of children with speech disorders: An example from childhood apraxia of speech. *Folia Phoniatrica et Logopaedica, 72*(2), 152–166. https://doi.org/10.1159/000500664

Bayley, N., & Aylward, G. (2019). *Bayley Scales of Infant and Toddler Development Screening Test* (3rd ed.). Pearson. https://www.pearsonassessments.com/store/usassessments/en/Store/Professional-Assessments/Cognition-%26-Neuro/Brief/Bayley-Scales-of-Infant-and-Toddler-Development-Screening-Test-%7C-Third-Edition/p/100000108.html

Benway, N. R., & Preston, J. L. (2020). Differences between school-age children with apraxia of speech and other speech sound disorders on multisyllable repetition. *Perspectives of the ASHA Special Interest Groups, 5*(4), 794–808. https://doi.org/10.1044/2020_PERSP-19-00086

Bravo, L. (2017). *Bla Bla Bla* (Version 2.0) [Mobile app]. App Store. https://apps.apple.com/us/app/bla-bla-bla/id430815432

Bzoch, K. R., League, R., & Brown, V. L. (2003). *Receptive-Expressive Emergent Language Test, Third edition (REEL-3)*. Pearson.

Carlock, G. S., Fischer, T., Lynch, M. E., Potter, N. L., Coles, C. D., Epstein, M. P., . . . Fridovich-Keil, J. L. (2019). Developmental outcomes in Duarte galactosemia. *Pediatrics, 143*(1), e20182516. https://doi.org/10.1542/peds.2018-2516

Caruso, A. & Strand, E. (1999). *Clinical management of motor speech disorders in children*. Thieme.

Clark, H. M., & Baas, B. S. (2021). CAS: Similar hoofbeats, but not a horse. *ASHA Leader, 26*(1), 46–53.

Davis, B., & Velleman, S. (2000). Differential diagnosis and treatment of developmental apraxia of speech in infants and toddlers. *Infant-Toddler Intervention, 10*(3), 177–192.

Dodd, B., Hua, Z., Crosbie, S., Holm, A., & Ozanne, A. (2002). *Diagnostic evaluation of articulation and phonology*. Pearson. https://www.pearsonassessments.com/store/usassessments/en/Store/Professional-Assessments/Speech-%26-Language/Diagnostic-Evaluation-of-Articulation-and-Phonology/p/100000295.html

Duchow, H., Lindsay, A., Roth, K., Schell, S., Allen, D., & Boliek, C. A. (2019). The co-occurrence of possible developmental coordination disorder and suspected childhood apraxia of speech. *Canadian Journal of Speech-Language Pathology and Audiology, 43*(2), 81–93.

Dunn, W. (2014). *Sensory Profile 2*. Pearson. https://www.pearsonassessments.com/store/usassessments/en/Store/Professional-Assessments/Motor-Sensory/Sensory-Profile-2/p/100000822.html

Ertmer, D. J. (2010). Assessing speech intelligibility in children with hearing loss: Toward revitalizing a valuable clinical tool. *Language Speech and Hearing Services in Schools, 42*(1), 52–58. https://pubs.asha.org/doi/full/10.1044/0161-1461%282010/09-0081%29

Fenson, L. (2007). *MacArthur-Bates Communicative Development Inventories*. Paul H. Brookes.

Fletcher, S. (1972). Time-by-count measurement of diadochokinetic syllable rate. *Journal of Speech and Hearing Research, 15*(4), 763–770. https://doi.org/10.1044/jshr.1504.763

Fudala, J. B., & Stegall, S. (2017). *Arizona Articulation and Phonology Scale, Fourth edition*. Western Psychological Services. https://www.proedinc.com/Products/14723/arizona4-arizona-articulation-and-phonology-scalefourth-edition.aspx

Glaspey, A. (2021). *Glaspey Dynamic Assessment of Phonology*. Academic Therapy Publications. https://www.academictherapy.com/detailATP.tpl?eqskudatarq=2244-6

Glennen, S. (2014). A longitudinal study of language and speech in children who were internationally adopted at different ages. *Language, Speech, and Hearing Services in Schools, 45*, 185–203. https://doi.org/10.1044/2014_LSHSS-13-0035

Goldman, R., & Fristoe, M. (2015). *Goldman-Fristoe Test of Articulation-3*. Pearson.

Gozzard, H., Baker, E., & McCabe, P. (2006). Children's productions of polysyllabic words. *ACQuiring Knowledge in Speech, Language and Hearing, 8*, 113–116.

https://www.academia.edu/22333231/Children_s_productions_of_polysyllables

Gozzard, H., Baker, E. & McCabe, P. (2008). Requests for clarification and children's speech responses: Changing "pasghetti" to "spaghetti." *Child Language Teaching and Therapy, 24,* 249–263. https://doi.org/10.1177%2F0265659008096292

Groenen, P., Maassen, B., Crul, T., & Thoonen, G. (1996). The specific relation between perception and production errors for place of articulation in developmental apraxia of speech. *Journal of Speech, Language, and Hearing Research, 39,* 468–482. https://doi.org/10.1044/jshr.3903.468

Hayden, D., & Namasivayam, A. K. (2021). *Verbal Motor Production Assessment for Children–Revised (VMPAC-R)* [Mobile application software]. https://vmpac-r.com/

Hayden, D., & Square, P. (1999). *Verbal Motor Production Assessment for Children.* Psychological Corporation [out of print].

Hodson, B. (2004). *Hodson Assessment of Phonological Patterns* (3rd ed.). Pro-Ed. https://www.proedinc.com/Products/11550/happ3-hodson-assessment-of-phonological-patternsthird-edition.aspx

Ingram, S. B., Reed, V. A., & Powell, T. W. (2019). Vowel duration discrimination of children with childhood apraxia of speech: A preliminary study. *American Journal of Speech-Language Pathology, 28*(2S), 857–874. https://doi.org/10.1044/2019_AJSLP-MSC18-18-0113

Iuzzini, J., & Forrest, K. (2010). Evaluation of a combined treatment approach for childhood apraxia of speech. *Clinical Linguistics and Phonetics, 24*(4–5), 335–345. https://doi.org/10.3109/02699200903581083

Iuzzini-Seigel, J. (2019). Motor performance in children with childhood apraxia of speech and speech sound disorders. *Journal of Speech, Language, and Hearing Research, 62*(9), 3220–3233. https://doi.org/10.1044/2019_JSLHR-S-18-0380

Iuzzini-Seigel, J. (2021, May 4). Assessment of childhood apraxia of speech [Webinar]. *SPEECHPATHOLOGY.COM.* https://www.speechpathology.com/slp-ceus/course/assessment-childhood-apraxia-speech-9705

Iuzzini-Seigel, Allison, K. M., & Stoeckel, R. (2022). A tool for differential diagnosis of childhood apraxia of speech and dysarthria in children: A tutorial. *Language, Speech, and Hearing Services in Schools.* https://doi.org/10.1044/2022_LSHSS-21-00164

Iuzzini-Seigel, J., Hogan, T. P., & Green, J. R. (2017). Speech inconsistency in children with childhood apraxia of speech, language impairment, and speech delay: Depends on the stimuli. *Journal of Speech, Language, and Hearing Research, 60*(5), 1194–1210. https://doi.org/10.1044/2016_JSLHR-S-15-0184

Iuzzini-Seigel, J., & Murray, E. (2017). Speech assessment in children with childhood apraxia of speech.

Perspectives of the ASHA Special Interest Groups, 2(2), 47–60. https://doi.org/10.1044/persp2.SIG2.47

Jenista, J. (1997). Russian children and medical records. *Adoption Medical News, 3*(7), 1–8.

Kahn, M. L., & Lewis, N. P. (2015). *Khan-Lewis Phonological Analysis* (3rd ed.). Pearson. https://www.pearsonassessments.com/store/usassessments/en/Store/Professional-Assessments/Developmental-Early-Childhood/Khan-Lewis-Phonological-Analysis-%7C-Third-Edition/p/100001242.html

Kaufman, N. (1995). *Kaufman Speech Praxis Test for Children.* Wayne State University Press.

Kent, R. D., Kim, Y., & Chen, L. (2021). Oral and laryngeal diadochokinesis across the life span: A scoping review of methods, reference data, and clinical applications. *Journal of Speech, Language, and Hearing Research,* 1–50. https://doi.org/10.1044/2021_JSLHR-21-00396

Kent, R., & Rountrey, C. (2020). What acoustic studies tell us about vowels in developing and disordered speech. *American Journal of Speech-Language Pathology, 29,* 1749–1778. https://doi.org/10.1044/2020_AJSLP-19-00178

Kilpatrick, D. A. (2019). *Phonological Awareness Screening Test (PAST).* https://www.thepasttest.com/

Levy, E. S., Chang, Y. M., Hwang, K., & McAuliffe, M. J. (2021). Perceptual and acoustic effects of dual-focus speech treatment in children with dysarthria. *Journal of Speech, Language, and Hearing Research, 64*(6S), 2301–2316. https://doi.org/10.1044/2020_JSLHR-20-00301

Lewis, B. A., Freebairn, L. A., Hansen, A. J., Iyengar, S. K., & Taylor, H. G. (2004). School-age follow-up of children with childhood apraxia of speech. *Language, Speech, and Hearing Services in Schools, 35*(2), 122–140. https://doi.org/10.1044/0161-1461(2004/014)

Lindamood, P. C., & Lindamood, P. (2004). *Lindamood Auditory Conceptualization Test* (3rd ed.). Pro-Ed. https://www.proedinc.com/Products/10980/lac3-lindamood-auditory-conceptualization-testthird-edition.aspx

Lipkin, P. H., & Macias, M. M. (2020). Promoting optimal development: Identifying infants and young children with developmental disorders through developmental surveillance and screening. *Pediatrics, 145,* e20193449. https://doi.org/10.1542/peds.2019-3449

Locke, J. L. (1980). The inference of speech perception in the phonologically disordered child. Part II: Some clinically novel procedures, their use, some findings. *Journal of Speech and Hearing Disorders, 45,* 445–468. https://doi.org/10.1044/jshd.4504.445

Maassen, B., Groenen, P., & Crul, T. (2003). Auditory and phonetic perception of vowels in children with apraxic speech disorders. *Clinical Linguistics & Phonetics, 17*(6), 447-467. https://doi.org/10.1080/0269 920031000070821

Maenner, M., Shaw, K., Bakian, A.V., Bilder, D., Durkin, M., Esler, A., . . . Cogswell, M. E. (2021). Prevalence and characteristics of autism spectrum disorder among children aged 8 years—Autism and Developmental Disabilities Monitoring Network, 11 sites, United States, 2018. *Morbidity and Mortality Weekly Report Surveillance of Summaries, 70*(11), 1–16. http://dx.doi.org/10.15585/mmwr.ss7011a1

Masso, S., McLeod, S., & Baker, E. (2018). Tutorial: Assessment and analysis of polysyllables in young children language. *Language, Speech, and Hearing Services in Schools, 49*, 42–58. https://doi.org/10.10 44/2017_LSHSS-16-0047

McLeod, M. (2020). Intelligibility in context scale: Crosslinguistic use, validity, and reliability. *Speech, Language and Hearing, 23*(1), 9–16. https://doi.org/10.1080/2050571X.2020.1718837

McLeod, S., & Crowe, K. (2018). Children's consonant acquisition in 27 languages. A cross-linguistic review. *American Journal of Speech-Language Pathology, 27*, 1546–1571. https://doi.org/10.1044/2018_AJSLP-17-0100

McLeod, S., Harrison, L. J., & McCormack, J. (2012a). *Intelligibility in Context Scale.* Charles Sturt University. http://www.csu.edu.au/research/multilingual-speech/ics

McLeod, S., Harrison, L. J., & McCormack, J. (2012b). The intelligibility in context scale: Validity and reliability of a subjective rating measure. *Journal of Speech, Language, and Hearing Research, 55*(2), 648–656. https://doi.org/10.1044/1092-4388(2011/10-0130)

McLeod, S., & Verdon, S. (2014). A review of 30 speech assessments in 19 languages other than English. *American Journal of Speech-Language Pathology, 23*(4), 708–723. https://doi.org/10.1044/2014_ajslp-13-0066

Monsen, R. B. (1981). A usable test for the speech intelligibility of deaf talkers. *American Annals of the Deaf, 126*, 845–852. https://doi.org/10.1353/aad.2012.1333

Morley, M., Court, D., & Miller, H. (1954). Developmental dysarthria. *British Medical Journal, 1*, 8. https://doi.org/10.1136/bmj.1.4852.8

Morris, S. R., Wilcox, K.A., & Schooling, T. L. (1995). The preschool speech intelligibility measure. *American Journal of Speech-Language Pathology, 4*(4), 22–28. https://doi.org/10.1044/1058-0360.0404.22

Murray, E., Iuzzini-Seigel, J., Maas, E., Terban, H., & Ballard, K. J. (2021). Differential diagnosis of childhood apraxia of speech compared to other speech sound disorders: A systematic review. *American Journal of Speech-Language Pathology, 30*(1), 279–300. https://doi.org/10.1044/2020_AJSLP-20-00063

Murray, E., McCabe, P., Heard, R., & Ballard, K. J. (2015). Differential diagnosis of children with suspected childhood apraxia of speech. *Journal of Speech, Language, and Hearing Research, 58*(1), 43–60. https://doi.org/10.1044/2014_JSLHR-S-12-0358

Nelson, N., Plante, E., Helm-Estabrooks, N., & Hotz, G. (2016). *Test of Integrated Language and Literacy Skills.* Brookes Publishing. https://products.brookespublishing.com/Test-of-Integrated-Language-and-Literacy-Skills-TILLS-Examiners-Kit-P1271.aspx

Newcomer, P. L., & Hammill, D. D. (2019). *Test of Language Development: Primary* (5th ed.). Western Psychological Services. https://www.wpspublish.com/told-p5-test-of-language-developmentprimary-fifth-edition

Nijland, L. (2009). Speech perception in children with speech output disorders. *Clinical Linguistics & Phonetics, 23*(3), 222–239. https://doi.org/10.1080/026992 00802399947

Osberger, M. J., Robbins, A., Todd, S., & Riley, A. (1994). Speech intelligibility of children with cochlear implants. *Volta Review, 96*(5), 169–180.

Overby, M., Belardi, K., & Schreiber, J. (2020). A retrospective video analysis of canonical babbling and volubility in infants later diagnosed with childhood apraxia of speech. *Clinical Linguistics & Phonetics, 34*(7), 634–651. https://doi.org/10.1080/02699206.2019.1683231

Overby, M., & Caspari, S. S. (2015). Volubility, consonant, and syllable characteristics in infants and toddlers later diagnosed with childhood apraxia of speech: A pilot study. *Journal of Communication Disorders, 55*, 44–62. https://doi.org/10.1016/j.jcomdis.2015.04.001

Overby, M. S., Caspari, S. S., & Schreiber, J. (2019). Volubility, consonant emergence, and syllabic structure in infants and toddlers later diagnosed with childhood apraxia of speech, speech sound disorder, and typical development: A retrospective video analysis. *Journal of Speech, Language, and Hearing Research, 62*, 1657–1675. https://doi.org/10.1044/2019_JSLHR-S-18-0046

Parks Warshaw, S. (2013). *Hawaii Early Learning Profile (HELP: 0-3).* VORT Corporation. https://www.vort.com/product.php?productid=5

Patel, R., & Connaghan, K. (2014). Park play: A picture description task for assessing childhood motor speech disorders. *International Journal of Speech-Language Pathology, 16*(4), 337–343. https://doi.org/10.3109/17549507.2014.894124

Potter, N. L. (2004). *Oral/speech and manual motor development in preschool children* (Publication No. 3155158)

[Doctoral dissertation, University of Wisconsin–Madison]. ProQuest Dissertations and Theses Global.

Potter, N. L., & Skinder-Meredith, A. E. (2022). Structural Functional Praxis Exam [Unpublished data].

Prizant, B., & Wetherby, A. (2003). *Communication and Symbolic Behavior Scales (CSBS)*. Brookes Publishing. https://brookespublishing.com/product/csbs/

Rvachew, S. & Brosseau-Lapré, F. (2021). Speech perception intervention. In A. L. Williams, S. McLeod, & R. J. McCauley (Eds.), *Interventions for speech sound disorders in children* (2nd ed., pp. 201–224). Brookes Publishing.

Sacrey, L.-A. R., Bryson, S., Zwaigenbaum, L., Brian, J., Smith, I. M., Roberts, W., . . . Garon, N. (2018). The Autism Parent Screen for Infants: Predicting risk of autism spectrum disorder based on parent-reported behavior observed at 6–24 months of age. *Autism: The International Journal of Research and Practice, 22*(3), 322–334. doi:10.1177/1362361316675120

Seikel, A., Konstantopoulos, K., & Drumright, D. (2020). *Neuroanatomy and neurophysiology for speech and hearing sciences*. Plural Publishing.

Shriberg, L. D., Austin, D., Lewis, B. A., McSweeney, J. L., & Wilson, D. L. (1997). The percentage of consonants correct (PCC) metric: Extensions and reliability data. *Journal of Speech, Language, and Hearing Research, 40*, 708–722. https://doi.org/10.1044/jslhr.4004.708

Shriberg, L. D., & Kwiatkowski, J. (1982). Phonological disorders III: A procedure for assessing severity of involvement. *Journal of Speech and Hearing Disorders, 47*, 256–270. https://doi.org/10.1044/jshd.4703.256

Shriberg, L. D., Potter, N. L., & Strand, E. A. (2009, November). *Childhood apraxia of speech in children and adolescents with galactosemia.* [Conference presentation]. American Speech-Language-Hearing Association National Convention, New Orleans, LA.

Shriberg, L. D., Strand, E. A., Fourakis, M., Jakielski, K. J., Hall, S. D., Karlsson, H. B., . . . Wilson, D. L. (2017). A diagnostic marker to discriminate childhood apraxia of speech from speech delay: IV. The Pause Marker Index. *Journal of Speech, Language and Hearing Research, 60*(4), S1153–S1169. https://doi.org/10.1044/2016_JSLHR-S-16-0149

Shriberg, L. D., Strand, E., Jakielski, K. J., & Mabie, H. L. (2019). Estimates of the prevalence of speech and motor speech disorders in persons with complex neurodevelopmental disorders. *Clinical Linguistics & Phonetics, 33*(8), 707–736. https://doi.org/10.1080/02699206.2019.1595732

Skinder, A., Strand, E., & Mignerey, M. (1999). Perceptual and acoustic analysis of lexical and sentential stress in children with developmental apraxia of speech. *Journal of Medical Speech Pathology, 7*, 133–144.

Skinder-Meredith, A., & Fish, M. (2022). Dynamic Multisyllabic Word Probe [Unpublished].

Skoog, K. & Maas, E. (2020). Predicting intelligibility: An investigation of speech sound accuracy in childhood apraxia of speech, *CommonHealth, 1*(2), 44–56. https://doi.org/10.15367/ch.v1i2.397

Soriano, J. U., Olivieri, A., & Hustad, K. C. (2021). Utility of the Intelligibility in Context Scale for predicting speech intelligibility of children with cerebral palsy. *Brain Sciences, 11*(11), 1540. https://www.mdpi.com/2076-3425/11/11/1540

Strand, E. A. (2017). Appraising apraxia: When a speech-sound disorder is severe, how do you know if it's childhood apraxia of speech? *The ASHA Leader.* https://doi.org/10.1044/leader.FTR2.22032017.50

Strand, E. A., & McCauley, R. J. (2019). *Dynamic Evaluation of Motor Speech Skill (DEMSS) manual.* Brookes Publishing. https://products.brookespublishing.com/Dynamic-Evaluation-of-Motor-Speech-Skill-DEMSS-Manual-P1100.aspx

Thoonen, G., Maassen, B., Gabreels, F., & Schneider, R. (1999). Validity of maximum performance tasks to diagnose motor speech disorders in children. *Clinical Linguistics & Phonetics, 13*(1), 1–23. https://doi.org/10.1080/026992099299211

Torgensen, J. K., & Bryant, B. R. (2004). *Test of Phonological Awareness, Second edition: PLUS (TOPA-2+).* Pro-Ed. https://www.proedinc.com/Products/11880/topa2-test-of-phonological-awarenesssecond-edition-plus.aspx

van den Bedem, N. P., Dockrell, J. E., van Alphen, P. M., Kalicharan, S. V., & Rieffe, C. (2018). Victimization, bullying, and emotional competence: Longitudinal associations in (pre)adolescents with and without developmental language disorder. *Journal of Speech, Language, and Hearing Research, 61*(8), 1–17. https://doi.org/10.1044/2018_JSLHR-L-17-0429

Wagner, R., Torgesen, J., Rashotte, C., & Pearson, N. (2013). *Comprehensive Test of Phonological Processing, Second edition (CTOPP-2).* Pearson. https://www.pearsonassessments.com/store/usassessments/en/Store/Professional-Assessments/Speech-%26-Language/Comprehensive-Test-of-Phonological-Processing-%7C-Second-Edition/p/100000737.html

Westby, C. (1980). Assessment of cognitive and language abilities through play. *Language, Speech, and Hearing Services in Schools, 11*, 154–168. https://doi.org/10.1044/0161-1461.1103.154

Wilson, B. N., & Crawford, S. G. (2007). *Developmental Coordination Disorder Questionnaire.* https://www.dcdq.ca/

Yorkston, K., Beukelman, D., & Hakel, M. (1996). *Sentence Intelligibility (SIT) Standard* [Electronic version].

https://www.madonna.org/payments/products/sit-standard

Yorkston, K., Strand, E., & Kennedy, M. (1996). Comprehensibility of dysarthric speech: Implications for assessment and treatment planning. *American Journal of Speech-Language Pathology*, *5*(1), 55–66. https://doi.org/10.1044/1058-0360.0501.55

Zuk, J., Iuzzini-Seigel, J., Cabbage, K., Green, J., & Hogan, T. (2018). Poor speech perception is not a core deficit of childhood apraxia of speech: Preliminary findings. *Journal of Speech, Language, and Hearing Research*, *61*, 583–592. https://doi.org/10.1044/2017_JSLHR-S-16-0106

APPENDIX 2–A
Case History for Young Children

Name _____ Date _____

Birth Date _____ Chronological Age _____

Family and developmental History

Family history of speech, language, and/or literacy disorders

Genetic testing results or other diagnosis

Pregnancy and birth history:

Age of attainment of motor milestones.

turning over _____ crawling _____

sitting _____ walking _____

Has your child been diagnosed with, or do you have concerns with any of the following areas related to development?

_____ Clumsy and poor coordination for fine motor and gross motor activities

_____ Possible autism spectrum disorder (ASD)

_____ Delayed auditory comprehension

_____ Delayed expressive language

_____ Dysarthria (weakness, limited range of motion, and lack of coordination of the structures used for speech)

_____ Feeding and swallowing concerns

_____ Drooling

_____ Sensory Issues (dislikes specific sounds, textures, touch, lighting, etc.)

_____ Behavioral Concerns (difficult to soothe, highly anxious in new situations, dislikes change in routine, frequent temper tantrums, aggressive behavior, etc.)

History of Vocalizations, Babbling, and First Words

As an infant was your child quiet with limited babbling? What sounds did they make?

Does it seem like your child doesn't have as many sounds as their peers?
What sounds does your child produce?
At what age did your child produce their first consonant?
At what age did your child say their first word?
At what age was your child able to say 10–15 different words that they use regularly?
Provide examples of how your child says their most frequently occurring words (e.g., "wawa" for *water*).
Does your child use a variety of intonation patterns? In other words, can they change their voice from loud to quiet, high to low, express different emotions?
Is it common for your child to say a word and then never say it again?
Does your child ever appear to be groping for sounds?
Does your child have difficulty combining different syllables?
Does your child have more difficulty with volitional than automatic nonspeech oral motor behaviors?
Does your child use idiosyncratic signs for functional communication?

APPENDIX 2–B
Observations of Vocalizations and Communication Attempts

Name _____ Date _____

Birth Date _____ Age _____

Phonetic inventory

:

Syllable shape repertoire:

Primary modes of communication: (e.g., gestures, vocalizations, word approximations)

Circle the communicative intents observed:

   request for help labeling

   request for items describing

   request for activities commenting

   request for attention expressing feelings

   refusing or rejecting items refusing or rejecting activities

Mark the characteristics observed during the evaluation.	
	Limited resonant (speech-like) vocalizations
	Limited phonetic inventory of consonants and vowels
	Predominant use of simple syllable shapes (V, CV, CVCV, VC)
	Early sound productions restricted to Early Eight (/p, b, j, n, w, d, p, h/)
	Use of gestures and signs
	Receptive language appears higher than expressive language

APPENDIX 2-C
Case History for Preschoolers and Young School Age

Child's name: _____ DOB: _____

Parent/Guardian's name (s): _____

Tell me about a typical day with your child.

Does your child have any other diagnosis besides apraxia of speech?

Does your child have any other/related medical concerns?

Does your child have any food restrictions?

Has your child had a standardized articulation test? If so, which one, and what were the results?

How does your child get your attention? Words? Sounds? Gestures? What type of gestures?

How does your child communicate wants and needs? Speaking? Gestures?

How many words does your child produce? Are they nouns, verbs, adjectives?

Circle yes (Y) or no (N) and add any additional relevant information.

Y N   Does your child imitate speech sounds?

Y N   Does your child combine two or more words in a phrase? (i.e., more cookie, car bye-bye)

Y N   Does your child count or say the alphabet?

Y N   Does your child use simple grammatical endings (verb -ing, plural -s)?

Y N   Does your child answer simple/follow commands (i.e., get your cup)?

Y N   Does your child take turns in conversation or play?

What are some words or attempts at words that your child says?

_____

_____

_____

continues

Appendix 2–C. *continued*

What sounds does your child make? (circle all)

Sound	Example Words	Sound	Example Words
p	pin, happy, cup	sh	ship, special, rush
b	bake, rabbit, knob	h	hut, forehead
t	tan, hotel, sat	ch	cheese, nachos, beach
d	dim, soda, food	j	jug, magic, age
k	cat, bucket, music	w	wood, away
g	gum, again, dog	y	yell, royal
f	fun, coffee, rough	l	look, color, fell
v	vote, oven, have	r	run, carrot, hair
th (voiceless)	thin, nothing, tooth	m	make, summer, same
th (voiced)	that, mother, breathe	n	new, sunny, mean
s	sunny, mercy, chase	ng	longer, song, ring
z	zip, easy, peas		

How intelligible is your child's speech to strangers? (circle one)

Unintelligible   25%–50%   50%–75%   75%–100%

Are there are any phrases they say? Do they put two words together? Three words?

_____

_____

_____

With whom does your child spend a majority of the day?

Does your child initiate play with others by using language (e.g., "do you want to play with me?")?

What kinds of play activities does your child engage in?

Does your child play computer/tablet/phone games? If yes, list games.

What are some shows/movies/toys your child especially enjoys?

What are some games or activities that seem to be especially motivating to your child?

Are there any other positive reinforcements or motivating techniques your child responds well to?

What are some words/phrases that you would like your child to work on or be able to say?

1. _____

2. _____

3. _____

4. _____

What letter sounds can your child identify, and what letter sounds can they say? Circle the ones you think they understand, and underline the ones they can say.

A	B	C	D	E	F
G	H	I	J	K	L
M	N	O	P	Q	R
S	T	U	V	W	X
Y	Z				

Does your child recognize sounds in words?

Does your child recognize letters in words?

Language—Mark Y for YES, N for no, and U for UNSURE.

_____ uses language to express emotion

_____ follows two- and three-part commands

_____ tells two events in chronological order

_____ understands concepts related to time (e.g., yesterday, today, tomorrow)

_____ counts to 10

continues

_____ names days of the week in order

_____ uses conjunctions (e.g., and, or, but)

_____ uses past tense and future tense appropriately

_____ asks *how* questions

_____ follows instructions given to a group

_____ understands *left* and *right*

Phonological Awareness—Mark Y for YES, N for no, and U for UNSURE.

_____ can your child tell you the beginning sounds of words (e.g., *popcorn* begins with *p*)?

_____ does your child know the beginning sounds of their name?

_____ can your child identify the first sound in a word (e.g., Which two words start with the same sound? Pot- talk- pig)

_____ can your child identify the last sound in a word (e.g., Which two words end with the same sound? cup- lip-run)

_____ can your child recognize simple rhymes (e.g., Which two words rhyme? fat-foot-cat)

_____ can your child make a rhyme?

_____ can your child clap the number of syllables in a multisyllabic word (e.g., *cowboy* has two parts, *cow* and *boy*)?

_____ can your child add or delete phonemes from a word (e.g., "say *cat* without the *c* sound . . . *at*")?

Is there any family history of reading disabilities? Yes/No/Unsure

Literacy/Writing—Mark Y for YES, N for no, and U for UNSURE.

_____ can your child identify the front of a book?

_____ can your child identify the back of a book?

_____ does your child show an interest in books?

_____ does your child enjoy being read to?

_____ does your child have a favorite book?

_____ does your child notice print in their environment? (business signs, house items)

_____ does your child understand that pictures in a book tell a story?

_____ does your child read or pretend to read?

_____ does your child make up stories?

_____ does your child know that adults read printed text when reading stories aloud?

_____ does your child know that reading occurs from top to bottom?

_____ does your child know that reading occurs from left to right?

_____ does your child ask and/or answer questions about a story?

_____ can your child predict events in a story using illustrations or already known facts?

_____ does your child recognize their name in print?

_____ does your child pretend to write?

_____ does your child use real letters when writing?

_____ does your child attempt to write real words, even if misspelled?

_____ does your child attempt to copy words?

_____ can your child write their first name?

APPENDIX 2–D
Structure-Function-Praxis-Motor Speech Exam
(Potter & Skinder-Meredith, 2022, unpublished)

Name _____ Date of Birth _____ Date of Exam _____

Examiner _____ Age _____

History regarding chewing, drooling, swallowing, oral aversion, sensory issues, TMJ issues, etc.

_____

_____

_____

Structure & Tone (observe at rest)

Structure (STR)	Comments	Within Functional Limits (WFL)	Deviant
Cranial/facial symmetry			
Lips			
Ears			
Eyes			
Mandible			
Dentition			
Occlusion			
Tongue (symmetry at rest)			
Length of lingual frenulum			
Hard palate			
Velum			

Observations Relating to Tone		Absent	Present
Drooling			
Open-mouth posture			

Oral Motor Function (OMF)

Structure	Performance		
Tongue—CN XII	WFL	Mild-Moderately Impaired	Severely Impaired
Protrusion "Stick out your tongue." Look for deviation to left or right and range of motion (ROM).			
Elevation "Can you touch your tongue to your nose?" (Or place a tongue depressor over the upper lip and say, "Touch the stick with your tongue.") Tongue tip should elevate to the upper lip without lower lip/jaw assistance.			
Tongue wag "Can you move your tongue like mine?" Model tongue movement from corner to corner for three complete back-and-forth sequences. Observe child's attempt for speed, coordination, and ROM.			
Lateral tongue strength "I'm going to try to push your tongue. Don't let me." With jaw approximately half open, have the child push against tongue depressor on each side. Note resistance.			
Lips—CN VII			
Pucker "Say (oo)" Look for symmetry and ROM.			

continues

Appendix 2–D. *continued*

Structure	Performance		
Lips—CN VII	WFL	Mild-Moderately Impaired	Severely Impaired
Retraction *"Say (ee)"* Look for symmetry and ROM.			
Pucker to retraction *"Say (oo-ee x 3)"* Look for symmetry, ROM, and speed.			
Strength of lips pressed together *"Bite your teeth together. Now press your lips together. I'm going to try to pull your lips apart, but don't let me."* Apply upward pressure against upper two quadrants and downward pressure against lower two quadrants to check for resistance with a tongue depressor or gloved finger. If any weakness is observed, note which quadrant—upper right (UR), upper left (UL), lower right (LR), lower left (LL).			
Jaw—CN V			
Symmetry, ROM, and stability during jaw opening and closing *"Open and close your jaw x 2."* Look for smooth movement, symmetry, appropriate excursion, and evidence of jaw sliding.			
Velum—CN IX and X			
Velar elevation during sustained "ah" *"Say ah for 5 seconds. I'll tell you when to start and stop."* Look for timing of movement, ROM, symmetry, and endurance.			
Velar elevation during staccato production of "ha" *"Say ha-ha-ha."* Look for timing of movement, symmetry, and ROM.			

Summary of findings: Include observations of symmetry and tone of structures at rest and observations of range of motion, symmetry, speed, strength, and coordination during movement tasks.

_____

_____

_____

_____

Assessment of Resonance, Phonation, Respiratory Support, and Articulation

Resonance

To assist with judgment of resonance use a listening tube or straw going from under one of the client's nostrils to the listener's ear or place a small mirror under the nostrils while they repeat the following stimuli. If the phrase is too difficult, have them repeat the syllable instead.

	Normal	Hypernasal	Nasal Emissions	Hyponasal
Buy Bobby a puppy Pa pa pa				
Seesaw, Seesaw, Seesaw Sa sa sa				
Mama made lemonade Ma ma ma				
Spontaneous speech				

continues

Appendix 2–D. *continued*

Phonation and Respiration

Use a stopwatch or sound editing software (e.g., Audacity) to time the number of seconds for each trial.

Phonation-Respiration Duration	Trial 1	Trial 2	Trial 3	Longest of Three Trials
Maximum exhalation duration (MED) Have a cup of water with a straw positioned so the low end is 5 cm below the surface of the water. You may need to plug the child's nose to avoid air escape. *"Blow through the straw and make bubbles for as long as you can in one breath. I'll go first."*				
Maximum phonation duration (MPD) *"Say /ah/ for as long as possible. I'll go first."*				

Phonation-CN X
*You can use your observations of sustained phonation from the last task, rather than having the child sustain phonation again.

Observations of Phonatory Quality and Control	Normal	Abnormally High Or Low Pitch	Reduced Pitch Range	Strained/ Strangled	Breathy	Rough	Tremor/ Flutter/ Pitch Instability
*Sustained Phonation** *"Say /ah/ steadily for as long as you can. I'll go first."*							

Observations of Phonatory Quality and Control	Normal	Abnormally High Or Low Pitch	Reduced Pitch Range	Strained/ Strangled	Breathy	Rough	Tremor/ Flutter/ Pitch Instability
Pitch Range *"Sing ah, then go as low as you can. Sing ah again and then go as high as you can. I'll go first."*							
Spontaneous Speech Observe the child's pitch range and voice quality during a connected speech sample.							

*If the child could speak in multisyllable utterances, note how many syllables they could say in one breath group and if they appear to be running out of breath by the end of their sentence or taking a breath in linguistically inappropriate places.

Normative Data on Maximum Phonation Duration (MPD) and Maximum Exhalation Duration (MED) Based on 20 males and 20 females per age group (Carlock et al., 2019; Potter, 2004).

Age in Years	MPD Mean (SD) in Seconds	MED Mean (SD) in Seconds
3–4	3.45 (1.23)	6.08 (2.61)
5–7	11.65 (4.09)	11.13 (6.00)
8–9	14.23 (4.96)	13.72 (6.18)
10–12	15.77 (6.02)	17.55 (7.75)

continues

Appendix 2–D. *continued*

Articulation-Diadochokinetic (DDK) Task

DDK	Trial 1	Trial 2	Trial 3	Highest DDK Rate of the Three Trials
/pʌ/	_____syllables/ _____seconds =___ syll/sec	_____syllables/ _____seconds =___ syll/sec	_____syllables/ _____seconds =___ syll/sec	=___ syll/sec
/tʌ/	_____syllables/ _____seconds =___ syll/sec	_____syllables/ _____seconds =___ syll/sec	_____syllables/ _____seconds =___ syll/sec	=___ syll/sec
/kʌ/	_____syllables/ _____seconds =___ syll/sec	_____syllables/ _____seconds =___ syll/sec	_____syllables/ _____seconds =___ syll/sec	=___ syll/sec
/pʌtʌkʌ/	_____syllables/ _____seconds =___ syll/sec	_____syllables/ _____seconds =___ syll/sec	_____syllables/ _____seconds =___ syll/sec	=___ syll/sec

DDK comparative data in syllables/second for ages 2–15 years (Kent et al., 2021)
These data represent a compilation of multiple studies of children without speech disorders. The ranges represent the lowest mean DDK rate to the highest mean DDK rate reported in these studies. (Outliers were removed from averages and ranges.)

Age in Years	/pʌ/ Mean (range)	/tʌ/ Mean (range)	/kʌ/ Mean (range)	/pʌtʌkʌ/ Mean (range)
2–3[a]	3.86 (3.46–4.74)	3.83 (3.38–4.56)	3.56 (3.36–3.75)	3.41 (2.82–4.23)
4–5	4.21 (3.62–4.92)	4.35 (3.54–4.82)	3.89 (3.00–4.76)	3.70 (2.86–4.47)
6–7	4.45 (3.93–5.56)	4.46 (3.42–5.88)	4.04 (3.33–4.74)	3.86 (2.91–4.74)
8–9	4.78 (4.54–5.88)	4.7 (4.30–5.88)	4.26 (4.12–4.49)	4.32 (3.85–5.19)
10–11	5.1 (4.63–5.56)	5.03 (4.66–5.56)	4.62 (4.50–5.00)	4.92 (4.22–5.46)
12–15	5.9 (4.76–6.06)	5.25 (4.46–6.06)	4.91 (4.39–5.40)	5.55 (4.35–6.66)

[a]Although data are available for young children, it is not always possible to elicit the productions in a reliable and valid manner.

DDK observations: In addition to comparing the child's DDK rates to the norms above, note observations on rhythmicity, articulatory accuracy, voicing errors, sequencing errors, addition of a segment, deletion of a segment, consistency of errors, and ability to complete task. You can also compare ease of producing AMRs to the SMR task.

_____

_____

Summary of observations of resonance, phonation, respiratory support, and articulation:

_____

_____

_____

_____

Examination for Nonverbal Oral Apraxia (NVOA):

Give verbal directions, then model if necessary.

0 = imitates immediately

1 = mild groping; or delayed but successful

2 = groping **or** sequential efforts (up to four tries), then success

3 = could not achieve imitation even though there is purposeful effort

4 = child does not/cannot attempt to do the task

	Blow out a candle	Smile	Puff out your cheeks	Smack your lips together	Clear your throat	Bite your lower lip
Score						

Sum NVOA Score _____ (0–24 possible)

Nonspeech Movement Sequencing (NSMS):

Give verbal directions, then model if necessary (same scoring as above)

	Smile, Blow, Smile	Smack your lips together, then clear your throat	Sip through a straw, then bite your lower lip	Open your mouth wide, then lick the back of your top teeth
Score				

continues

Appendix 2–D. *continued*

Sum NSMS Score _____ (0–16 possible)

Sum PRAXIS Score _____ (0–40 possible)

For comparison to children without a speech sound disorder, see the table below to note if the child fell within the normal range.

NVOA Average Scores With Standard Deviations and Ranges of Children With Typical Speech Development (GFTA-3 standard score of over 75)

Age/Sample	Boys	Girls
6- to 7-year-olds (boys *n* = 35; girls *n* = 30)	4.3 (3.6) Normal range 0–10	2.5 (1.96) Normal range 0–6
8- to 9-year-olds (boys *n* = 50; girls *n* = 36)	2.3 (2.5) Normal range 0–6	1.9 (2.5) Normal range 0–6
10- to 12-year-olds (boys *n* = 51; girls *n* = 59)	1 (1.3) Normal range 0–3	1 (1.3) Normal range 0–3

Summary statement for NVOA: include if the child's performance fell within the normal range or not and diagnostic impressions on the child's performance.

Dynamic Multisyllabic Word Repetition Probe
(Skinder-Meredith & Fish, 2022)

Target Word	Articulatory accuracy + if correct Transcribe or mark sounds that were incorrect, added, or omitted, if incorrect	Coarticulation + good smooth coarticulation – poor coarticulation – syllable segmentation	Lexical stress accuracy + correct – incorrect	If incorrect, is there improvement with backward chaining or other cuing methods? Y/N If so, note the method that was helpful.
Three-Syllable Words				
vacation /ve.ˈkeɪ.ʃən/				
medicine /ˈmɛ.də.sɪn/				
accident /ˈæk.sə.dənt/				
gigantic /dʒaɪ.ˈgæn.tɪk/				
beautiful /ˈbju.ɾɪ.fəl/				
character /ˈkæ.rə.ktɚ/				
computer /kəm.ˈpju.ɾɚ/				
magnified /ˈmæg.nə.faɪd/				
subtraction /səb.ˈtræk.ʃən/				
principal /ˈprɪn.sə.pəl/				

continues

Appendix 2–E. *continued*

Target Word	Articulatory accuracy + if correct Transcribe or mark sounds that were incorrect, added, or omitted, if incorrect	Coarticulation + good smooth coarticulation – poor coarticulation – syllable segmentation	Lexical stress accuracy + correct – incorrect	If incorrect, is there improvement with backward chaining or other cuing methods? Y/N If so, note the method that was helpful.
Four-Syllable Words				
avocado /a.və.ˈka.doʊ/				
macaroni /mæ.kə.ˈroʊ.ni/				
television /ˈte.lə.vɪ.ʒən/				
embarrassment /ɪm.ˈbæ.rəs.mənt/				
calculator /ˈkæl.kjə.leɪ.rɚ/				
celebration /sɛ.lɪ.ˈbreɪ.ʃən/				
experiment /ɛk.ˈspɛ.rɪ.mənt/				
impossible /ɪm.ˈpa.sə.bl̩/				
punctuation /pʌŋk.tʃu.ˈeɪ.ʃən/				
dictionary /ˈdɪk.ʃə.ne.ri/				
combination /kam.bɪ.ˈneɪ.ʃən/				

Target Word	Articulatory accuracy + if correct Transcribe or mark sounds that were incorrect, added, or omitted, if incorrect	Coarticulation + good smooth coarticulation – poor coarticulation – syllable segmentation	Lexical stress accuracy + correct – incorrect	If incorrect, is there improvement with backward chaining or other cuing methods? Y/N If so, note the method that was helpful.
Five-Syllable Words				
congratulations /kən.ˌɡræ.t͡ʃə.ˈleɪ.ʃənz/				
enthusiasm /ɛn.ˈθu.zɪ.jæ.zəm/				
evaporation /ɪ.væ.pə.ˈreɪ.ʃ<u>ən</u>/				
intimidating /ɪn.ˈtɪ.mə.deɪ.ɾɪŋ/				
unbelievable /ʌn.bə.ˈliː.və.bl̩/				
photosynthesis /foʊ.ɾoʊ.ˈsɪn.θə.sɪs/				
electricity /ɪ.lek.ˈtrɪ.sə.ɾi/				
imagination /ɪ.mæ.dʒɪ.ˈneɪ.ʃən/				
hippopotamus /hɪ.pə.ˈpɑ.ɾə.məs/				
pediatrician /pi.di.jə.ˈtrɪ.ʃən/				

APPENDIX 2–F

Sentential Stress and Intonation Probe

(Adapted from Skinder et al., 1999)

Directions: *I am going to say a sentence. I want you to repeat the sentence exactly like I said it.*

(Stress italicized words. Use appropriate statement versus question intonation, and add tone of voice variations when appropriate, e.g., excitement for "We won the game!" or displeasure for "Go away!")

- Intonation Contour: Mark + when the child matches the intonation contour and – when they do not.

- Primary Stress: Mark + when the child matches the stressed word(s) and – when they do not.

- WSD: Mark – if weak syllable deletion occurred and + if it did not.

	Intonation Contour	Primary Stress	Omission Of Unstressed Words Or Syllables
1. Have *you* seen my cat?			
2. *We* won the *game*!			
3. This is *so* boring.			
4. I wanna go *home*.			
5. Is it *time* to *go*?			
6. Look at *me*.			
7. *Please* stop doing that.			
8. Do *you* like pizza?			
9. *Go away*!			
10. I *like* you.			
TOTAL	/10	/10	/10

TOTAL: ___ /30 = ___ %

APPENDIX 2–G
Phonetic Transcription

Phonetic Symbols for American English Consonants, Vowels, and Diphthongs

Consonants	
Phonetic Symbol	**Sample Word**
/p/	pot
/b/	bike
/t/	toe
/d/	dough
/ɾ/ flap/tap[a]	butter /bʌɾɚ/
/k/	cup
/g/	game
/ʔ/ glottal stop[b]	mitten [mɪʔn̩]
/m/	me
/n/	new
/ŋ/	ring
/w/	wait
/j/	you
/f/	fine
/v/	van
/θ/	thing
/ð/	that
/s/	sing
/z/	zoo
/ʃ/	shoe
/ʒ/	rouge
/h/	him

continues

Appendix 2–G. *continued*

Consonants	
Phonetic Symbol	**Sample Word**
/tʃ/	chair
/dʒ/	jump
/l/	lake
/r/	run

ᵃThe flap/tap is an allophone of /t/ and /d/ typically used for intervocalic alveolar stops when the second syllable is not stressed.

ᵇThe glottal stop is dialectal and may occur when a /t/ or /d/ is unreleased and precedes a syllabic /n/ and occasionally syllabic /l/. Glottal stop substitutions can also occur as an error and should not be confused with omissions.

Pure Vowels	
Phonetic Symbol	**Sample Word**
/i/	team
/ɪ/	fit
/e/	pain
/ɛ/	pet
/æ/	hat
/u/	new
/ʊ/	push
/o/	coat
/ɔ/	ball
/ɑ/	hot
/ʌ/	fun
/ə/	again
/ɝ/	perfect
/ɚ/	super

Diphthongs	
Phonetic Symbol	**Sample Word**
/aɪ/	**high**
/aʊ/	**out**
/ɔɪ/	**boy**

When evaluating a child with an articulation disorder, it may be sufficient for the SLP to mark the substitution or distortion errors on the assessment form; however, when evaluating a child with suspected CAS, it is imperative for the SLP to be able to accurately transcribe the child's productions narrowly. The nature of the speech characteristics, such as vowel distortions, lengthening or shortening of phonemes, syllable stress errors, and gaps between syllables, make it essential for the SLP to accurately transcribe the child's speech using narrow transcription. An SLP completing a motor speech evaluation should be able to do the following:

- identify the phonotactic structure of words
- accurately transcribe speech phonetically
- recognize and transcribe vowel errors, including distortions
- use diacritical markers to describe nuances of the child's speech
- recognize gaps between syllables/words
- recognize glottal stops
- calculate the percentage of consonants and vowels correct

Each of these transcription skills is described below.

continued

Appendix 2–G. *continued*

Identification of the Phonotactic Structure of Words and Phonetic Transcription

When identifying the phonotactic structure of words, each consonant and vowel should be identified, along with the syllable breaks and stress assignment. The SLP should know what the correct phonotactic structure should be for the target word or phrase and be able to compare this to the child's actual production of that target. Following are examples of phonotactic structures and phonetic transcriptions of accurately produced English words, including syllable breaks (identified with "." between syllables) and stress assignment (identified with " ' " before the stressed syllable). Some words were left undone to practice. Answers can be viewed on the Online Book Companion.

Target Word	Phonotactic Structure	Phonetic Transcription
Brought	CCVC	/brɔt/
Touch		
Shopped	CVCC	/ʃapt/
Judged		
Bunny	'CV.CV	/'bʌ.ni/
Machine		
Pronounced	CCV.CVCCC	/prə.'naʊnst/
Subscribes		
Millions	CVC.CVCC	/'mɪl.yənz/
Earthquakes		
Confusing	CVC. 'CCV.CVC	/kən.'fju.zɪŋ/
Beautiful		
Evacuation	V.CVC.CV.'V.CVC	/ɪ.væk.ju.'e.ʃən/ or /ɪ.væk.ju.'e.ʃn̩/
Incredible		
Unbutton	VCCVCC	/ʌn.bʌ.ʔn̩/
Forgotten		

Diacritical Marks

When using narrow transcription, there are numerous diacritical marks that can be used to describe nuances in the child's speech that the phonetic transcription alone would not be able to describe. Only a few diacritical marks are listed below. Please refer to the Online Book Companion to hear audio files of these practice words to help better understand the meaning and use of these diacritical marks.

Diacritical Marks	Symbol Used	Phonetic Transcription
Syllable stress marker	ˈ	bunny [ˈbʌ.ni]
Syllabic consonants (e.g., /n, l, m/)	ˌ	Purple [ˈpɝ.pl̩]
Glottal stop	ʔ	Mitten [mɪ.ʔn̩]
Aspiration	ʰ	Top [tʰɑp]
Dentalization	◌̪	Top [t̪ɑp]
Lateralization	ˡ	Bus [bʌˡs]
Lengthening	ː	Top [tɑːp]
Nasalized	õ	Tap [tãp]
Syllable gap	..(short gap) ...(longer gap)	Baby [ˈbe..bi] [ˈbe...bi]
No audible release	◌̚	Tap [tɑp̚]
Extra short	ŏ	Bed [bĕd]
More rounded	◌̹	Saw [sɔ̹]
Less rounded	◌̜	Saw [sɔ̜]
Creaky voice	◌̰	Box [b̰ɑks]
Breathy voice	◌̤	Box [b̤ɑks]

Following are examples of productions of target words phonetically transcribed without diacritical marks and with diacritical marks. When you go to the Online Book Companion, you can listen to how each word would be produced without and with diacritical markers. The differences are meaningful and offer important information about how a child actually produces the target words.

continues

Appendix 2–G. *continued*

Target Word	Phonetic Transcription Without Diacritical Marks	Target Word	Phonetic Transcription With Diacritical Marks
Brought	[bap]	Brought	[bap̚]
Touch	[dʌ]	Touch	[d̪ʌ]
Bunny	[bʌ.ni]	Bunny	[ˈbʌ...ˈn̪ːi]
Machine	[din]	Machine	[dĩːn]
Confusing	[du.du]	Confusing	[ˈd̪u.d̪u]
Beautiful	[bu.bo]	Beautiful	[ˈbu...ˈbo]

Calculation of percentage of consonants and vowels correct

To calculate the percentage of consonants correct (PCC) or percentage of vowels correct (PVC), the following equation is used:

$$\text{PCC-R} = \text{Number of correct consonants (excluding distortions)} \div \text{Total number of consonants} \times 100.$$

$$\text{PVC-R} = \text{Number of correct vowels (excluding rhotics)} \div \text{Total number of vowels} \times 100.$$

To calculate the percentage of phonemes correct (PPC), the following equation is used:

$$\text{PPC-R} = \text{Number of correct phonemes (excluding rhotic vowels and distorted consonants)} \div \text{Total number of phonemes} \times 100.$$

For practice calculating Percentage Consonants and Vowels Correct, please go to the Online Book Companion and try the practice activities.

Percentage of Phonemes Correct		Number of Phonemes in Target Word		Number of Phonemes Produced Correctly by Child	
Target Word	Transcription	C	V	C	V
Brought	[bɑpʲ]	3	1	1	0
Touch	[d̪ʌ]	2	1		
Bunny	[ˈbʌ...ˈn̪ːi]	2	2	2	2
Machine	[dĩːn]	3	2		
Confusing	[ˈd̪u.d̪u]	6	3	0	1
Beautiful	[ˈbu...ˈbo]	5	3		
TOTALS		21	11		
	PERCENTAGES			% correct consonants	% correct vowels

When determining the percentage of phonemes correct, minor distortions or incorrect articulatory placements (e.g., dentalization of /n/ in "bunny;" nasalization of the /i/ in "machine") are counted as correct. The use of diacritics, however, is still important, because it provides important nuanced information about the way the child produces utterances (e.g., equal stress, syllable segmentation, nasalization).

Fundamentals of Treatment for Childhood Apraxia of Speech

When providing treatment for children with childhood apraxia of speech (CAS), there are several underlying principles to keep in mind. Although each child's profile will be unique, certain principles will remain consistent in treatment. These include the following:

- understanding the **principles of motor learning** that will guide treatment decisions
- providing opportunities for **repetitive practice**
- addressing **phoneme sequencing** and **coarticulation**
- selecting appropriate **target utterances** for treatment
- incorporating **multisensory cueing**
- providing sufficient **intensity of treatment**

Principles of Motor Learning and Their Application to Treatment of CAS

This section describes the *principles of motor learning* (PML) that guide treatment decisions when working with children with CAS. These principles correspond to the substantial amount of research on motor learning principles from the field of motor control and learning. Maas et al. (2008) offer a comprehensive discussion of the PML and their relationship to speech motor learning in adults and children. Research regarding PML in CAS treatment is somewhat limited; however, there have been some studies over the past several years that have helped guide speech-language pathologists (SLPs) in their application of PML to treatment of children with CAS.

In CAS treatment, children first need to acquire a skill, then work on retention and generalization of the skill. The organization of the sessions will look different depending on whether we are trying to support initial acquisition of a skill or help the child retain and generalize the skill. These principles, described by Schmidt and Lee (2005), suggest optimal conditions of practice that support the initial acquisition of motor skills, as well as retention (maintenance) and transfer (generalization) of these skills. Table 3–1 lists the PML that have the greatest impact on our treatment decisions. Each of these principles is discussed in greater detail in the rest of this chapter.

Pre-Practice

During *pre-practice*, the clinician draws the child's attention to aspects of the target utterances that require change. Several teaching and cueing strategies are incorporated into pre-practice,

Table 3–1. Principles of Motor Learning Guiding Treatment Decisions in Children With CAS

Principles of Motor Learning Related to Conditions of Practice	Descriptions
Pre-practice	Preparation for learning—providing cues and strategies to set the stage for learning to occur
Distribution of practice • Massed • Distributed	Length and frequency of sessions
Practice amount/number of trials • High # of trials • Low # of trials	Number of practice trials provided during a given session
Schedule of practice • Blocked • Random	Practicing one target skill repeatedly (blocked) or several target utterances in random order (random)
Variability of practice • Constant • Variable	Providing opportunities to vary the motor plan (e.g., rate, prosody, pitch)
Principles of Motor Learning Related to Conditions of Practice	**Descriptions**
Type of feedback • Knowledge of performance • Knowledge of results	Providing specific feedback or general feedback
Frequency of feedback • High frequency • Low frequency	How frequently the feedback is provided
Timing of feedback • Immediate • Delayed	Whether the feedback is provided immediately after the child's productions or after a delay

such as shaping, modeling, phoneme placement cues, probing for facilitating contexts, focused stimulation, or work on discrimination of correct and incorrect productions. During pre-practice, the clinician introduces relevant information about the target utterances and provides opportunities for the child to accurately achieve sensorimotor plans for those targets. This gives the child the sensory experience (tactile, kinesthetic, proprioceptive, and auditory sensations) of achieving several correct productions of the desired response prior to moving on to the practice phase. In essence, pre-practice sets the stage for the child to be successful during the practice portion of the session.

During the pre-practice portion, the clinician provides frequent and specific feedback about what the child did well and what the child needs to do differently. The clinician facilitates the child's *motivation* and *focused attention*. *Motivation* is enhanced when the clinician develops a rapport with the child and provides strategies and opportunities for the child to be successful in communicative attempts. Fun and engaging activities (that do not take too much time away from practice) also will make the learning more enjoyable and more motivating. To facilitate *focused attention*, the clinician provides cues that bring the child's attention to the clinician's face, so the child can see what is expected in terms of movement of the oral-facial structures. When a child is reluctant to look at the clinician's face, video modeling can be used as an alternative. The initial use of slower rate and tactile cues also helps the child focus attention internally on how the movement should feel through development of greater proprioception. Focused attention also helps the child develop an understanding of why they are there and what they are working on—movement. The words you choose when speaking to the child help bring the child's attention to movement (e.g., "I like the way you <u>moved</u> your tongue tip up to make the /t/ sound." "Your mouth moved just like my mouth!").

Distribution of Practice—Massed/Distributed

Distribution of practice refers to the frequency and duration of treatment sessions. Schmidt and Lee (2005) suggest that individuals achieve better performance using a *massed practice* schedule of more frequent sessions over a shorter period (e.g., four sessions per week for 8 weeks) than a *distributed practice* schedule of less frequent sessions over a longer period (e.g., twice-weekly sessions for 16 weeks). Research by Thomas et al. (2014), Murray et al. (2012), and Namasivayam et al. (2015) confirmed this recommendation, as children in their studies receiving massed practice treatment had better outcomes than those with distributed practice schedules. A study by Allen (2013) found that children with phonological impairments (not CAS) who received frequent sessions for a shorter time frame (i.e., three sessions per week for 8 weeks) demonstrated better performance than those who received less frequent intervention over a longer time frame (i.e., one session per week for 24 weeks).

Practice Amount—High/Low

Higher amounts of practice (number of practice trials within a given session) should lead to better treatment outcomes. Edeal and Gildersleeve-Neumann (2011) provided validation of the importance of frequent production of treatment targets in children with CAS. Their research found that when targets were practiced with higher frequency (100+ productions of each target within a session), there was faster improvement and greater generalization to untrained targets than when targets were practiced at a lower frequency (30–40 productions of each target within a session). In a more recent study by Maas et al. (2019), most of the subjects demonstrated better motor learning with higher amounts of practice of each target utterance (e.g., ≅14 practice opportunities versus ≅7 practice opportunities of each target utterance per session). These findings are important because they remind clinicians that it is critical to use treatment time efficiently, so the child has more practice opportunities.

Schedule of Practice—Blocked/Random

In *blocked practice*, the child would practice a specific target utterance for a specified number of trials before moving on to the next stimulus item. In *random practice*, the child would practice items in a random order. Maas et al. (2008) suggest that blocked practice may be more effective in promoting early learning of targets during the acquisition stage, whereas random practice facilitates retention and transfer of sensorimotor speech plans.

Maas and Farinella (2012) compared random versus blocked practice treatment schedules in children with CAS and found mixed results, with some subjects demonstrating better results with blocked and some showing an advantage with random practice schedules. It is likely that the child's response to blocked practice or random practice schedules is dependent on where the child was in the acquisition of the particular motor skill being addressed. Strand (2020) suggests using a *modified block* practice schedule "that begins with blocked practice and moves to shorter blocks and finally random practice" (p. 41). In a modified block schedule, a child practices multiple productions of one stimulus item in a block ("Hi mommy") before moving on to the next block with a different stimulus item ("Go home"). Within each block, the child works toward increasing accuracy of production with greater variability (e.g., loud, quiet, fast, slow, varied intonation patterns) and reduced cueing.

In the early stages of acquisition of a new sensorimotor plan, blocked practice of the target utterance is recommended. After the child is able to produce the target utterance more reliably without intensive cueing and with normal prosody, the utterance could be practiced along with other target utterances in a more randomized order. Consider a child who is working on eight targets: *"Hi mom," "Oh wow!" "Bye daddy," "Go home," "I do," "nigh nigh baby," "shhh,"* and *"all done."* The clinician may set up several activities for the session. During the first activity, the child can produce *"Hi mom"* each time a toy character gets off the school bus and greets the "mommy" figure until the child has achieved 30+ practice trials of *"Hi mom."* The "mommy" figure can then tell the toy characters that she has a surprise in the kitchen to elicit *"Oh wow"* for 20+ trials before moving on to the second activity to work on *"Bye daddy"* and *"go home."* Because of the child's earlier success and stability with *"I do"* (from a prior session) and *"Oh wow!"* the clinician will practice these two utterances in a random practice mode, shifting between the two targets in random order. The final two activities would elicit three new targets, *"nigh nigh baby," "shhh,"* and *"all done,"* along with two targets practiced earlier, *"go home"* and *"Hi mom,"* each practiced in a blocked schedule. A sample blocked and random practice schedule for a child with severe CAS is shown in Figure 3–1.

In reality, the clinician will be making decisions about using a blocked or random practice schedule based on the child's responses in the moment. The child may be producing target utterances in random order, but if the child begins to struggle with a specific target, the work on that target would shift to blocked practice before it is rotated back into the random practice schedule. For a child with severe CAS, a small number of stimulus items (perhaps five or six items) would be practiced during a treatment session using a blocked schedule. When the child's production of a stimulus item is stable in a blocked schedule, that stimulus item can be rotated into a set of stimuli to practice in a random schedule.

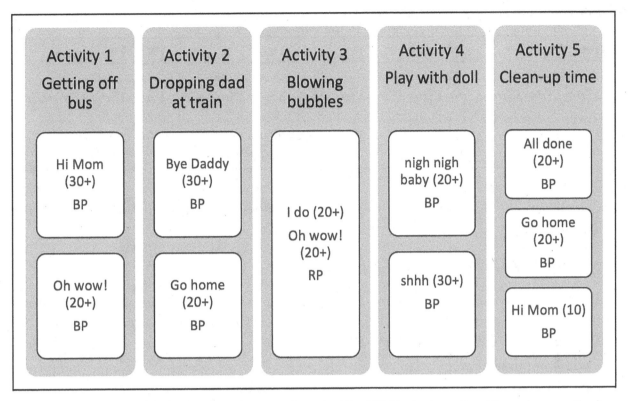

Figure 3–1. Sample blocked and random practice schedule. (*BP, blocked practice; RP, random practice.*)

The example in Box 3–1 provides a case study of a child who is struggling with CVC shapes. You will see the clinician shift from a blocked to a random practice schedule as the child's skills improve. In phonological intervention, working on final consonant deletion is a common goal, and it often is addressed by choosing stimuli with a variety of final consonants (e.g., hat, mom, moon, cup, back). For a child with CAS, however, final consonants may need to be addressed more methodically, with a focus on sensorimotor planning, first choosing a final consonant for which the child is stimulable, perhaps a bilabial continuent, such as

■ **Box 3–1.** Case Illustration of Blocked and Random Practice Schedule

Kamal is a 4-and-a-half-year-old boy with moderate-to-severe CAS. It was difficult for him to work on mixed targets within the same session, as he would overgeneralize from earlier productions. For example, when working on closing syllables with a final consonant, Kamal achieved early success with final /m/. When attempting to vary the final consonant by introducing a different target, such as final /f/ or /t/, Kamal demonstrated overgeneralization of the /m/ and would insert /m/ for all final consonants. Eventually, final /t/ was introduced in a blocked practice condition of practicing all final /m/ targets during one activity and all final /t/ targets in a separate activity. Over time, other targets with varied place, manner, and voicing features were added to expand Kamal's coarticulatory flexibility. Eventually he was able to demonstrate a high level of accuracy when we shifted to a random practice condition where different targets were practiced in random order (e.g., go home, off, go out, hi mom, enough, hey wait, go home, enough, hi mom, off, go out, hey wait). Table 3–2 illustrates the changes in practice schedule over time for Kamal's final consonant productions.

Table 3–2. Sample Practice Schedule Illustrating Movement From Blocked to Random Practice

Week 1	Week 2	Week 4	Week 6
Blocked practice	Blocked practice	Random practice	Random practice
Activity 1: Final /m/	Activity 1: Final /m/	Activity 1: Final /m/ and final /t/	Activity 1: Final /m/, /t/, and /f/
Activity 2: Final /m/	Activity 2: Final /t/	Blocked practice	Activity 2: Final /m/, /t/, and /f/
		Activity 2: Final /f/	

/m/, before moving on to other consonant phonemes with variations in place and manner of production.

Variability of Practice—Constant/Variable

Practice variability relates to practicing target stimuli in either a relatively constant manner/context (*constant practice*) or in varied manners/contexts (*variable practice*). A clinician can vary the manner of production of a target by changing

- rate of production
- loudness
- pitch
- tone of voice
- intonation

Contextual variability may include the following:

- using varied phonetic contexts to achieve variability in movement patterns
- varying sentential stress
- practicing targets in different settings
- practicing with a less familiar communicative partner
- shifting from single-word productions to phrase-/sentence-level productions

When first learning a challenging sensorimotor plan, a child benefits from practicing targets at a relatively constant rate and with relatively consistent vocal parameters (loudness, pitch, vocal quality, intonation, stress). After the child is able to produce the desired sensorimotor plan, practice should become more variable. Children can practice producing the targets using variable rates of production (normal or slow rate), volume (whispered, normal, and louder), pitch (like papa bear, mama bear, baby bear), vocal quality/tone of voice (using an angry, sad, happy, tired voice), intonation patterns (declarative statement versus yes/no question), or stress (placing stress on different words within the phrase/sentence). The clinician can introduce variability in practice by having the child produce target utterances in different settings (in treatment room, hallway, classroom, playground) and with different communicative partners (clinician, parents, siblings, familiar and less familiar peers and adults). Altering the manner and context of the practice will lead to better maintenance and generalization of skills.

Types of Feedback—Intrinsic/Extrinsic, Knowledge of Results/Knowledge of Performance

Schmidt and Lee (2005) divide feedback into two basic types: *inherent feedback* and *augmented feedback*. *Inherent feedback*, also known as *intrinsic feedback*, is derived naturally from the sensory information received from the movement itself. In the case of speech, intrinsic feedback for a learner would include the tactile, kinesthetic, and proprioceptive input received through the skin, muscles, and joints, as well as auditory feedback received from listening to the production and examining if the production matched the intended outcome. Because children with CAS may have a reduced ability to detect the somatosensory information received through tactile and proprioceptive input during the process of speaking, they tend to rely on auditory feedback and possibly faulty error detection of their speech. Thus, it is imperative that the clinician provides the child with *augmented feedback*, also termed *extrinsic feedback*, which is information provided by an outside source. Extrinsic feedback can be provided either as *knowledge of performance* (KP) or *knowledge of results* (KR). Schmidt and Lee describe KP as feedback about the movement itself ("Your tongue poked through your teeth that time. Try again with your tongue behind your teeth." "Nice job rounding your lips for that one!"). KR refers to knowledge about the accuracy of the movement, that is, whether the production was correct or incorrect ("That was correct." or "Not quite. Try it again."). KP feedback supports early attainment and acquisition of a sensorimotor plan; KR supports generalization and retention of the sensorimotor plan. It is key that the information provided as KP is clear and specific to the features of movement that need to be changed. When the learner has shown the capacity to produce the sensorimotor plan with a fairly high level of accuracy with KP, the clinician would shift the feedback to KR. Schmidt and Lee indicate that performance and generalization outcomes actually can be hindered if children become reliant on KP feedback.

Clinicians often fall into a pattern of providing praise (e.g., Very good!), almost as a knee-jerk reaction, even when the child's productions do not meet the expected goal. We often want to provide positive reinforcement but may be reinforcing incorrect productions. For example, the utterance is *"go home,"* and the child said, *"go ho."* It would be better to say, "You used good circle lips but forgot your humming lips at the end," than to say, "Good job! Try again with your 'mmmm' sound at the end." The difference is subtle but less confusing for the child. By providing specific KP feedback, we can provide reinforcement for what the child did well, while providing constructive feedback. Examples of KP feedback are shown in Table 3–3.

Table 3–3. Examples of Specific Feedback (Knowledge of Performance) in Treatment

Target Utterance	Child's Response	Therapist's Response
Hi mom.	/ha mam/	"I like how you used your breath for /ha/. This time, be sure to finish with 'smile lips' when you say, *hi - Ha-eeee*."
Hi mom.	/haɪ mam/	"You used your smile lips when you said *hi*. Great job!"
banana	/næ.nə/	"That word has three syllables. Try again. We'll tap it out together."
banana	/bə.næ.nə/	"Nice job! You got all your sounds that time."

Frequency of Feedback—High Frequency/Low Frequency

A second consideration with regard to feedback is the frequency with which the feedback is delivered, with feedback being more frequent during earlier stages of acquisition and decreasing gradually as the child improves. Maas et al. (2012) examined if reducing frequency of feedback would enhance motor learning in children with CAS; however, their findings were inconclusive. The authors suggest that a child's age or the severity of the child's speech challenges may factor into how well they are able to benefit from a reduced schedule of feedback during production activities. Teachers and therapists tend to want to provide positive reinforcement frequently to keep children motivated and feeling good about their work; however, we do not want children to become feedback dependent, so gradual reduction in feedback is recommended.

Timing of Feedback—Immediate/Delayed

Schmidt and Lee (2005) provide evidence related to optimal timing of feedback during motor learning. They warn against providing feedback too soon after the performance of the movement. When feedback is provided instantaneously upon completion of a target, the child does not have adequate time to reflect on the performance and compare the production to the desired output, which may hinder both acquisition and retention of the sensorimotor plan. Even a delay of 2 or 3 seconds before providing the child with feedback can support acquisition and retention of the sensorimotor plan.

In summary, SLPs can refine their treatment for children with sensorimotor speech challenges. Children's speech outcomes can be enhanced when clinicians understand the PML and consider these principles when making treatment decisions. Clinical judgment, of course, is required to analyze how individual students are responding to specific conditions of practice and conditions of feedback, and to vary the practice conditions as needed to meet the needs of specific clients. Table 3–4 provides a summary chart of the application of motor learning

Table 3–4. Summary of Principles of Motor Learning in Acquisition and Retention Phases of Treatment

Facilitating **Acquisition** of Skills	**Motor Learning Principles**	Facilitating **Retention** And **Transfer** of Skills
CONDITIONS OF PRACTICE		
High levels of cueing and feedback	*Pre-practice*	Not applicable
High number of trials per session	*Number of trials*	High number of trials per session
Blocked practice	*Schedule of practice*	Random practice
Constant practice	*Variability of practice*	Variable practice
CONDITIONS OF FEEDBACK		
High frequency	*Frequency of feedback*	Gradual reduction in frequency
Knowledge of performance	*Type of feedback*	Knowledge of results
Immediate feedback	*Timing of feedback*	Delayed feedback and summary feedback

principles to the current best practices for children with sensorimotor speech disorders. Further research will continue to shed light on how these principles can best be applied when working with children with CAS.

Repetitive Practice

In the previous section, the importance of incorporating high practice amounts to facilitate motor learning was discussed. One challenge facing clinicians is finding ways to keep children motivated, interested, and engaged when working on many of the same skills repeatedly. In this section, we discuss how to set up an environment to help children sustain attention, persistence, and willingness to engage in repetitive practice activities in the face of frustrations that often exist for individuals who struggle to communicate verbally.

Tips for Creating a Learning Environment That Promotes Repetitive Practice

Following are tips for creating a learning environment that will encourage a practice mindset for children:

- Provide a pleasant learning environment without unnecessary visual and auditory distractions.
- Provide seating that facilitates postural stability for the child.
- Sit facing the child and at the child's eye level to encourage the child to look at your face.
  - For infection control, consider a clear mask resistant to fogging or a modified shield that fills in the gap between the shield and the face, such as the Bend Shape mask or the Badger Shield, so the child can still see your face.
- For children who struggle to attend to the clinician's face, consider using video modeling (described in greater detail later in this chapter).
- Reduce the number of materials within the child's reach to help reduce distraction.
- Consider the child's age, attention span, frustration tolerance, persistence, and interests when planning intervention activities.
- Choose activities that are quick and simple, yet motivating and reinforcing, to increase practice opportunities (e.g., craft projects may be fun but are too time consuming).
- Have an efficient, organized manner for data collection (see Chapter 12).
- Have a visual representation of how many reps they need to produce before moving on. (e.g., token tower, count down on the hand and end with a high five after five reps of good productions, 10 × 10 grid to fill with stickers or stamps)

Repetitive Practice Activities to Support Varied Interests

Another important consideration in repetitive practice is finding activities that spark the child's interest. Children vary in what they find interesting and motivating. Making the treatment activities enjoyable for children will impact their willingness to put forth the effort necessary to achieve gains in treatment. Talk with the child and the family to find out what types of activities the client enjoys, ask colleagues about activities they have used successfully in treatment to elicit high numbers of responses within a session, and be creative. For instance, some children show their best work when they can be moving, while other children prefer quiet activities or the challenge of earning points. Table 3–5 describes several activities that elicit multiple repetitions of targets. The activities are simple and quick so children can spend most of their time working on speech, rather than using precious practice minutes setting up elaborate games and projects. Each of the activities is sorted based on the specific interests of the child.

Phoneme Sequencing, Syllable Shapes, and Coarticulation

The ability to combine sounds fluidly and to make minor adjustments in articulatory placement based on surrounding phonemes is referred to as *coarticulation*. The American Speech-Language-Hearing Association (ASHA, 2007) describes challenges in the planning and programming of speech movements for smooth coarticulation as a core deficit for children with CAS. Thus, it is important to **rethink our treatment goals** and to **rethink the way we talk to children about their goals** and the work they are doing. Strand (2020) suggests that rather than thinking and talking about specific phonemes, we think and talk about **speech movement sequences**. Thinking in terms of movement sequences is essential for addressing coarticulation in CAS treatment. Following are things to consider when addressing phoneme sequencing and coarticulation in children with CAS.

Addressing Syllable Shape Complexity

The term *syllable shape* refers to the ordering of consonant (C) and vowel (V) phonemes within a syllable. The words "*me*" and "*shoe*" have a syllable shape of CV, "*school*" and "*trip*" have a CCVC shape, and "*splashed*" and "*streets*" have a CCCVCC shape. Words with more than one syllable such as "*mommy*" and "*happy*" combine two CV syllables to form a CVCV shape, while "*hotdog*" and "*goodnight*" combine two CVC syllables to form a CVCCVC shape. Note that the phonemes, not the alphabetic letters used to spell the word, determine the syllable shape.

It is useful to think of short phrases in terms of syllable shape. For instance, "*Hi mom,*" when produced without a pause between the words, could be considered to have a CVCVC shape and "*Oh no*" to have a VCV shape. Remember that helping children develop smooth, accurate, and consistent coarticulatory transitions within words *and* between words will be a primary focus of treatment.

A child's ability to produce increasingly more complex syllable shapes is a progressive skill. Table 3–6 illustrates a progression of syllable shape development, along with sample words and phrases that are representative of these syllable shapes. This progression should be viewed as a reference rather than an absolute progression, as you often will be choosing target utterances with a variety of syllable shapes even within the same intervention session. For example, a child may be working on CVCVCV targets (e.g., banana, hi daddy, we go now) while also working on single-syllable targets with simple syllable shapes when addressing inclusion of final consonants (e.g., up, in, hot) or production of more challenging phonemes (e.g., show, shoe, see).

Table 3–5. Activities to Facilitate Repetitive Practice of Target Utterances

Activities That Get Children Moving	
Bowling	Place blocks on the floor either in the positions of bowling pins or a few inches apart in a row. The child names the target pictures several times before placing each picture against a block. When each block has a picture, the child can roll a ball and knock over the blocks. After the pictures are knocked over, say the target word several times again. *Variation: Use the target word in a carrier phrase such as "_____ fell down." or "I knocked over a _____."*
Basketball	The child takes a shot at making a basket after saying the target word or phrase 10 times. The basket may be a small basketball hoop attached to a door or a large laundry basket on the floor or on a raised surface.
Picture hop	Pictures are placed in a row approximately 1 foot apart. The child names each picture several times as they hop from picture to picture. *Variation: Each time the child hops onto a picture, have the child insert the word into a carrier phrase such as "I hopped on a _____."*
Treasure hunt	"Hide" the practice cards around the room and have the child use a flashlight to find the hidden cards. Once found, the child says the word five times. *Variation: Each time a picture is found, use the word in a carrier phrase such as "I found a _____." or "The _____ was hiding under/in/behind a _____." Hint: To reduce the time it takes to search for the pictures, portions of the pictures should be visible, and the children may "peek" while the pictures are hidden.*
Ball toss/roll	The child sits or stands several feet from the therapist. The child says the target word or phrase each time the ball is tossed or rolled back and forth.
Mailman	After naming each word several times, place the word card in an envelope to be delivered to a family member, stuffed toy or doll using a truck as the delivery vehicle. Name each picture again as it is delivered. *Variation: Use a carrier phrase such as "You got a _____." or "Here's a _____." when delivering the mail.*
Beanbag throw	Name each picture and turn it upside down on the floor. Throw a beanbag onto a picture, turn it over, and name it several times.
Move and say	Pictures are separated into two decks: target picture deck and action deck. The action deck contains written instructions or a picture of an action the child will perform while producing the target utterance. The child picks one card from each deck and produces the target word while performing the action shown on the action card (*e.g., the child says the target word "butterfly" while tapping his head; the child says the target word "bus" while hopping like a bunny*).
Hop to it	A target picture or toy is placed on the floor or table. The child stands a good distance from the picture/toy and hops as many times as it takes to reach it. The target utterance is produced before each hop. The distance the child stands from the picture/toy can be varied, allowing the child to guess how many hops it will take to reach the picture/toy.

continues

Table 3–5. *continued*

	Activities for Pretend Play
Go for a ride	Take dolls, toy characters, superheroes, or animals for a ride in a vehicle. Characters can be named (consider choosing names of familiar family, friends, classmates, neighbors). Multiple toys provide opportunities for repetitive practice of phrases (e.g., ____ on the bus; go in; open door). *Hint: For children working on CV and CVCV, reduplicated shapes (e.g., cow, moo, neigh neigh, baba), farm animal names and noises can be appropriate targets, while zoo animals can be appropriate targets for CVCV variegated, CVCVC, and other complex syllable shapes (e.g., hippo, rhino, zebra, monkey, alligator, penguin).*
Time to eat	Take those characters and animals to a restaurant or into the kitchen and give them something to eat. There will be plenty of opportunities to practice functional vocabulary and phrases/sentences (e.g., mommy eat apple; time to eat; I'm hungry; more cookies).
Doctor	Pretend these characters get sick or hurt. Again, so many opportunities exist to practice functional words and phrases (e.g., body parts; boo boo; sick; hurt; owie; I hurt my ___).
Take care of baby	Taking care of a doll provides opportunities to practice functional words and phrases related to bedtime routine, eating routines, and dressing routines.
	Activities to Show Your Creative Side
Block designs	After saying the target several times, the child earns a block with which to create a design.
Tall tower	After saying the target several times, the child earns a large block to create a very tall tower—knocking it over is the best part!
Dominoes	Tape two index cards with target words/pictures together at the edge so that you are able to stand them up in an inverted V or tent. Each time the child says the word correctly several times, place the card on the floor so it stands up. Each time a new card is completed, place it next to the last card so that the cards form a dominoes chain. At the end, knock them over and enjoy the chain reaction. *Variation: Phrases can be created using the two target pictures that are taped together (e.g., "boy," "toy" "The <u>boy</u> got a new <u>toy</u>.").* *Note: Using words that form compound words is a nice way of linking the two words together (e.g., "cow," "boy" "cowboy")*
Stickers	Divide a piece of paper into several boxes (one box for each target word/phrase). After saying each target several times, the child earns a sticker to place in each box.
Progressive drawing	Each time the child produces the target several times, the therapist draws "part" of a picture. Continue until the picture is complete. The child can try to guess what you are making as you go along.
Paper chain	Place a picture or write each practice word, phrase, or sentence on a 1-inch-wide strip of paper. After the child says the target several times, glue the paper ends together to create a circle. Thread each paper strip through the last and glue the ends until a paper chain is created. *Variation: Each time a new word is added to the chain, use a carrier phrase "I put on a _____." or "The _____ is attached to the _____."*

Table 3–5. *continued*

Earn it now, make it later	The child earns individual parts to an art project each time the target is produced several times. After all parts are collected, place them in a bag (along with the instructions) and send them home with the child to complete later.
Act it out	After reading a storybook, act out the story. In the repetitive line storybook, *Mr. Gumpy's Outing* (Burningham, 1971), the child has opportunities to act out the story by placing animal characters in a boat and taking them for a ride before the boat finally tips over.
Sing out	Sing songs to reinforce the target utterances being addressed in therapy, whether they be familiar children's songs or song lyrics you make up yourself.

Activities for the Mathematical Mind	
Large number die	Use blank dice (available from Super Duper Publications) and label them with numbers 5–10. The child says the target the number of times designated on the die.
Large number spinner	Make your own spinner with higher numbers. This can be done by applying blank stickers over the original numbers on the spinner with the new, higher numbers written on them. After spinning the spinner, the child produces the target the number of times indicated on the spinner.
100 (or 200 or 300 or . . .)	The child earns points for each correct production of the target. The numbers are added together. The child wins the game when the predetermined number is reached.
Double dice roll	Instead of one die, use two dice. Add up the numbers on the two dice and have the child produce the target that number of times.

Miscellaneous Activities	
Go Fish	Using two sets of pictures, play a game of Go Fish. The child asks you for pictures and then has to obtain pairs. This is a good activity for working on using the target words in phrases and sentences. *Variation: Have the child use the carrier phrase "Do you have a _____." or "I need a _____." each time it is his turn. Also practice saying "Go fish" and "Yes, I have a _____." and "No, I don't have a _____."*
Memory	Place two sets of picture cards face down on the floor. Pick up and name two pictures at a time and try to find matching pictures. Continue until all matching pictures have been found. *Variation: Each time a picture is turned over, use the carrier phrase "I got a _____." If the two pictures turned over match, the phrase "I got 2 _____." and "I got a match." can be used; if not "No match" or "They do not match." can be used.*
Guess the picture	Place two or more pictures on the table and ask the child to name each picture several times. The pictures are then turned over and mixed up. The child chooses a picture to turn over, but before it is turned over, the child guesses the picture. *Variation: For phrase-/sentence-level productions, the child can say, "I think the _____ is here." "I think this one is a _____." or "It's a _____."*

continues

Table 3–5. *continued*

Make a puzzle	Find a colorful picture from a magazine or print a picture that would be of interest to the child and carefully remove it from the magazine, so it stays intact. Glue several target pictures to the back of the magazine picture. Cut around each picture into squares or curved shapes to separate each target picture. The child names each target picture several times and then turns them upside down. The pieces fit together to form a puzzle and reveal the colorful magazine picture. The number of puzzle pieces used will vary depending on the visual-perceptual skills of each child.
Feely box	Place small objects in a box with a hole large enough for a child to insert a hand and feel around. Have pictures of each of the objects upside down on the table. The child turns over the pictures one-by-one and tries to locate the objects that match each picture by feeling around inside the box. *Variation: The pictures are turned right side up on the table. The child chooses an object from inside the box and, without looking at it, tries to identify what it is from among the pictures available.*
Production tracker	For a quick way to achieve 100 repetitions, create a transparent 10 × 10 grid in Word (to make 100 boxes) and overlay it on an image the child would find motivating (e.g., from a favorite TV show, a pet, a favorite place). Make an X or a ☑ in each square of the grid as the child practices their target stimuli.
Board game	Make a board game using a manilla folder and a free downloadable game template. In each space of the game, provide a direction (e.g., Say phrase 10 times with your hands in the air and a loud voice, say phrase 15 times with a happy voice, say phrase 12 times as a question). The phrases can be on index cards in different colors to match the colors on the game board. This allows you to change out the phrases without changing the game board. Personalize the game by using graphics of things the child is interested in, like sports, a princess castle, or Mario Bros.
Applications specific for apraxia and articulation	*There are many applications (apps) for articulation and specifically for CAS. These apps can be used during in-person sessions or during telepractice sessions by using the mirroring function on your tablet computer. Following are a few of these apps:* Apraxia Picture Sound Cards (APSC Pro)—$179.99. Over 1,000 pictures ranging in complexity from CV and VC words to four-syllable words. Includes data collection and analytics. Card sets can be customized and saved and shared with caregivers. Apraxia Rainbow Bee—$26.99. Targets CV, VC level through three-syllable words and sentence-level productions. Data tracking available. Custom words can be added. Apraxia Farm—$29.99. Targets words with increasingly complex syllable structures of one to four syllables in length. Data tracking available. Custom words can be added. Bla Bla Bla—Free. For young children who are working to increase vocalization. This is a sound-reactive app. The child produces a sound, and the character's mouth widens according to how loud the vocalization is. Boom Learning—Search the Boom Learning library for PROMPT Institute boom decks, which are stories that feature target utterances based on PROMPT's Motor Speech Hierarchy. You can also use search words to find other boom decks specifically developed for children with CAS.

Table 3–5. *continued*

Applications specific for apraxia and articulation	Linguisystems Apraxia Sound Cards—$24.99. This is the online version of the Linguisystems Apraxia Sound Cards. The app contains 240 pictured items to practice words with increasingly complex syllable shapes in single words, phrases, and sentences.
	Speech Box for Speech Therapy—cost depends on usage. Hundreds of photos sorted by phoneme and category. Custom pictures can be added and new categories can be created and individualized (e.g., by syllable shape or specific child's targets).
	Speech FlipBook—$9.99. The child hears and makes each sound individually and then blends them into CV, CVC, or CVCV real and nonsense words. You can limit the selections to real words only. Supports phonological awareness and phoneme production and sequencing.
	Speech Stickers—$14.99. The child practices C, V, VC, and CV sounds and syllables by imitating various models of the target stimuli that change in pitch and prosody.
	Speech Therapy for Apraxia—a set of four apps/$4.99 each. The stimuli for each set progress from simple CV syllables to more complex word shapes. An in-app purchase is required to use the progress tracking feature.
	Speech Tutor Pro—$54.99. Provides pictures, games, and video books for English consonants and vocalic /r/, as well as videos of the sagittal and coronal views for production of consonant phonemes and a few vowels. Picture decks can be created for individual clients, and a data collection feature is included. There is also a Speech Tutor app ($24.99) that provides the videos of phoneme production.
	Word FLiPS—$29.99. The online version of Super Duper Publications' Word FLiPS flipbook. Practice CV, CVC, and CVCV targets in real or nonsense words. Data tracking is available.
Other applications that elicit multiple practice opportunities	Cake Doodle—$0.99. The Cake Doodle app (and other "doodle" apps from Shoe the Goose) allows the user to create a cake and decorate it. The user adds each ingredient one at a time, bakes the cake, and adds decorations, thus offering multiple opportunities for practice of functional target utterances (e.g., put it in, put it here, more eggs, I need ___).
	My PlayHome Series—$2.99–$3.99. The My PlayHome series of apps from My PlayHome Software, Ltd., are enjoyable apps that offer the user opportunities to practice functional words and phrases related to home, school, and community. There are multiple characters in the apps, so the user has multiple opportunities to practice these target utterances.
	Pepi Play Series—$1.99–$2.99. Pepi Play apps provide the user many opportunities for repetitive practice of functional phrases related to real-life situations (e.g., self-care, going to the doctor, daily living).

Table 3–6. Progression of Syllable Shape Development

Syllable Shapes	Sample Words
V	ooh, oh, ah, eye, ow
C	mmm (yummy), sh (quiet), sss (snake)
CV	me, hi, whee, two, no
VC	up, eight, in, eat
VCV	icky, eeny, icy, owie I go, I see, oh no, oh boy
Reduplicated CVCV $C^1V^1C^1V^1$	mama, dada, booboo, baba
Consonant harmonized $C^1V^1C^1V^2$	mommy, daddy, puppy, baby
Variegated $C^1V^1C^2V^2$	many, happy, movie, doggy no way, boy go, hi cow, me too
Harmonized CVC	pop, mom, dad, nine
CVC	hot, bus, man, book
CVCVCV	banana, potato, tomato we go now, hi daddy, bye pony
CVCVC	button, donut, hopping, magic hi mom, my boat, go home, boy sit
CVCCVC	cupcake, goodnight, helping, basket get down, hot sun, sit down, run home
Double clusters	spoon, black, grape jump, tent, best, bats
Triple clusters	splash, string masks, jumped
Multisyllables	alligator, helicopter, jack-o-lantern refrigerator, watermelon

Establishing Flexible Phoneme Sequencing Skills

When establishing new syllable shapes, choose targets that incorporate consonant phonemes with different articulatory placement (e.g., bilabials, alveolars, velars), manner (e.g., nasals, stops, fricatives), and voicing (voiced, voiceless), as well as vowel phonemes with varied tongue height (high, mid, low) and tongue advancement (front, central, back). Establishing phonetic variety in terms of place, manner, and voicing is crucial to establishing flexible phoneme sequencing skills. Of course, early targets likely will include early developing phonemes (e.g., p, b, t, d, m, n, h, w); however, the goal is to continue to build the phoneme repertoire to develop maximum flexibility in phoneme sequencing.

Facilitate Targets With Final Consonants and Two Syllables Early in Treatment

The CVC and variegated $C^1V^1C^2V^2$ shapes are particularly significant points along the continuum of syllable shape development. Because the English language contains a high percentage of *closed syllables* (syllables that end in a consonant), developing the ability to produce final consonants in VC and CVC syllables has a positive and dramatic impact on a child's speech intelligibility. In addition, the number of words containing the variegated CVCV syllable shape vastly exceeds the number of words containing reduplicated or harmonized CVCV syllable shapes. The CVCV shape can also be the basis for early phrase development (e.g., my toy, hi ma, we go). Improvements in both articulatory control and expressive language are facilitated by spending time establishing flexibility and consistency at the variegated CVCV level.

Coarticulation and Efficiency

Depending on dialect or speaking context (casual versus formal), English speakers may adjust word productions in connected speech to increase efficiency. Phonemes may be shortened, omitted, or altered in some way in certain coarticulatory contexts, and your modeling should reflect these dialectic differences. Ladefoged (2001) describes several coarticulation rules for English allophones. Some that are important to consider when working on coarticulation are listed next.

When modeling target utterances for the child, be sure you are modeling the most efficient productions of the target utterances, keeping in mind these rules of coarticulation:

- Alveolar stops /t/ and /d/ are reduced or omitted when they occur between two consonants (e.g., *guest bedroom* produced as [gɛs bɛdrʊm]; *end late* produced as [ɛn leɪt]).

- Voiceless stops /p, t, k/ are aspirated in the initial position of a syllable (e.g., [pʰat] for *pot*, [tʰap] for *top*, [kʰʌp] for *cup*). By lengthening the duration of the aspiration during early stages of acquisition of initial voiceless stops, the child has time to coordinate the sensorimotor plan for transitioning from the voiceless phoneme to the voiced vowel that follows. As the child improves, the duration of the aspiration shortens, so the child's speech sounds more natural.

- The voiceless alveolar stop /t/ when followed by /n/ in the same word may be replaced by a glottal stop /ʔ/. The word "*mitten*," for example, would be produced as [mɪ.ʔn̩].

- When two identical consonants come next to one another, the first consonant is shortened, though not omitted. In the sentence, "*She has very white teeth,*" the /t/ in "*white*" is shortened but is not completely omitted, otherwise it would sound like "*why teeth.*"

- In words with an intervocalic "t" followed by a vowel in an unstressed syllable, as in "*butterfly*" or "*water*," the "t" will change to a quick, lightly voiced alveolar sound known as a flap or tap /ɾ/, as in [bʌ.ɾɚ.flaɪ]. When modeling the word "*butterfly*," the "tt" will sound like a quick tap rather than the full alveolar plosive /t/.

- In certain contexts, some English words are produced in a shortened manner, either by changing the vowel to a schwa, or by omitting a consonant. Examples are *and* produced as /ən/ or /n̩/ (salt /n̩/ pepper), *for* produced as /fɚ/ (one /fɚ/ you), *or* produced as /ɚ/ (apples /ɚ/ oranges), and *to* produced as /tə/ (went /tə/ the store). The rule does not apply to *all* productions of these words and is dependent on context and formality.

- In some syllables in English, the consonants /m, n, l/ may serve as the nucleus of the syllable; thus, the syllable will not require a vowel. This is referred to as a *syllabic consonant* and is marked phonetically with a line below the syllabic consonant /m̩/, /n̩/, and /l̩/, as in *rhythm* /ˈrɪðm̩/, *mitten* /ˈmɪ.ʔn̩/, and *bicycle* /ˈbaɪ.sɪ.kl̩/.

- When the phonemes /t/ and /d/ are followed by /j/, the sound changes to /tʃ/ or /dʒ/. Examples include *congratulations* /kən.græ.dʒə.ˈle.ʃənz/; *I'll meet you there.* /aɪl.mi.tʃu. ðɛɚ/; *Did you do it?* /dɪ.dʒu.du.ɪt/; *You can ride your bike.* /yu.kæn.raɪ.dʒɚ.baɪk/.

Juncture

Another way in which coarticulation can be supported is through *juncture*, or the manner of moving between two successive syllables in speech by pausing, joining the phonemes, or adding a new phoneme. Proper use of juncture can help distinguish between phoneme combinations that sound the same but have different meanings by using either *open juncture*, in which a short pause is inserted between words in the phrase, or *closed juncture*, in which there is no pause. For example, a short pause between the words in the phrase, "*That's tough,*" would help distinguish it from the phrase, "*that stuff,*" where the two words would be joined, without a pause between the words. Examples of open and closed juncture are shown in Table 3–7.

Words within phrasal units can be joined without pausing. This creates an opportunity for the final phoneme of a word to become the initial phoneme of the following word. This is common when the final consonant precedes a vowel (e.g., "*Mom's at home*" produced as /mam.zæt hoʊm/; "*Put on your coat*" produced as /pʊ.dan jɔɚ coʊt/; or "*Can I do it?*" produced as /kæ.naɪ du wɪt/). This type of juncture can be used to the child's benefit, especially for children who tend to omit final consonants. Using backward chaining, the child can practice "*Can I do it*" using the sequence shown in Box 3–2.

In some instances, phonemes are added between words and syllables to join the words or syllables together. For example, when moving from a retracted vowel to another vowel, the words or syllables are joined with a /j/. When moving from a rounded vowel to another vowel, the vowels are joined with a /w/. Examples are shown in Table 3–8.

Table 3–7. Open and Closed Juncture Phrases

Open Juncture: Pause Between Syllables	Closed Juncture: Syllable Joining
a nice house	an icehouse
stopped aching	stop taking
I scream	ice cream

■ Box 3–2. Backward Chaining Using Closed Juncture

/wɪt/

/du wɪt/

/naɪ du wɪt/

/kæ.naɪ du wɪt/

Table 3–8. Vowel-to-Vowel Juncture With Phoneme Addition

From Retracted Vowel to Another Vowel	From Rounded Vowel to Another Vowel
flying = /flaɪ.jɪŋ/	doing = /du.wɪŋ/
she is = /ʃi jɪz/	do over = /du wo.vɚ/
created = /kri.je.rɪd/	so it's = /so wɪts/

Target Utterance Selection

The careful selection of target utterances in treatment has a significant impact on treatment success for children with sensorimotor speech planning challenges. Some of these evidence-based treatment programs (described in greater detail in Chapter 4) provide guidance regarding the selection of target utterances. For instance, Dynamic Temporal and Tactile Cueing (DTTC; Strand, 2020) recommends selecting functional words and phrases that facilitate a variety of phoneme combinations to support sensorimotor planning. Rapid Syllable Transition Treatment (ReST; Murray et al., 2015) uses two- to three-syllable nonsense words to support smooth and accurate coarticulatory transitions and correct syllable stress assignment. Prompts for Restructuring Oral Muscular Phonetic Targets (PROMPT; Hayden, 2004) treatment protocols use a specific hierarchy of sensorimotor speech development to guide target utterance selection along with a focus on functional communication that will build language and socialization.

As clinicians, we should consider several factors when making decisions about target utterance selection, so we are working within the child's *zone of proximal development (ZPD)*. ZPD refers to tasks a learner is able to do with assistance. This zone falls between what the learner is able to do on their own and what they are not able to do, even with assistance. To work within a child's ZPD, several factors related to speech and language should be considered. The child's repertoire of phonemes and syllable shapes and their ability to vary lexical and phrasal stress influence the stimuli to be chosen for the treatment sessions. Additionally, other linguistic, social, and environmental factors have a substantial impact on the clinician's choice of treatment targets. In fitting within the framework of the World Health Organization's International Classification of Functioning, Disability, and Health (WHO ICF; WHO, 2007), ideally the target utterances should be motorically, cognitively, linguistically, and socially appropriate for each individual child. Figure 3–2 illustrates five primary factors that should influence the selection

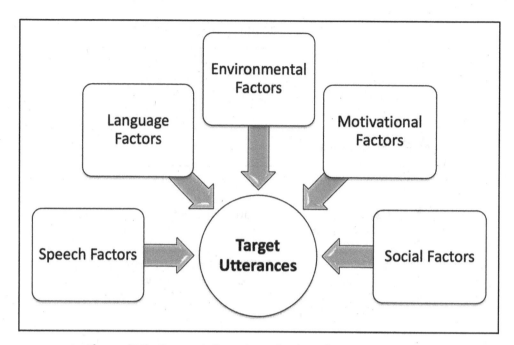

Figure 3–2. Factors influencing selection of target utterances.

of target utterances for children with CAS. When each factor is given consideration in the treatment planning and target selection process, there are increased opportunities to facilitate growth not only in the child's speech intelligibility but also in the child's expressive language, peer engagement, social development, and self-esteem.

    In keeping with the framework of the ICF, it is important to incorporate input from caregivers and consider this input alongside the speech-related factors that allow the child to work within their ZPD. Table 13–2 in Chapter 13 provides a parent questionnaire that can be used to solicit input from parents regarding important and functional words/phrases for their child. When reviewing the parent input, you may note that some of the functional words/phrases provided by the parents are well above the sensorimotor planning capacities of the child at this moment in time. Reassure the parents that you will work on those target stimuli for which the child will be able to be successful, and you will continue to expand to more complex targets in the future.

Influence of Current Speech Capacities on Target Utterance Selection

Five aspects of speech should be considered when selecting target utterances for treatment. They include the following:

- syllable shape complexity (syllable length and complexity, number of syllables)
- phonemes (consonant and vowel repertoire and stimulability)
- prosody (word and sentence stress patterns)
- flexibility and contextual limitations
- facilitating contexts

Each of these areas is discussed next.

Addressing Syllable Shape Complexity

When attempting to challenge the child's phoneme sequencing skills, Davis and Velleman (2000) recommend choosing words that contain phonemes within the child's repertoire. If the child is working on improving consistency in production of the VCV and CVCV syllable shapes, consider target utterances that contain phonemes within the child's repertoire. After the child has demonstrated greater consistency in production of these syllable shapes with well-established phonemes, it would be appropriate to introduce a new phoneme and incorporate that phoneme into CVCV words or phrases.

Addressing Specific Phonemes

Reduced consonant and vowel repertoires are a common characteristic of children with CAS; therefore, treatment also will support the child's attainment of new phonemes. According to Davis and Velleman (2000), new phonemes should be practiced in known syllable shapes, as challenging the child's sensorimotor skills for phoneme and syllable shape accuracy simultaneously could prove frustrating.

When deciding on phonemes to address in treatment, consider selecting phonemes for which the child demonstrates some stimulability. Early on in treatment, consider phonemes that are more visible, such as labials, alveolars, or phonemes that are easy to facilitate through tactile input (e.g., bilabials, vowels requiring lip retraction or lip rounding, or neutral vowels with a simple up-down jaw movement). A more thorough discussion of vowels is found in Chapter 5.

Addressing Prosody

When the child has begun to produce two-syllable words, prosody becomes an important consideration. Trochaic stress patterns, in which a stressed syllable is followed by a weak syllable (e.g., **po**tty, **ta**ble) are more common in English language than iambic stress patterns, in which a weak syllable is followed by a stressed syllable (e.g., a**lone**, for**got**). In English speech, trochaic words tend to be easier for children to produce than iambic words. When introducing two-syllable words into treatment, begin with words with trochaic stress before moving to words with iambic stress. As the child progresses, provide more opportunities for the child to practice a wider variety of prosodic patterns. More detailed information on prosody is found in Chapter 5.

Addressing Flexibility, Contextual Limitations, and Facilitating Contexts

Children with CAS often demonstrate contextual constraints in their phoneme production. For example, a child may be able to produce /b/ and /p/ but only in certain *facilitating contexts*, such as in the initial position when followed by the /a/ vowel (e.g., baba, papa). When choosing target utterances for treatment, consider the child's contextual limitations and choose targets with vowels in neighboring vowel spaces, as in *ball* or *buhbuh* for bubble, or try to expand to final position, as in *up* or *pop*. Research findings regarding facilitating contexts can help guide our choices in determining treatment targets. Table 3–9 describes some of the research findings related to facilitating contexts and provides suggestions for treatment targets based on this research.

Table 3–9. Research Findings Related to Facilitating Contexts

Research Reference	Research Finding	Potential Targets
Kehoe & Stoel-Gammon (2001)	Children produce final consonants in syllables more frequently when the final consonant follows a lax vowel /ɪ, ɛ, æ, ʊ, a, ə, ɚ/ than a tense vowel.	"hit" "mess" "book" "cup" "catch"
	Children attain voiceless obstruents /p, t, k, f, θ, s, ʃ, tʃ/ earlier than other phonemes in word final position.	
Velleman (2002)	Fricatives and velars may be easier to elicit in final position than initial position of words.	"back" "rug" "tough" "bus" "push"
	Children tend to produce the high front vowel /i/ in the second syllable of CV.CV words.	"mommy" "daddy" "baby" "bunny" "happy"
Theoretical construct of coarticulation	Use well-established initial consonants to facilitate the same consonants in the final position.	"home made" "bad day" "fish shop" "goes zoom" "big game" "truck key" "tough fish"
	Use well-established final consonants to facilitate the same consonants in the initial position.	
Davis & MacNeilage (1990, 1995)	Alveolar consonants tend to co-occur with high front vowels /i, ɪ/.	"tea" "sit" "lead"
	Labial consonants tend to co-occur with central vowels /a, ʌ, ə/.	"pup" "mama" "bah"
	Velars tend to co-occur with back vowels /u, ʊ, o, ɔ/.	"cook" "go" "goo"

Influence of Language on Target Utterance Selection

Children with CAS often demonstrate expressive language challenges. Therefore, it is important to consider the child's linguistic needs when selecting target utterances. Several linguistic factors should be considered when selecting target utterances for treatment of children with CAS.

Parts of Speech

When selecting targets for treatment sessions, be sure your selected targets represent a wide range of parts of speech. Typically, children's first 10 words represent labels for objects or people within the environment, with the next 40 words representing a mix of labels, action words, modifiers, and function words (Nelson, 1973; cited by McCormick & Schiefelbusch, 1984). Too often, however, nouns make up the bulk of vocabulary introduced as target words in a child's treatment, primarily because it is easier to find pictures that represent objects. An overrepresentation of nouns, however, limits opportunities for facilitation of phrases and sentences.

Semantic Relations

By selecting a range of vocabulary representing different parts of speech, the SLP provides the child with a vocabulary set from which to formulate a variety of early semantic relations (e.g., **my** puppy, puppy **in**, puppy **go**, **tiny** puppy, **no** puppy). Chosen phrases should mirror language development norms for how children learn to combine words. Chapter 6 of this book provides greater detail about the role of semantic relations in facilitating early phrase development in children.

Grammatical Morphemes

Consider the order of acquisition of grammatical morphemes (Brown, 1973) when selecting target utterances for treatment. The morphemes described by Brown include the following:

- *-ing* present progressive tense
  (e.g., "Daddy work*ing*." "I sleep*ing*.")
- "in" and "on" marking location
  (e.g., "baby *in* buggy" "go *on* swing")
- *-s* marking regular plural noun
  (e.g., "my doll*s*" "more bubble*s*")
- Early irregular past tense verbs
  (e.g., "Mommy *went* store." "I *ate* it.")
- *-'s* possessive noun
  (e.g., "mommy*'s* coat" "Go Daddy*'s* car.")
- "am," "is," "are," was," "were" uncontracted copula forms of *to be*
  (e.g., "My ball *is* big." "That *was* silly.")
- "a" and "the" making distinction between definite and indefinite referents
  (e.g., "here *the* ball" "that *a* book")
- *-ed* marking regular past tense verbs
  (e.g., "I jump*ed*." "Mommy help*ed* me.")
- *-s* third person regular tense verbs
  (e.g., "Cow sleep*s* here." Baby want*s* more.")
- "is," "has," "does" third person irregular verb forms
  (e.g., "Doggie *has* bone." "He *does*.")

- Uncontractible auxiliary verbs
  (e.g., "Mommy *is* cooking dinner." "I *am* going home.")
- Contractible copula forms
  (e.g., "It's my toy." "He's so funny.")
- Contractible auxiliary verbs
  (e.g., "Daddy's coming home." "Doggie's riding a bike.")

Influence of Environmental Factors on Target Utterance Selection

Carryover of the skills learned within the context of treatment is a primary goal for speech and language therapy; therefore, environmental factors related to the settings where children spend most of their time (home, school, community) need to be considered when choosing treatment targets.

Home Environment

The people, routines, and values within the home setting will influence the selection of target utterances for each child. Names of people and pets living within the home or with whom the child has regular contact are important targets. Ask parents and caregivers about family routines and regular activities of the child and family to determine targets that may be functional for the child within the home setting. Holiday celebrations, special events, and religious or cultural traditions also may influence the vocabulary to which the child is exposed in the home environment. Selecting targets that reflect the types of activities the child participates in within the context of the family serves important functions including the following:

- increases the functionality of the vocabulary
- increases opportunities for practice outside the context of therapy
- increases the child's motivation to use the vocabulary outside the context of therapy
- increases family members' awareness of the gains the child is making in therapy
- increases opportunities for praise and validation of the child's hard work

School Environment

Selecting target utterances that provide opportunities for children to participate more fully at school is important. Being able to produce more utterances with greater clarity in the school environment supports children in the following ways:

- increases opportunities for children to show what they know
- increases opportunities for interaction with peers
- increases self-esteem
- increases peer acceptance
- reduces reliance on adults as communicative partners. A study by Rice et al. (1991) showed that children with limited communication skills tended to initiate language far less than their normal peers and directed their language to adults far more frequently than to their peers.

Target vocabulary for young children may include names of teachers and favorite class-mates, terms used within specific thematic units, and toys and activities with which the child plays regularly. A fourth-grade child with CAS may have a speech goal of improving production of multisyllabic words. If the child is preparing to give an oral report to the class on the topic of tigers, it would be beneficial to practice words from the report such as "habitat," "predator," "Africa," and "nocturnal." The desire to speak clearly when presenting this report may facilitate motivation to practice these words and is more functional than practicing an arbitrary list of words during treatment.

Community

Children's communicative needs vary depending on the types of activities in which they participate and the places they go within their communities. Children may participate in recreational activities and social activities, attend birthday parties, visit favorite restaurants, or attend a place of worship within their community. Choosing target utterances that support the child's ability to communicate within a wide range of settings within the community, such as being able to order a meal at a favorite restaurant, serves an important function for the child.

Influence of Motivation on Target Utterance Selection

Children will make greater progress if they are motivated to work hard in therapy. Research has shown a strong correlation between emotion and learning. Children are more apt to experience positive emotions in connection with activities that interest them. When children experience strong positive emotions within the learning process, their ability to attain and retain the information is increased (Vail, 1993). Although some children may love to engage in imaginative play with animal toys, superheroes, or dolls, others may prefer expressing themselves through art, building, or movement activities. Asking a child who loves to run, swing, and climb to sit at a table and place animal puzzle pieces into a puzzle could prove to be frustrating for both the child and the clinician and lead to less positive learning outcomes. Find out from the child, family, or teachers what motivates and interests the child. Consider these interests when selecting target utterances for treatment.

Influence of Socialization on Vocabulary Selection

Another overriding goal for the treatment of children with communicative disorders is to facilitate opportunities for improved social language development. It is important to consider the social implications when selecting target utterances.

Language Functions

Verbal communication opens opportunities for increased social interaction for children. Typically developing children naturally use language for a wide range of communicative functions. Several communicative functions are listed in Table 3–10, along with suggested target words or phrases to facilitate the use of the specific communicative functions. Although this is not an exhaustive list, it does provide another tool for considering how we, as SLPs, determine

Table 3–10. Communicative Functions and Corresponding Target Utterances Sample Worksheet

Communicative Function	Targets To Elicit Communicative Function
Greeting/closing	Hi, hello, Hey, Goodbye, Bye, See ya later
Requesting objects	More _____, I want _____, Can I have _____
Requesting actions	Go get _____, Do this
Requesting attention	Look at me, Watch this
Rejecting	No, I don't want _____, All done
Asking for information	Where is _____? How do you _____?
Requesting assistance	Help me, I need help, Can you _____?
Asking permission	Can I _____? May I _____?
Disagreeing	I don't think so, That's not right, Not me
Protesting	Stop, Don't _____, No
Sharing information	Guess what, Let me tell you about_____
Commenting	Me too, Mine's faster, Cool, Yucky, Sorry
Responding to questions	Yes, Yeah, Uh huh, Mmm Hmm, No, Uh Uh, I don't know
Self-advocacy	I need a break, Stop that, That hurts, My turn, Go away, Not now

which target utterances to incorporate into our treatment sessions. A blank worksheet that lists communicative functions with blank spaces to fill in targets to elicit those functions is included in Appendix 3–A.

Children will be more likely to utilize a wider range of communicative functions if they have the vocabulary with which to do so. For example, if a child is not using the greeting function, it may be appropriate for the child to practice producing *"Hi," "Hey,"* or *"Hello"* in treatment. A child who becomes easily frustrated may not have the words at their disposal that allow to protest or express feelings. Teaching words or phrases like *"no," "stop," "too hard," "I'm mad,"* or *"all done"* helps give the child ways to protest and express feelings.

Conversational Skills

Target utterances can be selected to facilitate a child's ability to participate more fully in conversations. The three primary interactions used between conversational partners include the following:

- asking appropriate questions to gain new information about the conversational partner
- making comments to let the partner know you are listening and interested
- providing new information about yourself, either spontaneously or in response to a specific question

To support a child's ability to ask appropriate questions, treatment targets may include *"what," "where," "who," "when,"* and *"why"* or *"do you," "is it," "can I."* Teaching words and phrases like *"cool," "wow," "too bad,"* or *"I'm sorry"* can facilitate the use of commenting. *"Not me,"* or *"me too"* would support a child's ability to provide new information about themselves in the context of a conversation. Chapter 8 provides more detailed information to support social language skill development and conversational skills as children get older.

Practice Activity in Selecting Target Utterances

A child with CAS is described in this section. The child's phoneme repertoire and syllable shape variety along with language information, environmental influences, specific interests, and social skills/needs are listed in a Target Utterance Selection Considerations Worksheet in Table 3–11. All this information influences target utterance selection and should be considered when making decisions about the target words and phrases that will be practiced during intervention. Table 3–12 displays a completed Intervention Plan Worksheet, which illustrates how the various influential factors are considered collectively in planning treatment activities and choosing stimuli for a lesson. A blank Target Utterance Selection Considerations form and an Intervention Plan Worksheet form are provided in Appendix 3–A.

Target Utterances During Play

When working with a child in a school, a clinic, or the home, favorite toys and activities can be used to elicit meaningful and functional target utterances. Box 3–3 provides a few examples of simple target utterances that can be incorporated into treatment when playing favorite and familiar games and activities. Of course, the choice of targets will be based on the child's phonemic and phonetic capabilities. Notice how the target utterances incorporate vocabulary from various parts of speech, rather than primarily focusing on object labels.

Table 3–11. Target Utterance Selection Considerations Worksheet Sample Form

TARGET UTTERANCE SELECTION CONSIDERATIONS WORKSHEET	
Name: Lisa B.	
Age: 3 years, 6 months	
Speech →	Phoneme repertoire: /b, d, m, n, h/; /u, o, a, ʌ/ Word shapes: CV; CV.CV reduplicated
Language →	Single words
Environmental →	Lives with mother, father, and baby sister, Jessica. Visits grandparents weekly
Interests →	Balls, farm animals, dolls, toy people, outdoor play
Social →	Requests, rejects, labels, responds to, but does not ask questions; robust gestural system

Table 3–12. Intervention Plan Worksheet Sample Form

<table>
<tr><td colspan="3" align="center">**Intervention Plan Worksheet**</td></tr>
<tr><td colspan="3">Name: Lisa B.</td></tr>
<tr><td colspan="3">Date: 1-27-2023</td></tr>
<tr><td>**Word Shape(s)**</td><td>**Social/Pragmatic Goals**</td><td>**Vocabulary; Phrase Structures**</td></tr>
<tr><td>CV

Harmonized CV.CV

V (using diphthongs)</td><td rowspan="2">Greet/close; comment; request</td><td rowspan="2">bee, me, ow, mommy, daddy, baby, bubble, more, high, uh oh

Facilitate phrases if possible (e.g., "Hi/bye mommy/daddy/baby." "more bubble(s)")</td></tr>
<tr><td>**Phoneme(s) C and V**

/b, d, m, h/

/i, e, o, ɔ, ɑ, ʌ, ʊ,/</td></tr>
<tr><td>**Materials**</td><td colspan="2" align="center">**Activities**</td></tr>
<tr><td>Baby Bumblebee song book</td><td colspan="2">Sing "Baby Bumblebee" song. Facilitate production of /i/ vowel in "me" and "bee" and the diphthong /aʊ/ for "ow"</td></tr>
<tr><td>Animal Families (baby, mommy and daddy animals)</td><td colspan="2">Build a zoo and sort the animals. Facilitate harmonized CV.CV by labeling "baby," "mommy," and "daddy" animals</td></tr>
<tr><td>Bubbles</td><td colspan="2">Play with bubbles. Facilitate harmonized CV.CV for "bubble" /bʌ.bo/, diphthong /aɪ/ for "high," /ɔ/ for "more"</td></tr>
</table>

■ **Box 3–3.** Examples of Target Utterances for Various Play Activities

Playing With Toy Food or in a Toy Kitchen

eat; I eat; you eat; mommy eat; more ___; tea; I do; cup; bowl; pour; stir; open; cut; hot; dirty; wash; in; on; here you go; apple; banana; cookie; *names of other foods/drinks*; water/wawa; beep/ding (sound of timer going off); pan; pot; yum/yummy; yuck; yucky; turn on; ready; all done; all gone

Playing With Puzzles

out; in; me; you; help/help me/I need help; no; here/go here; put; put here; piece; not there; turn/turn it; I do it; Let me do it; *labels of puzzle piece pictures*

Games for Young Children (e.g., Lucky Ducks by Pressman)

duck; ducky; duck in; my turn; your turn; you do; I do; in water; put in; wet; on; turn on; push; colors (red; yellow; purple; blue); yay; match; not match; *number words for counting*

Bubbles

bubbles; pop; blow; again; up; down; in; out; wet; sticky; yucky; big; small/tiny; I do; you do; wow; uh oh; oh no; messy; all done

Playground/Park

up; go; I do/I do it; by myself; help/help me; whee; push; high; low; fast; slow; too fast; up; down; sit; swing; slide; spin; climb; go; jump; run; ball; bird; tree; ow; ouch; hurt; boo boo

Multisensory Cueing and Feedback

Providing multisensory cues and specific feedback is one of the cornerstones of the successful provision of treatment for children with CAS. The SLP may be following the best treatment practices: selecting appropriate vocabulary, creating opportunities for multiple repetitions of target words, and providing an intensive treatment schedule. However, if the cues being provided to the child from trial-to-trial in treatment are not carefully selected based on each of the child's responses and patterns of errors, progress will not be realized.

It is hypothesized that children with CAS may have poor *feedforward programs* (anticipatory sensorimotor plans) and thus rely on auditory feedback (Terband et al., 2009) to increase accuracy of speech productions. A study by Iuzzini-Seigel et al. (2015) compared speech production parameters in children with CAS, speech delay, and typically developing speech when auditory masking was introduced during speaking. The auditory masking made it difficult for children to employ auditory feedback to monitor their speech productions. Their findings further supported the premise that children with CAS are more reliant on auditory feedback than typically developing or speech delayed children. Looking in the rearview mirror at an utterance that already has been produced, however, is an inefficient way to facilitate better speech production. In addition, many children with CAS, particularly those children with CAS and language impairment, have been found to have poorer speech perception skills than typically developing children or children with CAS only (Zuk et al., 2018). Because reliance on auditory feedback is inefficient in the process of speech, and because many children with CAS evidence poor speech discrimination skills, it is essential that SLPs provide cueing (including visual, tactile, and proprioceptive) that facilitates greater internal representations of the sensorimotor speech plans so they are not reliant on auditory feedback for accurate productions of target utterances. A wide variety of cues that help children gain greater sensorimotor control of speech are described in the next sections.

Primary Types of Cues

Use of multisensory cueing is a common theme of many therapy techniques for CAS. All sensorimotor-based treatment programs for CAS encourage the child to watch and listen to the clinician model the target utterances and attempt to imitate the model. If the child does not respond correctly, other types of cues are provided. The cues provided may include the following:

- **visual** (a visual model or image of the way the mouth looks during production of the target utterance)
- **auditory** (an auditory model of the target utterance)
- **tactile/kinesthetic/proprioceptive** (what the child feels during production of the target utterance)
- **metacognitive** (an associative cue that helps the child focus on a specific aspect of the target utterance)

Visual Cues

Visual cues show the child how the mouth looks during production of the target utterance. The child receives a visual cue when they watch the clinician's face while the clinician is modeling a target utterance or when they observe themself in a mirror during production of the utterance. Static photos or drawings of a specific lip or tongue position and videos of target utterance productions also may serve as visual cues.

Auditory Cues

Auditory cues are those cues that allow the child to listen to a verbal model of the target utterance.

Somatosensory (Tactile, Kinesthetic, and Proprioceptive) Cues

Tactile cues relate to the sense of touch on the skin. During speech, we receive tactile input from the articulators contacting one another (e.g., lip contact when producing bilabials; tongue to alveolar ridge contact while producing alveolars). In treatment, clinicians can provide tactile cues to increase the child's awareness of the feel of the articulators during specific articulatory configurations.

Kinesthetic awareness is the body's internal sense of movement. *Proprioception* is the internal sense that helps a person recognize the amount of effort or force with which the body is moving, the speed of movement, and how the different body parts are moving in relation to one another in space. By reducing the rate of speech production or by holding an articulatory posture slightly longer, you increase kinesthetic and proprioceptive awareness of speech movements, the positioning of the articulators, and the relationship of the articulators to one another in space.

Metacognitive Cues

Metacognitive cues provide the child ways to think about speech movements either through specific instruction or through some type of associative cue. Metacognitive cues encompass many of the cues described in this chapter. They include such strategies as providing phonetic placement cues ("Lift the back of your tongue to make the 'k' sound"), tapping out syllables of a word to reduce syllable deletion, and using metaphors ("Be sure to use your 'humming sound' at the end") to facilitate the use of a specific phoneme or combination of phonemes.

For metacognitive cues to be effective, the child must already have an internal representation of the sensorimotor plan. The cues simply provide a way for the child to access the sensorimotor plan. It has been our experience that when metacognitive cues are paired with visual, auditory, and/or tactile cues early in treatment, the clinician can begin to fade from the more salient visual, auditory, and tactile cues to the less salient metacognitive cues. For example, the clinician can pair a direct model for the word *"go"* with a tactile cue to facilitate lip rounding, as well as a metaphor cue *"be sure to use your circle lips,"* then begin to fade the model and the tactile cue and provide only the metaphor cue to trigger an accurate response from the child. By laying down a variety of metacognitive cues for a child, the child eventually develops greater internal access to these cues and can call upon them as needed to achieve an accurate production.

The Use of Multisensory Cues in Treatment of CAS

Clinicians typically provide a variety of cues to facilitate accurate production of target utterances. The cues provided by the SLP help a child learn to focus their attention on the specific change(s) required to eventually achieve accurate production of all aspects of the speech movement. Determining the most salient aspect of the speech movement depends on where the breakdown in speech accuracy is occurring. For example, a child who is reducing a two-syllable word (bunny) to a single syllable (bu) may benefit from a metacognitive cue (two blocks) as a reminder to incorporate both syllables in the target word. The child who pronounces "bunny" as "nunny" may benefit from a tactile cue to the lips to facilitate lip closure for the /b/ and reduce the assimilation.

Table 3–13 provides a way of sorting the cues based on which sensory system(s) is being engaged during the cueing process. During the evaluation and diagnostic treatment processes, the SLP can determine which types of cues are most beneficial for a specific child.

Descriptions of Multisensory Cues

Each of the cues listed in Table 3–13 is described in the following sections to better understand how the various cues are applied in the context of treatment.

Direct Imitation and Delayed Imitation

The clinician models the target for the child prior to the child producing the target.

Modeling provides both auditory and visual cues that fire up mirror neurons when the clinician secures the child's visual attention prior to modeling the target. Initially, the child will imitate the target immediately following the model (direct imitation). As the child progresses, a delay of 1 to 3 s after the model can be added prior to the child producing the target (delayed imitation). This delay can be achieved by one of the following:

- producing the model but signaling for the child to wait before producing the target utterance

- embedding the model in the context of the instruction (e.g., "*Puppy* is the next word." or "Let's say '*bye*' to all the animals. *Bye* cow. Now you try it.")

For children who are easily visually distracted, a box or wide tube can be placed around the face of the clinician, so the child is encouraged to look only at the clinician's face and not become distracted by other things in the treatment space. Some children, including but not limited to children with autism, may have trouble focusing on the face (particularly the eyes) of the person modeling. Using a shield to hide the eyes of the person modeling (e.g., a folder or index card) may encourage better visual attention to the clinician's mouth.

Video Modeling

With *video modeling*, rather than watching the clinician in real time, the child views videos of people modeling the target utterances. Some children may find it easier to attend to video models. The video modelers are not limited to the clinician but can include the parents and

Table 3–13. Multisensory Cues for Treating Children With CAS

Cueing Technique	Associated Sensory Systems			
	Visual (child sees a model of production)	**Auditory** (child hears a model of production)	**Tactile-Kinesthetic-Proprioceptive** (child is provided with tactile input)	**Metacognitive** (child is provided with an associative cue)
Rate reduction		√	√	
Simultaneous production	√	√		
Direct imitation and delayed imitation	√	√		
Mirror	√	√		
Mime	√			
Backward chaining	√	√		
Forward chaining	√	√		
Hand cues for place, manner, voicing				√
Manual signs				√
Graphic cues				√
Tapping/clapping syllables				√
Blocks/chips				√
Metaphors				√
Phonetic placement cues				√
Mouth pictures and videos	√	√		
Visual syllable words				√
Tactile-kinesthetic-proprioceptive cues			√	
Visual biofeedback (ultrasound biofeedback, electropalatography, video modeling)	√			√

other family members. An added benefit of video modeling is that the videos can be viewed during the treatment sessions as well as outside the sessions during home practice.

Simultaneous Production

The child and clinician produce the target utterance simultaneously.

During simultaneous production, the clinician and the child produce the target utterance together at the same time. The DTTC approach (Strand, 2020), described in greater detail in Chapter 4, utilizes simultaneous production as a way of facilitating the correct production of challenging targets when direct imitation alone does not elicit an accurate production. It is the difference between "Say it after me" (direct imitation) and "Say it with me" (simultaneous production). Simultaneous production is used only to achieve initial acquisition of the target utterance for a few productions and then is faded and replaced with a less salient cue, such as direct imitation or miming.

Miming

The child watches the clinician while the clinician produces the target utterance without voice.

Although simultaneous production engages both the visual and auditory systems, miming engages only the visual system, making it a less salient cue. If a child is producing the target accurately with simultaneous production, the clinician may continue to model the word along with the child, but without voice, to see if the child is able to maintain accurate productions when the auditory cue is removed.

Rate Variations

Rate variations involve cueing the child to say the utterance at a reduced rate of speech and gradually increasing the rate until the sound combinations can be produced accurately at a normal rate.

Children can be cued to reduce their rate by doing one of the following:

- during direct imitation or simultaneous production, the clinician models the target utterance at a reduced rate
- the clinician reminds the child to use a reduced rate by incorporating associative cues, such as
  - hand signals
  - verbal reminders
  - picture cues (e.g., turtle or snail)
  - pacing board

Although rate reduction is beneficial for facilitating correct productions of targets within the practice setting, it is essential to gradually increase rate to approximate a normal rate of speech. The gradual increase of rate provides the learner with greater opportunities for generalization of the target in other settings and in the context of typical conversational speech.

There is a phenomenon in the acquisition of sensorimotor skills known as "*speed-accuracy trade off*, meaning simply that when performers attempt to do something more quickly, they typically do it less accurately" (Schmidt & Lee, 2005, p. 33). Some children, especially children with severe CAS, may not be able to achieve a rate of speech that matches their typically developing peers without substantial reduction in accuracy and intelligibility. Helping children establish a rate of speech that still allows for the best possible speech intelligibility may be required for children with more profound speech challenges.

Mirror

The child watches in the mirror while producing the word.

Having a child observe themselves in a mirror while producing the target may be beneficial, particularly for establishing sounds and sound sequences that are highly visible. The mirror serves to facilitate the use of appropriate movement gestures and to inhibit the use of incorrect movement gestures. For example, a child working on lip rounding during production of /w/ can watch themselves in the mirror to facilitate lip rounding for /w/. A child who tends to protrude his tongue when producing /l/ may use the mirror to inhibit tongue protrusion during /l/ production. It is essential that the child not become dependent upon the mirror for cueing, as the auditory and tactile/kinesthetic feedback should serve a greater and greater role in facilitating stronger internal representations of correct versus incorrect production of target utterances. Nevertheless, in initial stages of practice, the mirror can be helpful in facilitating or inhibiting articulatory movement gestures for accurate speech production.

Backward Chaining

The clinician models a multisyllabic word, a word containing an initial or final cluster, or a phrase by starting at the end of the utterance, producing the final sound, syllable, or word first, and moving from the back of the word to the front of the word in progressively longer units.

The use of backward chaining has been suggested by Chappell (1973) and Velleman (2003). Table 3–14 illustrates the use of backward chaining for facilitating correct production of consonant clusters, multisyllabic words, and sentences. When using backward chaining, it is essential to model the correct stress and intonation of the syllables and words in the utterance. In the examples that follow, the words and syllables in bold type would receive greater relative stress than the other words and syllables in the utterances.

Table 3–14. Examples of Backward Chaining

Backward Chaining to Elicit Cluster	Backward Chaining to Elicit Multisyllabic Word	Backward Chaining to Elicit Multisyllabic Word In Sentence
ick	ber	la
tick	tober	brella
stick	October	umbrella
		my umbrella
		got my umbrella
		forgot my umbrella
		I forgot my umbrella.

Forward Chaining

The clinician presents a multisyllabic word or a word containing an initial or final cluster by starting at the beginning of the word, producing the initial sound or syllable, then moving from the front to the back of the word.

Children may benefit from practicing portions of the word in smaller segments and adding sounds or syllables as they are able to manage the increased word shape complexity. If the target word is *ladybug*, the child may practice producing "lay," then "lady," then "ladybug." For a word with a final cluster such as *hops*, the child may practice producing "hop" and then be cued to add the /s/ to the end of the word to produce the target word, "hops," correctly. Table 3–15 provides other examples of forward chaining.

Preston et al. (2019) describe a combination of both backward and forward chaining in a Speech Motor Chaining procedure for children with speech sound disorders, including children with CAS. A five-step process of moving from a CV or VC target to a self-generated sentence is used as the child attains various CV and VC combinations of challenging target phonemes. For example, a child working on /r/ may have a motor speech chain with these targets (ra, rot, rotten, rotten food) and then a self-generated sentence with "rotten food" or these targets (or, for, before, just before) and a self-generated sentence with "just before."

The focus of chaining is facilitating flexible movement patterns—that is, moving from the challenging phoneme into and out of adjacent vowels with varied tongue height and advancement or consonants with varied place/manner/voicing. It is best to work from the contexts that are most facilitative to least facilitative for the particular child. Table 3–16 provides examples of building flexible movement gestures when working on challenging phonemes. The child works from the most facilitative context, in this case /ts/ followed by a vowel, toward more challenging contexts (e.g., /ts/ followed by /g/, as they differ in place, manner, and voicing). In the case of the /sk/ cluster, the child begins by moving from a vowel to /sk/ (most facilitative context) toward /k/ to /sk/, which is a challenging context for the child.

Hand Cues

The clinician uses specific finger/hand positions or hand motions representing a specific articulatory placement, lip shape, or manner of production of a phoneme or series of phonemes to cue the child to produce that phoneme or sequence of phonemes accurately.

Table 3–15. Examples of Forward Chaining

pull	police	policeman
but	butter	butterfly
base	baseball	baseball bat
bat	batter	battery
soup	super	Superman
spy	spider	Spiderman
me	meaty	medium

Table 3–16. Examples of Chaining Movement Gestures for /s/ Clusters

Target /ts/	/ts/ to V	/ts/ to /s/	/ts/ to /j/	/ts/ to /w/
It's	It's a It's a new day.	It's so It's so cool!	It's your It's your turn.	It's way It's way too hard.
/ts/ to /n/	**/ts/ to /m/**	**/ts/ to /tʃ/**	**/ts/ to /h/**	**/ts/ to /g/**
It's nice It's nice to meet you.	It's my It's my turn.	It's chilly It's chilly in here.	It's her It's her coat.	It's going It's going to rain.
Target /sk/	**V to /sk/**	**/z/ to /sk/**	**/t/ to /sk/**	**/n/ to /sk/**
School	to school Go to school now.	his school I like his school.	night school He went to night school.	in school We are in school all day.
/m/ to /sk/	**/p/ to /sk/**	**/l/ to /sk/**	**/f/ to /sk/**	**/k/ to /sk/**
Some schools Some schools are not open yet.	keep school Keep school closed this week.	until school One minute until school begins.	tough school He did a tough school project.	like school Do you like school?

Any hand position or hand motion that is meaningful to the child and offers the necessary reminders for production of a speech movement or movement sequence is appropriate. Hand positions and hand motions can be used to reference individual consonant or vowel phonemes or can be combined to facilitate accurate production of movement sequences for production of consonant clusters, syllables, or entire words. Hand cues can be provided alone or while modeling or miming the target utterance. Refer to Table 3–17 for suggestions of hand cues that help to facilitate accurate phoneme *placement* (e.g., child substitutes /ti/ "tea" for *key*) or *lip shape* (e.g., facilitating lip rounding for accurate production of /u/). Table 3–18 provides suggestions of hand cues to facilitate the child's accurate *manner* of production (e.g., child substitutes /toʊp/ for *soap*). The suggested hand cues provided here tend to be transparent—that is, they suggest the place or manner of production of the specified phonemes. Some materials for children with speech disorders recommend hand cues that are more arbitrary and do not relate to the placement or manner of articulatory production. Try different gestural cues until you find cues that are meaningful for the individual child.

The cues described in Tables 3–17 and 3–18 provide suggestions for gestures that have been beneficial in the treatment of children with CAS. Some children, however, benefit from bigger, more robust gestures. For example, the vowels /o/ and /u/ may be cued by shaping two hands together like a broad circle and extending them forward from the face. The vowel /i/ may be cued by pointing your fingertips toward the corners of the mouth and moving both arms sideways away from the mouth, whereas the /a/ vowel would be cued by pointing your fingertips toward the lower lip and dropping the arms straight down toward the chest. Marshalla (2009a, 2009b) has created YouTube videos, Pam's Place Cues—Vowels and Pam's Place Cues—Consonants, that demonstrate hand gestures for many consonant and vowel phonemes (https://www.youtube.com/watch?v=4te9DY1jTc8; https://www.youtube.com/watch?v=lBclowP9uds). They may be helpful when trying to establish hand signals for your students.

Table 3–17. Suggested Hand Cues to Reference *Place/Shape* of Articulation

Phonemes	Suggested Hand Cues
/p/, /b/, /m/	Place index finger along lip line.
/t/, /d/, /n/	Place the tip of index finger at the center of philtrum.
/k/, /g/	Place four fingertips under chin near throat.
/f/, /v/	Bite lower lip and place the tip of index finger at the center of lower lip.
/h/	Place an open palm in front of open mouth.
/s/, /z/	While smiling widely, place index finger and thumb at the corners of lips.
/ʃ/, /ʒ/, /tʃ/, /dʒ/	Protrude lips and place index finger and thumb at the pads of cheeks.
/l/	Place index finger just below the center of upper teeth.
/r/	Place index finger and thumb near the back of throat.
/i/	Place index fingers at opposite corners of lips while smiling.
/u/	Place index fingers at opposite corners of lips while shaping lips in a tight circle or gesture with index finger in a circular motion around lips.
/oʊ/	Place index fingers at opposite corners of lips while shaping lips in a more open circle or gesture with index finger in a circular motion around lips.
/ɑ/	Place index finger at the center of chin and lower jaw.

Table 3–18. Suggested Hand Cues to Reference *Manner* of Articulation

Phonemes	Suggested Hand Cues
/p/, /b/	Hold the tips of all fingers and thumb together near the corner of lip and release them quickly to represent a puff of air.
/m/	Place index finger at the side of nose while modeling /m/.
/t/, /d/	Hold the tips of thumb and index finger together near the center of lips and release quickly.
/n/	Place index finger at the side of nose while modeling /n/.
/k/, /g/	Place four fingertips at the back of throat and quickly release them forward while producing these phonemes.
/f/, /v/	Bite lower lip and then move index finger back and forth along the edge of the lower lip.
/h/	Place one hand flat against chest and one open palm (either the therapist's or the child's) in front of open mouth to feel the sensation of air.
/s/, /z/	Slide index finger along the length of upper lip or up the length of forearm.
/ʃ/, /ʒ/	Protrude lips and place index finger and thumb at the pads of cheeks moving fingers forward while producing these phonemes.
/tʃ/, /dʒ/	Hold the tips of all fingers and thumb together near the side of cheek and release them quickly to represent a puff of air.

Manual Signs

The clinician signs words just prior to or while the child is producing the words.

When a manual sign has been linked to a verbal model repeatedly, the verbal model can be faded, and the sign will still act as a cue to trigger the child's motor memory for how the target is produced. Phrases or specific words within phrases may be signed to the child as the child is speaking. Manual signs may be particularly effective for children who tend to omit function words (e.g., articles, prepositions) or morphological markers (e.g., present progressive "ing,").

Graphic Cues

The clinician incorporates letters, written words, or phrases denoting specific sounds or words in treatment.

Using graphic cues can remind a child who is able to recognize and make sense of the written information to insert sounds where they are needed in words. Written words can help draw a child's attention to a specific phoneme or sequence of phonemes within a word. Target phrases can be written on sentence strips to support accurate productions of the target phrase. For prereaders, graphic cues can be used to support later literacy development. More detailed information regarding ways to support early literacy development within the context of speech praxis treatment is included in Chapter 7. When using graphic cues, using bold type, underlining, highlighting, or enlarging certain phonemes can be used to bring a child's attention to specific elements of the target utterance. Some learners also respond to alternative spellings to help sound out the words. Examples are shown in Box 3–4.

Syllable Cues

The clinician and/or the child taps or claps out the number of syllables in the word or phrase or uses blocks or other tokens to denote those syllables.

Syllable cues are used when a child omits syllables from multisyllabic words or words from phrases by alerting the child to the correct number of syllables. Simply clapping hands for each syllable or tapping on the table, your knees, or a drum may provide a salient enough cue to facilitate inclusion of all syllables within the target word or phrase. Blocks or chips provide similar cues. Different-sized blocks can be used to denote syllables versus whole words or to differentiate stressed from weak syllables. For example, in Figure 3–3, the child is practicing the target word "*banana*" in the carrier phrase "*I ate a _____,*" with large blocks used to denote whole words and small blocks to denote individual syllables of the word banana.

When using syllable cues, be sure to model normal prosody to avoid robotic sounding productions.

■ Box 3–4. Examples of Graphic Cues

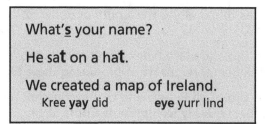

What'**s** your name?

He sa**t** on a ha**t**.

We created a map of Ireland.
Kree **yay** did   **eye** yurr lind

Metaphors

Rather than modeling the target word for the child, the clinician cues the child to produce a particular phoneme using a term that describes some feature of the phoneme.

Bleile (2006) uses the term *metaphor* as an analogy for production of a specific phoneme. Choosing metaphors that reflect a manner of production or an articulatory placement increases the saliency and meaningfulness of the cue. Table 3–19 provides examples of metaphors for many phonemes.

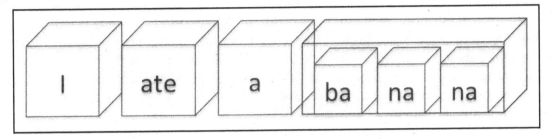

Figure 3–3. Using blocks to denote words and syllables.

Table 3–19. Suggested Metaphors Associated With Specific Phonemes

Phoneme	Metaphor	Phoneme	Metaphor
/b/	Submarine sound Noisy lip popper	/s/	Shy snake sound Quiet skinny air
/p/	Popcorn sound Quiet lip popper	/z/	Buzzing bee sound Noisy skinny air
/m/	Yummy food sound Humming lips	/ʃ/	Sleeping baby sound Quiet big air
/w/	Crying baby sound Lip squeezer	/tʃ/	Choo-choo train sound Big air popper
/d/	Drumbeat sound Noisy tongue tapper	/dʒ/	Noisy choo-choo sound Big air popper
/t/	Tick-tock clock sound Quiet tongue tapper	/θ/, /ð/	Brave snake sound
/n/	Noisy nose sound	/r/	Growling bear sound
/l/	Singing sound Teeth hugger	/k/	Coughing sound Quiet throat sound
/f/	Windy sound Quiet lip biter	/g/	Drinking sound Noisy throat sound
/v/	Car engine sound Noisy lip biter	/h/	Panting dog sound Warm air sound

Phonetic Placement Cues

The clinician provides a verbal description of how the specific phonemes are produced. Phonetic placement cues are often combined with gestural cues and other types of cues.

Phonetic placement cues are not specific to apraxia treatment but are commonly used in the treatment of articulation disorders. The clinician describes to the child how the speech sound is produced. For example, when producing the /f/ sound, the child can be told to "Bring the lower lip up to meet the top teeth then blow." The choice of wording of the cues will be dependent on what aspect of the movement the child needs to change. For instance, if a child is working on /s/ production, your phonetic placement cues will be different if the child is substituting /t/ for /s/ than if the child has a lateral lisp. Phonetic placement cues are one of the most commonly used cues in CAS treatment, so becoming adept at explaining movement of the articulators in ways that children can understand is essential for skilled treatment. It is important to talk to the child about jaw height, tongue, and lip positions and movements, and degree of tension or tightness of the oral musculature to help the child be successful in understanding the movement expectations.

Mouth Pictures and Videos

Pictures or videos of the mouth can be used to illustrate how specific sounds are produced.

There is an abundant number of mouth shape pictures available that illustrate the lip shape, jaw height, and tongue position for vowel and consonant phonemes through online sellers such as Etsy (https://www.etsy.com) and Teachers Pay Teachers (https://www.teacherspayteachers.com). Reading and apraxia materials that provide pictures of mouth shapes associated with specific phonemes include *Lindamood Phoneme Sequencing Program for Reading, Spelling, and Speech* (Lindamood & Lindamood, 1998), *Phonic Faces* (Norris, 2003), *Say and Do Sound Production Flip Book and Activities for Apraxia and More!* (Perkins Faulk & Priddy, 2005).

Videos of specific phoneme production can be viewed using the Sounds of Speech application ($3.99) from the University of Iowa Research Foundation. A preview of the application is found at https://apps.apple.com/us/app/sounds-of-speech/id780656219. This application displays a moving schematic of a sagittal section of the head and neck, showing the movements of the articulators and the relationships of the lips, teeth, tongue, pharynx, velum, and vocal folds during production of each phoneme of English. A video showing a frontal view of a person producing each phoneme also can be viewed on the website along with a written description of the place, manner, and voicing required to achieve accurate articulatory production of the phonemes. The Speech Tutor by Synapse Apps LLC ($24.99) and Speech Sounds Visualized by Pullman Regional Hospital (by monthly or annual subscription) are two apps that can be used on a tablet computer to help children visualize movement of the articulators during production of phonemes.

Syllable Pictures

Words containing two or more syllables can be simplified for children by using separate pictures that denote the individual syllables of the target word.

If a child can recognize and produce the individual syllables of a word as separate words, the production of the whole word often is much easier. Compound words lend themselves well to this technique and are the most basic example of using separate pictures to denote a new word. Words such as doghouse, cupcake, or football can be shown as two separate pictures that, when linked together, create a new word. Pictures also can be used to denote syllables of two- and three-syllable words that are not compound words (e.g., *movie*—a cow for "moo" and the letter V; *hamburger*—a ham, someone who is cold "brrr," and a bear "grrr;" *circus*—a nicely dressed man "sir" and a person giving another a kiss "kiss"). In some cases, not all the syllables need to be drawn, only the ones that are challenging for the child. For example, the medial syllable, "le," in "elephant," and the initial syllable, "com," in "computer," are weak and, thus, more likely to be omitted. Quickly drawing a person singing for "le" or a person signaling for a dog to "come" may be all that is needed to elicit inclusion of the omitted syllables. Figure 3–4 shows examples of syllable pictures for compound words and 2+ syllable words. Tables 3–20 and 3–21 provide lists of compound words and two- and three-syllable words that may lend themselves to syllable picture cues.

Tactile-Kinesthetic Cues

Tactile cues provided by the clinician to facilitate accurate and efficient articulatory movements.

When children do not respond to models, phonetic placement cues, or other metacognitive strategies and cues, tactile cues may be beneficial. Tactile cues offer a way to increase the child's tactile, kinesthetic, and proprioceptive awareness of the movement gestures. Two programs commonly described in CAS treatment literature that incorporate tactile cueing are DTTC (Strand, 2020) and PROMPT (Hayden, 2004). Both programs are described in greater detail in Chapter 4. Placement of your hand or fingers under a child's chin can support appropriate jaw opening for specific vowels. The fingers can be used to support lip closure for bilabials or lip rounding and retraction for vowels. Be sure to watch yourself in the mirror as you say the words in a natural way to determine the correct jaw height, lip rounding/retraction, or lip tightness/tension for the specific target utterance, as these movements will vary depending on adjacent phonemes. Keep in mind, of course, that the trajectories of jaw movements are wider in younger children than adults.

Fading of Multisensory Cues

Although providing cues is essential to improving sensorimotor speech skills, the ultimate goal is to fade cues over time, so the child takes greater responsibility for the clarity of their own speech. Fading cues also reduces the child's dependence on cues. To help the child take greater responsibility over accurate speech production, the clinician can use the following strategies:

- transition from using more salient to less salient cues (e.g., moving from tactile cue to direct model to metaphor)
- shift from using multisensory cues to simpler cues (e.g., moving from combined visual, tactile, auditory cues to an auditory cue alone)
- gradually fade cues over time (e.g., moving from verbal model to no model)

A more detailed discussion of adding and fading of cues is found in the discussion of DTTC in Chapter 4.

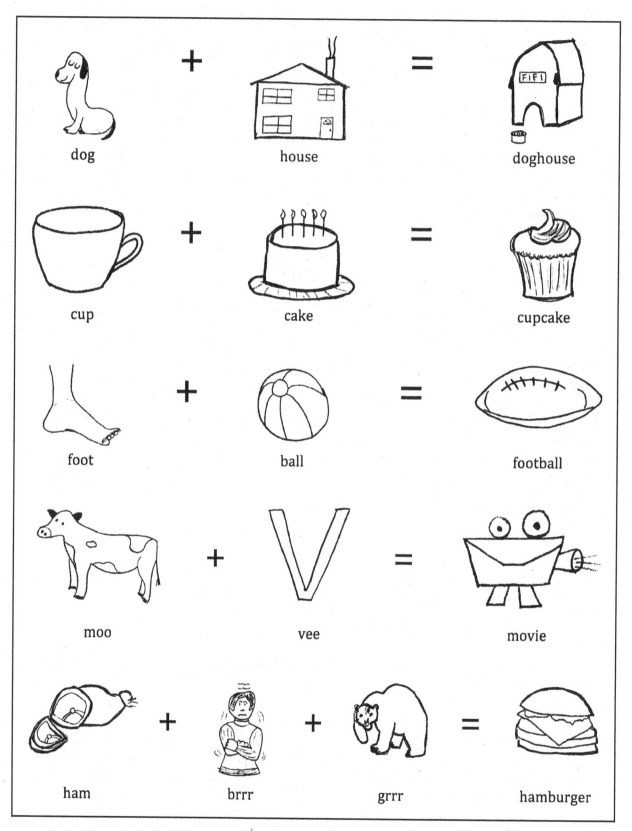

Figure 3–4. Syllable pictures for compound words and two- to three-syllable words.

Table 3–20. Compound Words for Syllable Pictures

Airplane	Backpack	Baseball
Bathroom	Bedroom	Birdhouse
Cowboy	Cupcake	Downstairs
Flashlight	Football	Haircut
Homework	Inside	Notebook
Outside	Pancake	Ponytail
Popcorn	Raincoat	Sidewalk
Snowman	Something	Suitcase
Toothbrush	Upstairs	Watermelon

Table 3–21. Two- and Three-Syllable Words for Syllable Pictures

Also	Always	Answer
All sew	All ways	Ann sir
Baby	Baking	Before
bay bee	bay king	bee four
Believe	Body	Candy
bee leave	bah D	can D
Careful	Christmas	DVD
care full	Chris miss	D V D
Enjoy	Explain	Friday
in joy	X plane	fry day
Going	Hamburger	Hiding
go wing	ham brrr grrr	hi ding
Label	Lady	Neighbor
lay bull	lay D	neigh brrr
Number	Okay	Paper
numb brrr	O K	pay purr
Pilot	Purple	Radio
pie lit	purr pull	ray D O
Snowing	Snowy	Tiny
snow wing	snow whee	tie knee
Tomato	Tomorrow	Video
toe may toe	two ma row	V D Yo

Intensity of Services

Much of the focus of research in speech-language pathology literature has been on trying to determine if specific treatment methods work. Far less research has focused on determining the amount of treatment required to facilitate improvement. Treatment intensity commonly is conceptualized as the number of treatment minutes per week/month for a given period of time (e.g., 90 min per week for 6 months). The critical elements regarding how many properly administered teaching episodes will be occurring within a session and the quality of the teaching episodes are eliminated from this simplistic model of treatment intensity (Warren et al., 2007). For a broader view of treatment intensity, several clinical questions can be considered including the following:

- **What is the optimal treatment dose?** *Dose* is defined as "the number of properly administered teaching episodes during a single intervention session" (Warren et al., 2007, p. 71). A *teaching episode* is "the sequence of events from initial elicitation of a target through the child's final attempt before switching to another target" (Maas et al., 2019, p. 3168). For example, a child is working to establish accurate production of the target phrase, *"stop it."* During a single teaching episode, the child may practice the target utterance five times before the target is produced correctly and a new teaching episode of *"stop it"* is begun. Those five production attempts are considered a single teaching episode. Thus, during a session, the number of production attempts will be higher than the number of teaching episodes.

- **What dose form is being used?** *Dose form* is defined as "the typical task or activity within which the teaching episodes are delivered" (Warren et al., 2007, p. 71). Whereas *dose* is a *quantitative* factor, *dose form* is a *qualitative* factor in treatment and an extremely important factor in the effectiveness of treatment. What types of tasks and activities you do during intervention are typically based on which intervention program is being used and your underlying theoretical foundations. A more thorough discussion of a variety of evidence-based intervention programs for CAS is found in Chapter 4. In short, it is important to become familiar with a variety of programs so you can choose which program is most appropriate for a given child based on a number of factors (e.g., age, severity, specific challenges).

- **What is the appropriate dose frequency?** *Dose frequency* is defined as "the number of times a dose of intervention is provided per day and per week" (Warren et al., 2007, p. 72). It encompasses both the *number of sessions per week* and *session duration* (e.g., one weekly 30-min session [low intensity] versus four weekly 30-min sessions [high intensity]). Researchers who have made suggestions regarding dose frequency for children with CAS typically recommend between two and four sessions per week with a high frequency of teaching episodes per session (Murray et al., 2015, Namasivayam et al., 2015; Strand, 2020).

- **What is the anticipated total intervention duration?** *Total intervention duration* is described as "the time period over which a specified intervention is presented" (Warren et al., 2007, p. 71). In treatment studies for children with CAS, the typical treatment duration is a specified number of weeks (e.g., 3, 6, 12 weeks). In reality, however, the treatment duration is far greater than the short durations used in research and will vary based on factors including the severity and complexity of the child's communication challenges, as well as the child's response to treatment.

- **What is the most desirable clinician-child ratio?** *The clinician-child ratio* refers to the ratio of the number of clinicians to clients. When a child is seen by the SLP individually, the clinician-client ratio would be 1:1; a dyad would be 1:2; and a small group could be 1:3 or 1:4. Theoretically, a smaller clinician-client ratio, as in individual treatment, would allow for a higher dose of teaching episodes. This would provide greater treatment intensity and would be preferable. There may be factors and situations, however, that would warrant dyad or small-group treatment. These factors may include motivation (a child may be more motivated to practice when working with a peer), individual communication profiles (a child may have needs in the area of social communication that warrant dyad or group treatment to meet social/pragmatic goals), and stage of development (a child may be working on generalization).

When you multiply *dose* by *dose frequency* by *total intervention duration*, you arrive at a *cumulative intervention intensity* (Warren et al., 2007). For example, a child receiving two, 60-min sessions per week with ~50 teaching episodes per session for 50 weeks would have a cumulative intervention intensity of 5,000 teaching episodes over 50 weeks. Table 3–22 provides examples for calculating cumulative intervention intensity.

Making Clinical Decisions About Treatment Intensity

Many researchers and experts in motor learning and CAS agree that to improve sensori-motor planning, intensive treatment is required (Maas et al., 2008; Strand & Skinder, 1999;

Table 3–22. Calculating Cumulative Intervention Intensity

Treatment Method	Dose	Dose Frequency	Total Intervention Duration	Cumulative Intervention Intensity
Language stimulation	~20 teaching episodes	Two sessions per week, 50 min each	30 weeks	1,200 teaching episodes
DTTC[a]	~60 teaching episodes	Three sessions per week, 30 min each	30 weeks	5,400 teaching episodes
PROMPT[a]	~50 teaching episodes	Two sessions per week, 50 min each	30 weeks	3,000 teaching episodes
ReST[a] practice portion	100 teaching episodes	Two sessions per week, 60 min each	10 weeks	2,000 teaching episodes

Note. DTTC, Dynamic Temporal and Tactile Cueing; PROMPT, PROMPTS for Restructuring Oral Muscular Phonetic Targets; ReST, Rapid Syllable Transition Treatment.

[a]These treatment programs are described in greater detail in Chapter 4.

Strode & Chamberlain, 2006). Strand (2008) recommends short, frequent treatment sessions for children with severe CAS (e.g., three to five 20- to 30-min sessions per week). Namasivayam et al. (2015) found individual motor speech treatment delivered two times per week was more effective in improving the articulation and functional communication of children with CAS than treatment delivered one time per week. Although dose frequency for children with moderate or severe CAS would be high, we may expect an older child with CAS who has made substantial progress in prior treatment and whose speech intelligibility is improving to continue to make progress with lower dose frequency. The critical element of dose cannot be overlooked when making decisions about treatment intensity. You want to be sure you are applying treatment methods that provide ample opportunities for practice to develop strong sensorimotor plans.

Clinical decisions about treatment intensity often are made based on factors that are unrelated to the child's needs, such as length of a class period at school, typical length of a treatment session at the clinic site, or the distance the child needs to travel to attend speech. In fact, decisions about treatment intensity should be more dependent on the child's developmental profile and individual needs. Things to consider may include the following:

- severity of the child's speech praxis challenges
- age of the child
- attention capacities of the child
- physical stamina of the child
- types of goals being addressed in speech and language treatment
- coexisting needs that may require other types of treatment (motor, cognitive, learning, medical, social, emotional)

Sample Cases

Five different children are described in this section. A summary is provided regarding the speech and language skills and needs of each child. Following the case summary section, a table is provided that compares and contrasts the number of service minutes per week and how those minutes are distributed (e.g., length of sessions, group versus individual) for each child.

Child 1

Name: Jayden

Age: 3 years, 7 months

Diagnosis: CAS; expressive language disorder

Summary: Jayden demonstrates specific deficits in speech praxis that severely impact his speech intelligibility. He has a limited phonetic inventory that impacts his expressive communication skills. He is speaking primarily in single words. His expressive vocabulary is quite delayed for his age, though this appears to be linked to his limited phonetic inventory. His receptive language and cognitive skills appear to be on target for his age. He is beginning to display frustration with his challenges in expressing his ideas, leading to frequent temper tantrums at home and occasional noncompliance during the initial evaluation. He is playful, engaging (typically gesturally), and well-liked by his peers in preschool.

Recommendations: It is recommended that Jayden receive intensive speech and language treatment services to upgrade speech intelligibility and expressive language. Short, frequent treatment sessions are recommended.

Child 2

Name: Kara

Age: 6 years, 4 months

Diagnosis: CAS

Summary: Kara has been receiving speech and language treatment services since the age of 2 years, 6 months. At age 3 years, Kara was diagnosed with CAS. She received intensive speech and language treatment, including four 30-min sessions per week in her school district preschool itinerant speech program and two 45-min sessions per week privately. She made excellent progress. Her current goals reflect her need to improve phoneme sequencing for multisyllabic words, increase accuracy of final consonant clusters, and increase consistency of /l/ production at single-word and sentence levels.

Recommendations: It is recommended that Kara receive twice-weekly speech and language treatment services to continue to upgrade speech intelligibility and address residual articulation issues.

Child 3

Name: Mateo

Age: 8 years, 8 months

Diagnosis: CAS; receptive and expressive language disorder

Summary: Mateo has been enrolled in speech and language treatment since age 2 years. His initial diagnosis was Developmental Delay. At age 3 years, Mateo entered a special education preschool class and received 90 min per week of speech and language treatment and 60 min per month of occupational therapy. He was diagnosed at age 4 years with severe CAS and began receiving an additional 60 min per week of private treatment to address his speech praxis needs. While he has made good progress, his overall speech intelligibility remains moderately impaired. His current speech goals reflect his need to increase accurate production of fricative phonemes; increase consistency of CVCVC, CVCCVC, CCVC, and CVCVCV syllable shapes; and stabilize the accuracy of phoneme sequences at the phrase and sentence levels. Current receptive language goals reflect Mateo's need to improve his ability to follow verbal instructions of increasing length and complexity, increase comprehension of conceptual terms, and improve comprehension of higher-level question forms. Expressively, Mateo is working to increase mean length of utterance, increase expressive vocabulary, and improve grammar. Social language goals involve increasing initiation of language with peers and using his language for a wider range of communicative functions.

Recommendations: It is recommended that Mateo receive intensive speech and language treatment services to upgrade speech intelligibility, receptive language, expressive language, and social communication skills. Establishing an alternative means of communication, such as a voice output communication device, should be initiated so Mateo has a way to communicate intelligibly when communicative breakdowns occur or when interacting with unfamiliar listeners.

Child 4

Name: Maribella

Age: 5 years, 11 months

Diagnosis: Autism spectrum disorder; CAS

Summary: Bella began receiving speech and language therapy at the age of 2 years, 6 months and was diagnosed with autism at age 3 years. Over the past year, Bella has begun to use more verbal language and improve her verbal imitation skills. This recent surge in verbal language allowed for completion of a motor speech evaluation. The recent motor speech assessment confirmed CAS. Because Bella is beginning to demonstrate stronger imitation skills recently, verbal communication will be addressed through individual treatment. However, dyad and small-group treatment will continue to be important to upgrade social pragmatic language skills.

Recommendations: It is recommended that Bella receive intensive speech and language treatment services to facilitate improved speech praxis skills, receptive language, expressive language, and social interaction.

Child 5

Name: Henry

Age: 6 years, 2 months

Diagnosis: Dysarthria; CAS; receptive and expressive language disorder

Summary: Henry has been receiving speech and language treatment in addition to other related services (occupational and physical therapy) since approximately 18 months of age. He exhibits a severe speech and language impairment. His combined dysarthria and CAS make his speech attempts highly inconsistent and labored. His phoneme and syllable shape repertoires are quite limited. Manual signs are approximations, as limb apraxia is evident. Recently, his SLP has introduced Picture Exchange Communication System, though he is not using it spontaneously at this time. The school and family are in the process of an augmentative communication evaluation and hope to choose a voice output communication device soon. Henry is enrolled in a self-contained special education classroom and spends the majority of time each school day either in this classroom or with one of his related service providers. He is included in the first-grade general education classroom for selected activities (e.g., calendar time, art, music, special events). Henry continues to receive physical and occupational therapy to address gross and fine motor strength, stability, and coordination issues.

Recommendations: It is recommended that Henry receive intensive, direct speech and language treatment services, plus weekly consultation to help his school staff facilitate improved communication skills aimed at increasing spontaneity, variety of communicative functions, and the expression of a wider range of ideas. Focus of treatment will be to establish a consistent means of functional, multimodal communication.

These case examples illustrate the need for flexibility in program planning for children with CAS. Although intensive, individual treatment is a rule of thumb, it is essential to consider multiple factors when making decisions about treatment schedules, as shown in Table 3–23.

Table 3–23. Intensity and Distribution of Speech and Language Treatment Services for Five Children With CAS

Child	Monday	Tuesday	Wednesday	Thursday	Friday
Jayden	30-min 1-to-1 to address speech praxis	30-min 1-to-1 to address speech praxis	30-min 1-to-1 to address speech praxis		30-min dyad to address use of newly acquired skills with a peer
Kara	30-min 1-to-1 or dyad to address articulation		30-min 1-to-1 or dyad to address articulation		
Mateo	30-min 1-to-1 to address speech praxis and use of augmentative and alternative communication (AAC)	30- to 45-min small group or dyad to address language and social interaction	30-min 1-to-1 to address speech praxis and use of AAC	30-min 1-to-1 to address speech praxis and use of AAC; 30-min consultation to classroom staff to support use of AAC device	30- to 45-min small group or dyad to address language and social interaction
Bella	30-min 1-to-1 to address speech praxis	30- to 45-min small group or dyad to address language and social interaction	30-min 1-to-1 to address speech praxis	30- to 45-min small group or dyad to address language and social interaction	30- to 45-min small group or dyad to address language and social interaction
Henry	30-min 1-to-1 or dyad to address functional, multimodal communication		30-min 1-to-1 or dyad to address functional, multimodal communication (co-treatment with occupational therapist)	30-min 1-to-1 or dyad to address functional, multimodal communication	30-min consultation with classroom staff to support use of AAC

Putting It All Together

The final section of this chapter is a discussion of ways in which SLPs can integrate the information from earlier sections of this chapter. We refine our clinical skills by making thoughtful decisions during planning and treatment to increase effectiveness in facilitating initial acquisition of skills, as well as retention and transfer. There are many things to consider simultaneously related to conditions of practice, conditions of feedback, treatment context, and complexity of the task to be sure we are providing services that are effective and efficient.

Rvachew and Brosseau-Lapré (2012) describe the importance of working at the child's *optimum challenge point*, a concept earlier described by Guadagnoli and Lee (2004). It is the point where the task is neither too difficult nor too easy for the child and is a moving target from moment to moment in treatment. There are a range of variables that come into play to facilitate working at the child's optimum challenge point. As clinical skills become more refined, the SLP is able to manipulate these variables in real time to keep the child working at the optimum challenge point. At any point within a session, the clinician can vary the following:

- complexity/difficulty of the task
- level of cueing
- amount and type of feedback
- treatment context

When a child is struggling to maintain a relatively high level of accuracy, the clinician will make the task easier, provide more cues, provide more frequent and descriptive feedback, and/or maintain a familiar treatment context. Likewise, when the child is performing at a very high level of accuracy, the clinician can increase the level of task difficulty, provide fewer cues, offer less frequent and less descriptive feedback, and/or vary the context of treatment. Table 3–24 lists several variables that can be adjusted by the SLP in real time to keep the child working at an optimum challenge point and get the most out of treatment. By manipulating one or more of these variables from moment to moment within the treatment session, the clinician is able to facilitate higher levels of skill acquisition and help the child attain better retention and transfer of skills acquired in therapy. Ideally, the clinician is providing the most appropriate intensity of service, planning the sessions carefully, and then manipulating these variables in "real time" to provide the best quality service possible for the child.

Table 3–24. Modifying Variables in Treatment to Achieve Optimum Challenge Point

How to Reduce Level of Challenge	Variable	How to Increase Level of Challenge
Choose a target with a less complex syllable shape, e.g., instead of "*mom*," try "*ma*."	Syllable shape complexity	Choose a target with a more complex syllable shape, e.g., instead of "*ma*" try "*mommy*" or "*mom*."
Choose target phonemes that are less challenging, e.g., instead of fricative, try a stop, nasal, or glide.	Phonemic complexity	Choose target phonemes that are more challenging, e.g., instead of a stop, try a fricative.
Reduce the diversity of phonetic contexts, e.g., instead of "*bye dad*," try "*bye bye*."	Phonetic contexts	Increase the complexity of phonetic contexts by manipulating the number of variations in place, manner, and voicing within the same utterance, e.g., instead of *pop up*, try *hop down*.

Table 3–24. *continued*

How to Reduce Level of Challenge	Variable	How to Increase Level of Challenge
Decrease rate of production of target utterance.	Rate of production	Increase rate of production of target utterance.
Decrease length of utterance, e.g., instead of "I want more pizza," try "I want pizza" or "more pizza."	Utterance length	Increase length of utterance, e.g., instead of "I want more pizza" try "I want more pepperoni pizza, please."
Reduce grammatical complexity, e.g., Instead of "Do you like cookies?" try "I like cookies."	Grammatical complexity	Increase grammatical complexity, e.g., instead of "I want pizza," try "Do you want pizza?" or "Mommy wants pizza."
Provide more salient cues, e.g., instead of a direct model, use simultaneous production and a tactile cue.	Cueing	Provide less salient cues, e.g., instead of a direct model, use a gestural cue or a metaphor. Fade cues and move toward elicited productions, e.g., production of the target utterance in response to a question or a fill-in-the-blank sentence.
Increase frequency of feedback.	Feedback frequency	Reduce frequency of feedback.
Instead of knowledge of results, provide more specific feedback in the form of knowledge of performance.	Type of feedback	Instead of knowledge of performance, provide less specific feedback in the form of knowledge of results.
Move from less structured to more structured activities, e.g., practice the targets in a simple, structured game.	Level of structure	Move from structured to less structured activities, e.g., try eliciting target utterances in a play activity.
Provide practice opportunities in a familiar setting, e.g., treatment room, "work-area" in the child's home.	Setting	Provide practice opportunities in less familiar or less structured settings, e.g., classroom, hallway, playground.
Reduce environmental distractions, e.g., competing visual and auditory noise.	Distractions	Increase distraction during practice, e.g., practice while tossing a ball back and forth or building a block tower.
Practice with the primary therapist or other familiar practice partner or caregiver.	Communication partners	Provide opportunities to practice with less familiar partners, e.g., a different therapist, a peer, a less familiar person in the school or clinic, a person in the community.

References

Allen, M. M. (2013). Intervention efficacy and intensity for children with speech sound disorder. *Journal of Speech, Language, and Hearing Research, 56,* 865–877. https://doi.org/10.1044/1092-4388(2012/11-0076)

American Speech-Language-Hearing Association. (2007). *Childhood apraxia of speech* [Technical report]. Available from www.asha.org/policy/

Bleile, K. (2006). *The late eight.* Plural Publishing.

Brown, R. (1973). *A first language: The early stages.* Harvard University Press.

Burningham, J. (1971). *Mr. Gumpy's outing.* Henry Holt Publishing.

Chappell, G. E. (1973). Childhood verbal apraxia and its treatment. *Journal of Speech and Hearing Disorders, 38,* 362–368. https://doi.org/10.1044/jshd.3803.362

Davis, B. L., & MacNeilage, P. F. (1990). Acquisition of correct vowel production: A quantitative case study. *Journal of Speech and Hearing Research, 33,* 16–27. https://doi.org/10.1044/jshr.3301.16

Davis, B. L., & MacNeilage, P. F. (1995). The articulatory basis of babbling. *Journal of Speech and Hearing Research, 38,* 1199–1211. https://doi.org/10.1044/jshr.3806.1199

Davis, B. L., & Velleman, S. L. (2000). Differential diagnosis and treatment of developmental apraxia of speech in infants and toddlers. *Infant-Toddler Intervention: The Transdisciplinary Journal, 10,* 177–192.

Edeal, D. M., & Gildersleeve-Neumann, C. E. (2011). The importance of production frequency in therapy for childhood apraxia of speech. *American Journal of Speech-Language Pathology, 20,* 95–110. https://doi.org/10.1044/1058-0360(2011/09-0005)

Guadagnoli, M. A., & Lee, T. D. (2004). Challenge point: A framework for conceptualizing the effects of various practice conditions in motor learning. *Journal of Motor Behavior, 36,* 212–224. https://doi.org/10.3200/JMBR.36.2.212-224

Hayden, D. A. (2004). *P.R.O.M.P.T. Prompts for restructuring oral muscular phonetic targets, introduction to technique: A manual.* PROMPT Institute.

Iuzzini-Seigel, J., Hogan, T. P., Guarino, A. J., & Green, J. R. (2015). Reliance on auditory feedback in children with childhood apraxia of speech. *Journal of Communication Disorders, 54,* 32–42. https://doi.org/10.1016/j.jcomdis.2015.01.002

Kehoe, M. M., & Stoel-Gammon, C. (2001). Development of syllable structure in English speaking children with particular reference to rhymes. *Journal of Child Language, 28,* 393–432. https://doi.org/10.1017/S030500090100469X

Ladefoged, P. (2001). *A course in phonetics* (4th ed.). Harcourt.

Lindamood, P. C., & Lindamood, P. D. (1998). *The Lindamood Phoneme Sequencing Program for Reading, Spelling, and Speech.* Pro-Ed.

Maas, E., Butalla, C. E., & Farinella, K. A. (2012). Feedback frequency in treatment for childhood apraxia of speech. *American Journal of Speech-Language Pathology, 21,* 239–257. https://doi.org/10.1044/1058-0360(2012/11-0119)

Maas, E., & Farinella, K. A. (2012). Random versus blocked practice in treatment of childhood apraxia of speech. *Journal of Speech, Language, and Hearing Research, 55,* 561–578. https://doi.org/10.1044/1092-4388(2011/11-0120)

Maas, E., Gildersleeve-Neumann, C., Jakielski, K., Kovacs, N., Stoeckel, R., Vradelis, H., & Welsh, M. (2019). Bang for your buck: A single-case experimental design study of practice amount and distribution in treatment for childhood apraxia of speech. *Journal of Speech, Language, and Hearing Research, 62,* 3160–3182. https://doi.org/10.1044/2019_JSLHR-S-18-0212

Maas, E., Robin, D., Austermann Hula, S., Freedman, S., Wulf, G., Ballard, K., & Schmidt, R. (2008). Principles of motor learning in treatment of motor speech disorders. *American Journal of Speech-Language Pathology, 17,* 277–298. https://doi.org/10.1044/1058-0360(2008/025)

Marshalla, P. (2009a). *Pam's place cues for consonants.* https://www.youtube.com/watch?v=lBclowP9uds

Marshalla, P. (2009b). *Pam's place cues for vowels.* https://www.youtube.com/watch?v=lBclowP9uds

McCormick, L., & Schiefelbusch, R. (1984). *Early language intervention.* Charles E. Merrill.

Murray, E., McCabe, P., & Ballard, K. J. (2012). A comparison of two treatments for childhood apraxia of speech: Methods and treatment protocol for a parallel group randomised control trial. *BMC Pediatrics, 12.* https://doi.org/10.1186/1471-2431-12-112

Murray, E., McCabe, P., & Ballard, K. J. (2015). A randomized controlled trial for children with childhood apraxia of speech comparing Rapid Syllable Transition Treatment and the Nuffield Dyspraxia Programme (3rd ed.). *Journal of Speech, Language, and Hearing Research, 58*(3), 669–686. https://doi.org/10.1044/2015_JSLHR-S-13-0179

Namasivayam, A. K., Pukonen, M., Goshulak, D., Hard, J., Rudzicz, F., Rietveld, T., . . . Van Lieshout, P. H. H. M. (2015). Treatment intensity and childhood apraxia of speech. *International Journal of Language*

& *Communication Disorders, 50*(4), 529–546. https://doi.org/10.1111/1460-6984.12154

Nelson, K. (1973). Structure and strategy in learning to talk. *Monographs of the Society for Research in Child Development, 38*, 1–135; cited by McCormick & Schiefelbusch (1984).

Norris, J. (2003). *Phonic faces manual* (2nd ed.). Baton Rouge, LA: Elementory LC. https://www.elementory.com/info.html

Perkins Faulk, J., & Priddy, L. (2005). *Say and do sound production flip book and activities for apraxia and more!* Super Duper Publications.

Preston, J. L., Leece, M. C., & Storto, J. (2019). Tutorial: Speech motor chaining treatment for school-age children with speech sound disorders. *Language, Speech, and Hearing Services in Schools, 50*, 343–355. https://doi.org/10.1044/2018_LSHSS-18-0081

Rvachew, S., & Brosseau-Lapré, F. (2012). *Developmental phonological disorders: Foundations of clinical practice.* San Diego, CA: Plural Publishing.

Rice, M., Sell, M., & Hadley, P. (1991). Social interactions of speech and language-impaired children. *Journal of Speech and Hearing Research, 34*, 1299–1307. https://doi.org/10.1044/jshr.3406.1299

Schmidt, R. A., & Lee, T. D. (2005). *Motor control and learning: A behavioral emphasis* (4th ed.). Human Kinetics.

Strand, E. A. (2008, July). *Principles of speech motor learning* [Paper presentation]. Childhood Apraxia of Speech Association of North America (CASANA) 2008 National Conference on Childhood Apraxia of Speech, Williamsburg, VA, United States.

Strand, E. A. (2020). Dynamic temporal and tactile cueing: A treatment strategy for childhood apraxia of speech. *American Journal of Speech-Language Pathology, 29*, 30–48. https://doi.org/10.1044/2019_AJSLP-19-0005

Strand, E. A., & Skinder, A. (1999). Treatment of developmental apraxia of speech: Integral stimulation methods. In A. J. Caruso & E. A. Strand (Eds.), *Clinical management of motor speech disorders in children* (pp. 109–148). Thieme.

Strode, R., & Chamberlain, C. (2006). *The source for childhood apraxia of speech.* LinguiSystems.

Terband, H., Maassen, B., Guenther, F. H., & Brumberg, J. (2009). Computational neural modeling of speech motor control in childhood apraxia of speech (CAS). *Journal of Speech, Language, and Hearing Research, 52*, 1595–1609. https://doi.org/10.1044/1092-4388(2009/07-0283)

Thomas, D. C., McCabe, P., & Ballard, K. J. (2014). Rapid syllable transitions (ReST) treatment for childhood apraxia of speech: The effect of lower-dose frequency. *Journal of Communication Disorders, 51*, 29–42. https://doi.org/10.1016/j.jcomdis.2014.06.004

Vail, P. L. (1993). *Emotion: The on off switch for learning.* Modern Learning Press.

Velleman, S. L. (2002). Phonotactic therapy. *Seminars in Speech and Language, 23*(1), 43–56.

Velleman, S. L. (2003). *Childhood apraxia of speech resource guide.* Thomson Delmar Learning.

Warren, S. F., Fey, M. E., & Yoder, P. J. (2007). Differential treatment intensity research: A missing link to creating optimally effective communication interventions. *Mental Retardation and Developmental Disabilities Research Reviews, 13*, 70–77. https://doi.org/10.1002/mrdd.20139

World Health Organization. (2007). *International classification of functioning, disability and health, children and youth version.* http://www.who.int/classifications/icf/en/

Zuk, J., Iuzzini-Seigel, J., Cabbage, K., Green, J. R., & Hogan, T. P. (2018). Poor speech perception is not a core deficit of childhood apraxia of speech: Preliminary findings. *Journal of Speech, Language, and Hearing Research, 61*, 583–592. https://doi.org/10.1044/2017_JSLHR-S-16-0106

APPENDIX 3–A

Communicative Functions and Corresponding Target Utterances Worksheet

Communicative Function	Targets to Elicit Communicative Function
Greeting/closing	
Requesting objects	
Requesting actions	
Requesting attention	
Rejecting	
Asking for information	
Requesting assistance	
Asking permission	
Disagreeing	
Protesting	
Sharing information	
Commenting	
Responding to questions	
Self-advocacy	

Target Utterance Selection Considerations Worksheet

TARGET UTTERANCE SELECTION CONSIDERATIONS WORKSHEET	
Name:	
Date:	Age:
Speech	
Language	
Environmental	
Interests	
Social	

Intervention Plan Worksheet Sample Form

Intervention Plan Worksheet		
Name:		Date:
Word Shape(s)	**Social/Pragmatic Goals**	**Vocabulary; Phrase Structures**
Phoneme(s) C and V		
Materials	**Activities**	

Evidence-Informed Decision-Making in Treatment of Childhood Apraxia of Speech

When making decisions about the most appropriate treatment programs for our clients, we look for evidence to help guide our treatment decision-making process. Figure 4–1 illustrates an evidence-based triangle that is commonly referred to in *evidence-based practice (EBP)*, along with the more recent evidence-based diamond model (Higginbotham & Satchidanand, 2019). *Evidence-informed decision-making (EIDM)* incorporates *internal evidence* into the decision-making process. Higginbotham and Satchidanand recommend considering these four components of EBP when making decisions about treatment: (a) **external evidence** (best available evidence from scientific literature); (b) **clinical expertise** and expert opinion; (c) **client/caregiver perspectives and preferences** based on cultural circumstances, priorities, and values; and (d) **internal evidence** (data collected by the treating clinician).

Looking at internal evidence is a relatively new, but critical, perspective in discussions of EIDM. Olswang and Bain (1994) suggest that careful data-keeping and analysis is an essential component of EIDM and that the clinician should consider the following when reviewing the data:

- if the client is responding to the treatment program
- if significant change is occurring
- if the treatment is responsible for the change
- how long specific therapy targets should be treated

There are a variety of ways to collect and analyze data depending on the child's goals. A more detailed discussion of data-keeping in treatment of childhood apraxia of speech (CAS) can be found in Chapter 12.

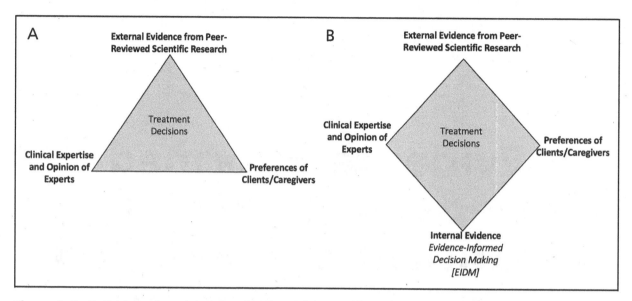

Figure 4–1. A. Evidence-based practice triangle model. **B.** Evidence-based practice diamond model. (Adapted from "From triangle to diamond: Recognizing and using data to inform our evidence-based practice," by J. Higginbotham and A. Satchidanand, *ASHA Journals Academy*, April 2019. Used with permission from Jeff Higginbotham.)

As more research in CAS treatment becomes available, the review of external evidence should be given substantial consideration when making treatment decisions. When analyzing external evidence, you will want to determine the *level of evidence* available for various treatment approaches you are considering. Table 4–1 provides a summary of levels of evidence for different types of research designs, with systematic reviews/meta-analysis of multiple randomized control trial (RCT) studies having the strongest evidence and expert opinion without research justification having the weakest evidence. Within those studies, even in RCTs, other factors such as number of participants, bias, and the criteria used to choose the participants need to be taken into consideration when determining the strength of the research. For each level of evidence, one example from peer-reviewed journals is listed.

Because children with CAS have difficulty with sensorimotor planning and programming, most treatment programs designed for children with CAS are sensorimotor-based treatment programs that incorporate at least some of the principles of motor learning described in Chapter 3 and emphasize some of these common features, including the following:

- providing frequent and intensive practice, particularly for children with moderate-to-severe CAS

- focusing on addressing sensorimotor planning and programming

- focusing on movement sequences, not individual phonemes, by addressing coarticulation in simple (e.g., CV, VC) to gradually more complex (e.g., CCVC, CVCVC) syllable shapes

- shaping those movement sequences into the most accurate productions possible

- building an expanding list of functional words and phrases

- gradually helping the child develop a complete repertoire of consonants and vowels

Table 4–1. Levels of Research Evidence

Level of Evidence	Description	Example in CAS Literature
1a	Meta-analysis of >1 randomized control trials	None available
1b	Single randomized control trial	Murray, E., McCabe, P., & Ballard, K. J. (2015). A randomized controlled trial for children with childhood apraxia of speech comparing Rapid Syllable Transition Treatment and the Nuffield Dyspraxia Programme (3rd ed.). *Journal of Speech, Language, and Hearing Research.* https://doi.org/10.1044/2015_JSLHR-S-13-0179
2	Well-designed control studies without randomization (e.g., case control or cohort study, single-case experimental design, quasiexperimental study)	McNeill, B. C., Gillon, G. T., & Dodd. B. (2009). Effectiveness of an integrated phonological awareness approach for children with childhood apraxia of speech (CAS). *Child Language Teaching and Therapy, 25,* 341–366. https://doi.org/10.1177/0265659009339823
3	Case reports, correlational	Lundeborg, I, & McAllister, A. (2007). Treatment with a combination of intraoral sensory stimulation and electropalatography in a child with severe developmental dyspraxia. *Logopedics Phoniatrics Vocology, 32,* 71–79. https://doi.org/10.1080/14015430600852035
4	Opinion of respected authorities, expert committee reports	American Speech-Language-Hearing Association. (2007). *Childhood apraxia of speech* [Technical report]. https://www.asha.org/policy/.

Note. Adapted from *Key steps in infusing evidence into CE course content: Step 2,* by American Speech-Language-Hearing Association, n.d., https://www.asha.org/ce/for-providers/ebcestep2/; *EBP and speech sound disorders: An anthology of 120 peer reviewed studies of phonological intervention 1978–2008* [Paper presentation], by E. Baker and S. McLeod, November 2008, American Speech-Language-Hearing Association Convention, Chicago, IL, United States; "Introduction," by A. L. Williams, S. McLeod, and R. J. McCauley, 2021, in *Interventions for speech sound disorders in children,* by A. L. Williams, S. McLeod, & R. J. McCauley (Eds.), pp. 1–22,). Copyright 2021 by Paul H. Brookes.

- providing multisensory cues for early success and fading these cues over time
- addressing prosody
- monitoring and treating the child's other communication needs (e.g., receptive and expressive language, social language, phonological awareness, fluency)

Some of the programs described in this chapter are more appropriate for younger children or children at the earlier stages of motor speech development, while other programs are more appropriate for older children who are working to refine their speech or acquire later-developing phonemes. It is important to keep in mind that no program is meant to be a "one-size-fits-all" program to use with all children with a CAS diagnosis. Rather, treatment decisions should be based on several factors, including the following:

- the individual child's profile across a variety of parameters (cognitive, linguistic, motor, social, emotional, attentional)
- the specific needs of the child
- the child's specific goals
- the child's changing needs over time
- the child's ability to tolerate more structured or drill-based treatment programs

By becoming familiar with a variety of evidence-based treatment programs, as well as the strength of the evidence that supports these programs, the clinician can begin to consider the current needs of each individual child and use the programs and strategies that best match the needs of the child at that point in time. A survey of clinicians who self-identified as having expertise in working with children with CAS found that many clinicians were unfamiliar with approaches for which there was strong supporting research evidence, such as Dynamic Temporal and Tactile Cueing (DTTC; Randazzo, 2019). In addition, some treatments for which there is no research evidence in CAS treatment were commonly used by many speech-language pathologists (SLPs) (e.g., nonspeech oral motor exercises; NSOMEs). These survey results reinforce the need for SLPs to become more familiar with the research evidence supporting treatment of CAS.

The process illustrated in Figure 4–2 can help provide guidance when you are determining what treatment program or evaluation method would be most effective for your clients. Rather

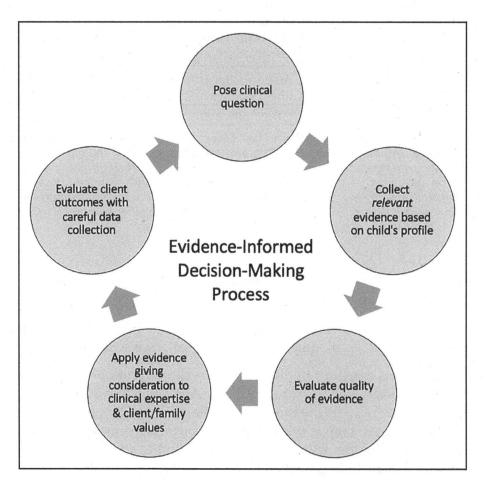

Figure 4–2. Evidence-informed decision-making process.

than fitting each child with a CAS diagnosis into a particular program, you can consider a child's specific profile and make an informed decision by critically evaluating the evidence that is most relevant for that child, applying the evidence, then evaluating the outcomes based on data collection. The cyclical process suggests that with each client, you may be posing the same or new questions again during the process of treatment depending on the child's response to treatment and/or new challenges that need to be addressed.

Several programs that offer research evidence to support their effectiveness are described in the next sections of this chapter. References are provided for each of the programs at the end of the chapter, so clinicians may read more detailed information about how to implement each of these programs. The programs described are listed in order of developmental appropriateness. That is, those programs appropriate for younger children or children with more limited speech are listed first, and those appropriate for children at later stages of speech and language development are listed later in the chapter. In addition, some programs that have preliminary evidence regarding their effectiveness in CAS treatment are listed toward the end of the chapter.

Prompts for Restructuring Oral Muscular Phonetic Targets

Prompts for Restructuring Oral Muscular Phonetic Targets (PROMPT) is a tactually grounded, sensorimotor, cognitive-linguistic intervention model grounded in Dynamic Systems theory, for the treatment of children (6 months and above) and adults with speech sound disorders. PROMPT, developed by Deborah Hayden (Chumpelik, 1984), is a motor-based approach that emphasizes the importance of focusing on functional language within the context of social interaction (Hayden, 2004a, 2004b). Therefore, target utterances would match or slightly exceed the child's motor, linguistic, cognitive, and social level of functioning (Hayden, 2006).

PROMPT assessment and treatment is unique among motor speech treatment approaches in that it requires the treating clinician to assess and treat the child across the physical-sensory, cognitive-linguistic, and social-emotional domains. Thus, target utterances and intervention activities would strive to balance and support (to the highest level possible for that child) the child's motor speech, cognitive-linguistic, and social-emotional levels of functioning. In addition, intervention activities would be functional and promote turn-taking and social interaction. The theoretical underpinnings of PROMPT align nicely with the World Health Organization's International Classification of Functioning, Disability, and Health: Children and Youth Version (ICF-CY) Activities and Participation component (World Health Organization, 2007).

During evaluation of the physical-sensory domain of the motor speech system, the PROMPT-trained clinician assesses the movements of the speech articulators and determines the coordination of these movements within speech synergies (i.e., jaw-lip, lip, tongue-jaw, tongue-lip, etc.). The Motor Speech Hierarchy (MSH; Figure 4–3) illustrates the sequential development of functional synergies of the motor speech subsystems, including breath support, control of phonation, mandible, lips, tongue, sequenced movements, and prosody. Further, the type and level of tactile/kinesthetic/proprioceptive (TKP) input required to facilitate flexible and refined development of speech motor control is determined. Evaluation and observation of the client's cognitive-linguistic skills and social/emotional skills provide further information that will influence the treatment goals and intervention activities.

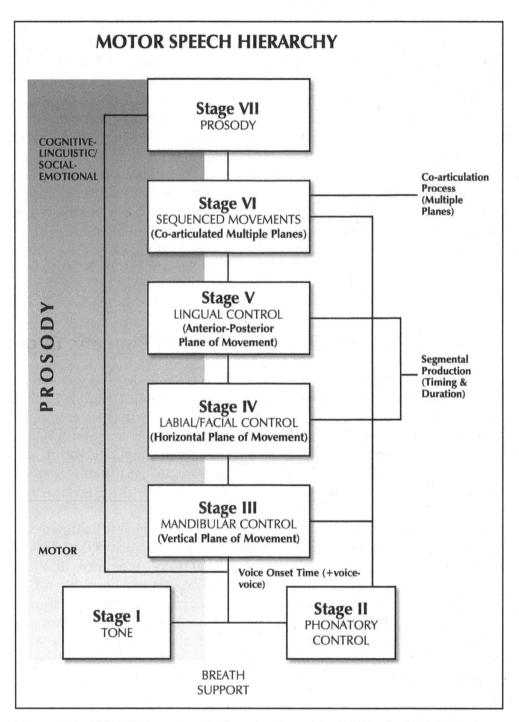

Figure 4–3. PROMPT Motor Speech Hierarchy. (Copyright 1994 by the PROMPT Institute. All rights reserved.)

To support motor speech development, the PROMPT-trained clinician provides "dynamic" TKP input to the mandibular-labial-facial-lingual subsystems (e.g., phonation, mandible, labial-facial, lingual). The TKP is delivered to develop and refine functional speech synergies for the stable and intelligible production of phonemes, words, and phrases. Tactile prompts are provided externally to

- the jaw (to facilitate the accurate degree of jaw opening, provide jaw stability, and reduce extraneous jaw excursions)

- the muscles of the face, including the cheeks and lips (to facilitate independent lip closure, rounding, and retraction)

- the tissue under the chin (mylohyoid) to facilitate placement, width, and timing of contraction in the tongue musculature)

- the throat to indicate and facilitate voicing

- the side of the nostril to indicate nasality for /m, n, ŋ/

Prompts are faded as the child develops greater control over the planning and execution of speech movements and coarticulation.

The TKP prompts used by a PROMPT-trained clinician are designed to support the following skills:

- *stabilization of the motor system* by always providing support to the head and providing support to the trunk and jaw when necessary

- *mobilization of the motor system* to facilitate articulatory movements and separation of jaw movement from tongue movement and jaw movement from lip movement

- *utilization of appropriate muscle movements* by providing sensory input to the articulatory muscles for accurate placement, timing, and coarticulation

- *reduction or inhibition of ineffective movements* to limit overretraction or overprotrusion of the lips and overextension of the jaw (Hayden, 2008)

The PROMPT Institute has created some online story-based materials that can be purchased through Boom Learning. Each story contains target utterances designed to facilitate development at different stages on the MSH. For example, at Stage III, the focus would be on mandibular control in the vertical plane. Target utterances may include *hop, hop on, on top, help mom, all done, papa, apple up*. At Stage IV, the focus would be on labial/facial control with target utterances such as *Oh no, Bo, Bo knows, uh oh, Mimi, you ate, eat food, feed me*.

Several studies have examined the effectiveness of PROMPT in children and adults with a variety of speech sound disorders. Two studies specifically examine the effectiveness of PROMPT in children with CAS. Dale and Hayden (2013) examined the efficacy of PROMPT in four children with CAS. The study examined the effectiveness of PROMPT overall and also compared the effectiveness of PROMPT when TKP cues were used versus when TKP cues were not used as part of PROMPT. The findings suggest that PROMPT was effective in improving production of trained and untrained targets and in facilitating greater speech intelligibility in children with CAS. Modest evidence was established that TKP cues add to the effectiveness of PROMPT in children with CAS. In another study, Kadis et al. (2014), used magnetic resonance imaging to examine cortical effects of PROMPT treatment in children with CAS. They found that eight of nine children receiving PROMPT intervention exhibited thinning of the left posterior superior temporal gyrus (Wernicke's area) following PROMPT treatment. PROMPT also has been effective in treatment of children with other types of speech sound disorders, including a recent RCT study showing that 10 weeks of twice-weekly "PROMPT intervention was associated with notable improvements in speech motor control, speech articulation, and word-level speech intelligibility" (Namasivayam et al., 2021, p. 613) but not on sentence-level speech intelligibility or functional communication for children with motor speech delay. The URL to the PROMPT website, where you can find more information about PROMPT, including available workshops, is listed in Table 4–4 (later in this chapter).

Nuffield Centre Dyspraxia Programme 3rd Edition (NDP3)

The Nuffield Centre Dyspraxia Programme 3rd Edition: NDP3 (Williams & Stephens, 2004) is a program designed to address the motor planning and programming challenges of children ages 3–7 years with CAS who exhibit a wide range of levels of severity. It can be adapted to children younger than 3 years and older than 7 years. NDP3 is a "bottom-up" approach to treatment that begins by helping children establish accurate motor programs for individual vowel and consonant phonemes and then systematically build from simple to increasingly complex syllable shapes, phrases, sentences, and connected speech. An integral feature of the NDP3 approach is the pictorial resources that accompany the treatment hierarchy. Throughout the program hierarchy, children are provided with pictorial and other specific cues and feedback to support the attainment of a full phoneme repertoire and increasingly complex phonotactic structures. The picture resources facilitate the child's ability to "lay down accurate phonological representations, which in turn support the development of accurate motor programs" (P. Williams, personal communication, April 2, 2015). The program supports the following skills:

- expansion of a child's phonetic inventory
- coordination of the connection of consonants and vowels into accurate CV and VC syllables (e.g., /aʊ/ + /t/ = out; /b/ + /i/ = bee) and increasingly complex syllable shapes (e.g., /s/ + wing = wing; /g/ + round = ground)
- gradually working to join syllables to form multisyllable words—blending worksheets are provided to facilitate transitioning between sounds and syllables using pictures to represent each unit (e.g., tie + knee = tiny; bay + bee = baby)
- facilitation of accurate syllable stress once bisyllable and multisyllable words are introduced
- development of phonological awareness skills to address blending and segmentation of syllables and phonemes

An important conceptual underpinning of NDP3 is the provision of frequent practice opportunities to support the development of accurate motor programs. The worksheets encourage repetitive practice at all levels. Although the program is built on a hierarchical framework that could be conceptualized as a "brick wall" (as illustrated in Figure 4–4), in which individual phonemes form the base and increasingly complex sequences are built on each subsequent layer, NDP3 also allows for, and encourages working at, more than one level within the same session. For example, a child may be working on (a) establishing accurate production of /ʃ/ in isolation, (b) incorporating well-established CVCV words in simple carrier phrases, and (c) producing voiceless plosives in final positions of CVC words in separate activities within a single session.

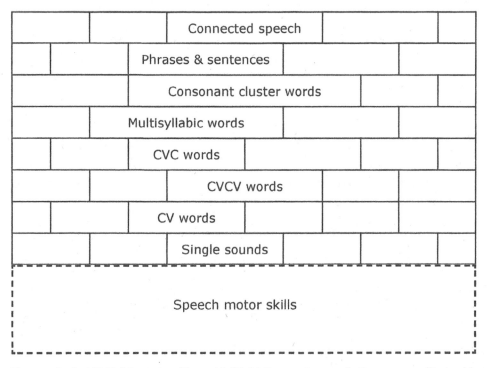

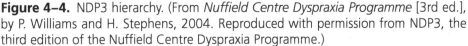

Figure 4–4. NDP3 hierarchy. (From *Nuffield Centre Dyspraxia Programme* [3rd ed.], by P. Williams and H. Stephens, 2004. Reproduced with permission from NDP3, the third edition of the Nuffield Centre Dyspraxia Programme.)

Phonological awareness skills are incorporated naturally throughout the stages of the program by including activities to address blending of syllables and phonemes, segmentation of syllables in CVCV and multisyllabic words, and segmentation of individual phonemes at the CVC level. Input training activities also can be incorporated into the program for children who struggle with auditory discrimination.

The RCT conducted by Murray et al. (2015) provides evidence that NDP3 is an effective program for facilitating articulatory accuracy, consistency, smooth articulatory transitions, and syllable stress assignment in children with CAS. A more recent RTC (McKechnie et al., 2020) looked at the impact of NDP3 treatment when provided using an Android tablet (rather than using the worksheets and picture cards from the program) under two conditions. In both conditions, children received four weekly, face-to-face sessions for 3 weeks. In the first condition, high-frequency knowledge of performance (KP) and knowledge of results (KR) feedback was provided during each session. In the second condition, high-frequency KP and KR feedback was provided one session per week, and only high-frequency KR feedback was provided during the other three sessions each week to simulate a dosage of one weekly session per week and three at-home practice sessions using a tablet-based treatment protocol. Both groups in the study demonstrated significant improvement in speech outcomes 4 months posttreatment, providing additional, preliminary evidence of the effectiveness of NDP3 in children with CAS. Sample worksheets are shown in Figures 4–5 through 4–10. Additional sample picture cards (which are brightly colored in the NDP3 program's materials) are shown in Figures 4–11 through 4–13. The URL to the NDP3 website, where you can find more information about NDP3, including available workshops and materials, is listed in Table 4–4.

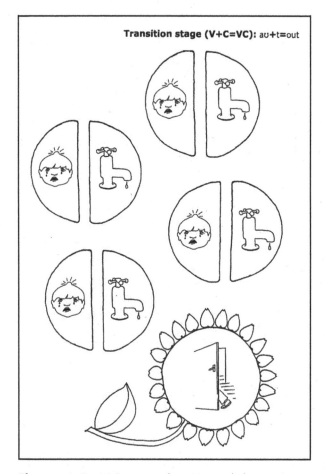

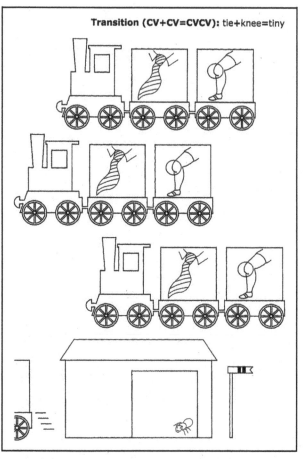

Figure 4–5. NDP3 sample VC worksheet. (From *Nuffield Centre Dyspraxia Programme* [3rd ed.], by P. Williams and H. Stephens, 2004. Reproduced with permission from NDP3, the third edition of the Nuffield Centre Dyspraxia Programme.)

Figure 4–6. NDP3 sample CVCV worksheet. (From *Nuffield Centre Dyspraxia Programme* [3rd ed.], by P. Williams and H. Stephens, 2004. Reproduced with permission from NDP3, the third edition of the Nuffield Centre Dyspraxia Programme.)

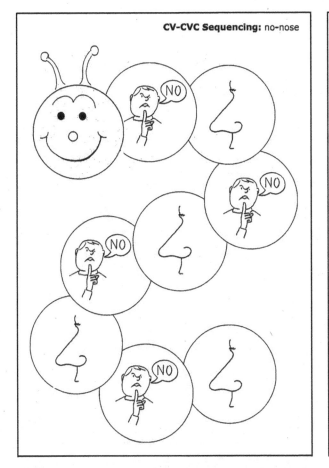

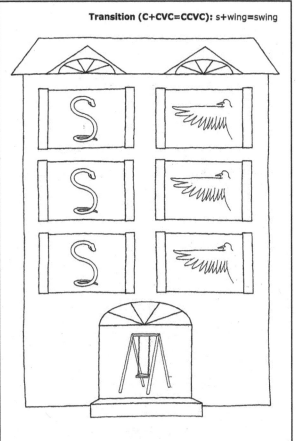

Figure 4–7. NDP3 sample CV-CVC sequencing worksheet. (From *Nuffield Centre Dyspraxia Programme* [3rd ed.], by P. Williams and H. Stephens, 2004. Reproduced with permission from NDP3, the third edition of the Nuffield Centre Dyspraxia Programme.)

Figure 4–8. NDP3 sample transition C+CVC=CCVC. (From *Nuffield Centre Dyspraxia Programme* [3rd ed.], by P. Williams and H. Stephens, 2004. Reproduced with permission from NDP3, the third edition of the Nuffield Centre Dyspraxia Programme.)

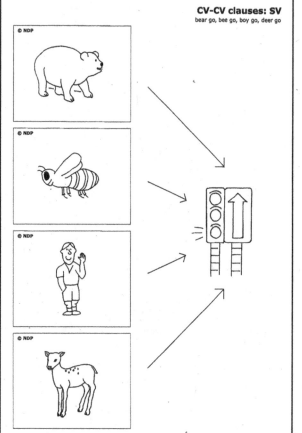

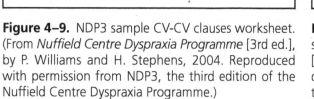

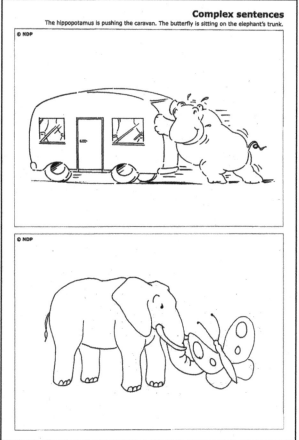

Figure 4–9. NDP3 sample CV-CV clauses worksheet. (From *Nuffield Centre Dyspraxia Programme* [3rd ed.], by P. Williams and H. Stephens, 2004. Reproduced with permission from NDP3, the third edition of the Nuffield Centre Dyspraxia Programme.)

Figure 4–10. NDP3 sample complex sentences worksheet. (From *Nuffield Centre Dyspraxia Programme* [3rd ed.], by P. Williams and H. Stephens, 2004. Reproduced with permission from NDP3, the third edition of the Nuffield Centre Dyspraxia Programme.)

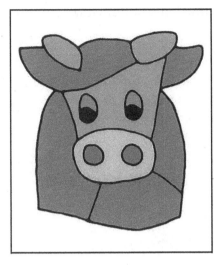

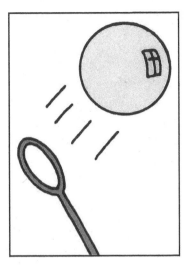

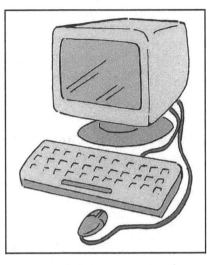

Figure 4–11. NDP3 "moo" picture card. (From *Nuffield Centre Dyspraxia Programme* [3rd ed.], by P. Williams and H. Stephens, 2004. Reproduced with permission from NDP3, the third edition of the Nuffield Centre Dyspraxia Programme.)

Figure 4–12. NDP3 "bubble" picture card. (From *Nuffield Centre Dyspraxia Programme* [3rd ed.], by P. Williams and H. Stephens, 2004. Reproduced with permission from NDP3, the third edition of the Nuffield Centre Dyspraxia Programme.)

Figure 4–13. NDP3 "computer" picture card. (From *Nuffield Centre Dyspraxia Programme* [3rd ed.], by P. Williams and H. Stephens, 2004. Reproduced with permission from NDP3, the third edition of the Nuffield Centre Dyspraxia Programme.)

Dynamic Temporal and Tactile Cueing

DTTC was developed by Edythe Strand and first described by Strand and Skinder (1999) as a form of integral stimulation (Rosenbek, 1985; Rosenbek et al., 1973). This integral stimulation approach was adapted by Strand for use with children with CAS. Children as young as 2 or 3 years of age may be appropriate candidates for DTTC, as long as they exhibit an intent to communicate and are able to attend to the clinician's face and to the task for short periods of time. According to Strand (2020), DTTC is intended for "children with more severe CAS and is not intended for long-term use" (p. 33). For children with severe CAS, the intended dosage for DTTC is at least three to four sessions per week.

DTTC is based on the assumption that the primary impairment in children with CAS is difficulty with planning and programming *movement gestures* for speech (Caruso & Strand, 1999; Davis et al., 1998): that is, they have difficulty with accurate coordination of articulatory movements to allow for a continuous flow of movement from one phoneme to another during production of an utterance.

Strand (2020) describes several core elements of DTTC:

- focusing on coarticulation of speech *movements* rather than focusing on individual phonemes
- helping the child develop a focus and intention to improve movement accuracy
- increasing proprioceptive awareness by maximizing proprioceptive input
- maximizing the number of practice trials of the target utterances during the session

- choosing carefully selected, meaningful, and functional utterances to practice during the sessions

- using auditory and visual modeling to facilitate imitation

- providing additional cues and strategies as needed (e.g., reducing rate of production, using simultaneous production, providing clear and specific feedback, gradually lengthening the time between the clinician's model and the child's production) in a dynamic manner to facilitate accurate productions at a normal rate and with varied prosody

- gradually fading cueing to facilitate greater independence in production of speech

When utilizing the DTTC approach, the following sequence is recommended:

1. Initially, the child produces an utterance immediately following the clinician's model while watching the clinician (direct imitation).

2. If the child is inaccurate, slow, or clumsy in production of the target, the clinician will produce the utterance with the client (simultaneous production), modeling the target utterance at a reduced rate (rate variations). Additional cues may be added as needed, such as a tactile cue or a phonetic placement cue, to support accurate production of the target utterance. As the child develops greater accuracy and maintains that accuracy at a normal rate and with varied prosody, the clinician begins to fade the cues and returns to direct imitation.

3. When the child can produce the utterance correctly (again, at normal rate and with varied prosody), the clinician slowly begins to increase the temporal interval between the model and the child's production (delayed imitation) of the target until the child can achieve accurate production of the target without a model. Figure 4–14 illustrates the sequence and dynamic nature of DTTC treatment beginning with Direct Imitation and transitioning to either Delayed Imitation (if the child's responses were accurate) or Simultaneous Production (if the child is incorrect) and working on specific target utterances until the child is able to produce the target utterances correctly spontaneously at a normal rate and with varied prosody.

The efficacy of DTTC for children with severe CAS has been demonstrated in three single-case experimental design studies: Strand and Debertine (2000), Strand et al. (2006), and Bass et al. (2008). Other research by Edeal and Gildersleeve-Neumann (2011), Maas et al. (2012), and Maas and Farinella (2012) examined various principles of motor learning using a DTTC framework in children with CAS. Maas et al. (2019) used a modified DTTC approach to examine practice amount and distribution. These studies are described in greater detail in Chapter 3. A more recent study by Lim et al. (2019) found training school teaching assistants in using DTTC with children with CAS was an effective means of providing treatment at school.

The following script in Box 4–1 encompasses approximately 5 minutes of a speech therapy session using DTTC. The script illustrates how cues can be delivered and faded in a dynamic manner following each of the child's responses.

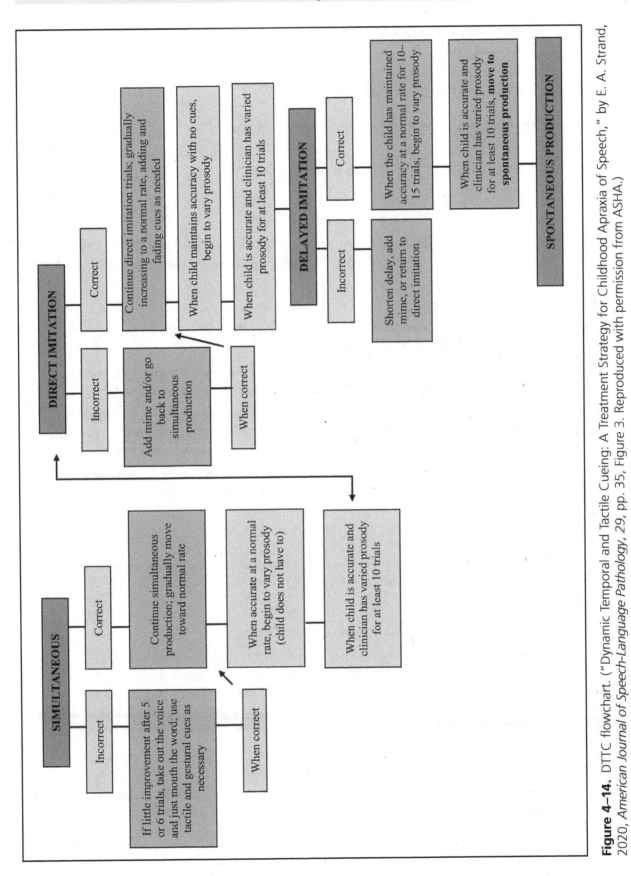

Figure 4–14. DTTC flowchart. ("Dynamic Temporal and Tactile Cueing: A Treatment Strategy for Childhood Apraxia of Speech," by E. A. Strand, 2020, *American Journal of Speech-Language Pathology, 29,* pp. 35, Figure 3. Reproduced with permission from ASHA.)

■ Box 4–1. Script Illustrating the Use of DTTC in Treatment

[The child is placing small cars at the top of a slide behind a gate. The child's job is to release the cars, and the clinician's job is to open the gate.]

Clinician: "Let me know when you're ready for the gate to *open*."

[*Open* is the target utterance. The clinician secures the child's visual attention prior to modeling the target word (Cueing technique: Direct imitation)]

Child: [oʊ ə]

Clinician: "*Open*." That's a tricky word. Let's say it together."

[The clinician secures the child's visual attention and produces the word at a reduced rate using prolonged vowels simultaneously with the child. (Cueing techniques: Rate reduction and simultaneous production)]

Clinician: "Open." **Child:** [oʊ.pə]

Clinician: "Let's try again. Be sure to finish the word. It has the 'nnn' noisy nose sound at the end. *Opennn.*" (Cueing techniques: Metaphor and model)

Clinician: "Let's say it together. Open." **Child:** [oʊ.pə] [The clinician produces the word along with the child. (Cueing techniques: Rate reduction and simultaneous production.)]

Clinician: "I didn't hear the 'nnn' noisy nose sound at the end." (Feedback: Knowledge of production. Cueing technique: Metaphor). "*Opennn.* Lift your tongue at the end." (Cueing techniques: Delayed imitation and phonetic placement cue) "Let me help you with this one."

[The clinician produces the word along with the child but adds a tactile prompt to cue the child for the final /n/. (Cueing techniques: Simultaneous production, rate variation, and tactile cue.)]

Clinician: "Open."

Child: [oʊ.pən]

Clinician: "Great! You used your noisy nose sound!" (Feedback: Knowledge of production) [The clinician opens the gate, and the car is released.] "Let's say it together again."

Clinician: "*Open, open open.*"

Child: [oʊ.pən, oʊ.pən, oʊ.pən] [The clinician opens the gate.]

Clinician: "Great! You remembered your noisy nose sound every time." (Feedback: Knowledge of production; Cueing technique: Metaphor) [After the child has produced the target utterance *open* correctly three to five times with the combined simultaneous production and tactile cueing (which was the required level of cueing to achieve a correct response), the clinician will begin to fade the cues systematically. On the next attempt, the clinician will omit the tactile cue but use simultaneous production.]

Clinician: "Here's another car. We need to . . . *open, open, open.*"

Child: [oʊ.pən, oʊ.pən, oʊ.pən] (Cueing technique: Simultaneous production with increased rate of production).

[The clinician opens the gate, releasing another car.]

Clinician: "That's perfect!" (Feedback: Knowledge of results).

■ **Box 4–1.** *continued*

[Because the child was able to produce the utterance with simultaneous production at a normal rate, the clinician will model the target word *open* just prior to the child producing the word.]

Clinician: "Let me know when you want the gate to *open*." (Cueing technique: Direct imitation)

Child: [oʊ.pən] [The child produces the word correctly but uses a slow rate of production.]

Clinician: "You did it!" (Feedback: Knowledge of results).

[To facilitate a normal rate of production, the clinician will mime the target word *open* as the child produces it to establish an increased rate. The clinician holds up three fingers to indicate the word should be produced three times and mimes "*open*" while the child produces it. (Cueing technique: Miming)

Child: [oʊ.pən, oʊ.pən, oʊ.pən]

Clinician: [The clinician opens the gate.] "Very nice!" (Feedback: Knowledge of results.) "We've got three more cars. Which one goes down the ramp next?"

Child: [The child points to the preferred car.]

Clinician: "Let me know when we should *open* the gate, okay?" (Cueing technique: Delayed imitation) [The clinician holds up three fingers to indicate three trials.]

Child: [oʊ.pən, oʊ.pə, oʊ.pə]

Clinician: "Try again. Be sure to put your 'nnn' noisy nose sound at the end of each word like this, *opennn*." (Feedback: Knowledge of results. Cueing techniques: Metaphor and direct imitation.)

Child: [oʊ.pən, oʊ.pən, oʊ.pən]

Clinician: [The clinician opens the gate.] "Correct! You remembered to lift your tongue at the end!" (Feedback: Knowledge of performance).

The preceding script illustrates several important concepts related to the DTTC model, including the following:

- The *level of cueing*, *frequency of feedback*, and *type of feedback* were varied after *each* of the child's responses.

- Initially the feedback was delivered after each response and later after a set of responses (*intermittent feedback*).

- Initially the feedback was delivered in the form of specific feedback (*KP*) and later as nonspecific feedback (*KR*).

- The child's rate of production was reduced to achieve initial success and then was increased as the child became more successful to facilitate generalization.

- A variety of cues were added as needed (simultaneous production, miming, direct imitation, phonetic placement, metaphors, and tactile cues; see Chapter 3 for descriptions of these cues) to establish initial success.

- Cues were faded as the child became more successful (simultaneous production to direct imitation to delayed imitation); see Chapter 3 and then added back again (delayed imitation to direct imitation) when the child's productions were inaccurate to support errorless learning.

The URLs to the Strand (2020) tutorial for DTTC as well as an in-depth, online course regarding Assessment and Treatment of CAS using DTTC from Child Apraxia Treatment (Once Upon a Time Foundation) are listed in Table 4–4.

Motor Speech Treatment Protocol

The Motor Speech Treatment Protocol (MSTP; Namasivayam et al., 2015) incorporates principles of motor learning (e.g., mass and distributed practice opportunities, feedback provided related to both KP and KR) in combination with multisensory cueing strategies (visual, auditory, tactile) and gradual manipulation of a delay between the clinician's model and the child's performance. The target utterances progress from simple to more complex and are "practiced in structured play activities using functional words and phrases that are meaningful to the child and family" (p. 533).

During MSTP sessions, the child's caregiver is present and is an active participant in the treatment process. After homework is reviewed, the targets are introduced to the child, followed by practice of the treatment targets in three or four more naturalistic activities (e.g., shared book reading, game, or craft). Throughout the sessions, the caregiver is provided with opportunities to practice treatment strategies that will support the child's speech practice at home.

Research by Namasivayam et al. (2015) investigated the effects of treatment dose frequency on 37 children with CAS undergoing MSTP intervention during a 10-week treatment block. The results of the study indicated that children receiving higher treatment dose frequency (2 times/week) had significantly better outcomes than children receiving lower treatment dose frequency (1 time/week) in articulation and functional communication. Although articulation and functional communication improved in the higher dose frequency group, neither group showed significant improvement in overall speech intelligibility at the single-word or sentence level after 10 weeks of treatment. It may be that children with CAS need more than a 10-week block of time to demonstrate improved overall intelligibility. In the Namasivayam et al. article, a fidelity checklist is included that provides supervising clinicians a structured way to determine if the treating clinician is adhering to the MSTP protocol. This fidelity checklist could be beneficial for use with other motor speech treatment programs.

Integrated Phonological Awareness Intervention

The Integrated Phonological Awareness (IPA) intervention was designed to facilitate improved speech and phonological awareness development in preschool and early elementary-age children with speech disorders who have accompanying phonological awareness challenges. According to McNeill and Gillon (2021), "words containing target speech sounds or patterns are used as stimuli during phonological awareness activities to strengthen phonological representations that drive speech production" (p. 111).

McNeill et al. (2009) and Hume et al. (2018) examined the effects of an IPA program to simultaneously address speech production, phonemic awareness, and letter-sound knowledge. An underlying assumption of the treatment was that strengthening phonological representations in children with CAS could facilitate improvements in speech production, phoneme awareness, and sound-letter association. Phonological awareness tasks included activities to strengthen sound-letter associations, blending, segmenting, and phoneme manipulation. The clinicians chose words for the phonological awareness activities that shared characteristics of the speech targets. For example, if the child was working on suppression of cluster reduction of /s/ initial clusters (e.g., stop, spot, stick), the child would practice production of /s/ clusters (to strengthen speech) and also work on blending and segmenting the individual sounds in these /s/ cluster targets (to strengthen phoneme awareness). The findings of these studies suggest that IPA facilitates improved phonological awareness and speech development in some children with CAS. Gillon and McNeill (2007) have provided a thorough online resource manual describing IPA and providing suggestions of activities for treatment, as well as a website to locate picture resources for IPA. The URLs for these information sources can be found in Table 4–4.

Rapid Syllable Transition (ReST) Treatment

ReST was designed to facilitate improvement in the following core features of CAS described by the American Speech-Language-Hearing Association (ASHA, 2007):

- phoneme accuracy and consistency
- appropriate lexical stress
- speed and fluidity of transitions from one syllable to the next

In the ReST model, these three features are referred to as "sounds," "beats," and "smoothness" (McCabe et al., 2020). To achieve these goals, ReST incorporates intensive practice (≥100 trials per session) in production of two- to three-syllable phonotactically permissible pseudo-words (e.g., CVCV /'ba.də/; CVCVCV /bə.'da.fi/) in single words and in carrier phrases (e.g., "I want a ['ba.də]." "Go to the [bə.'da.fi]"). By using pseudo-words, the learner is able "to practice motor planning and programming on word-like forms without interference from previously incorrectly learned plans" (Thomas et al., 2014, p. 2). Because of the nature of the program, ReST is recommended for children ages 4–13 years with mild-to-severe CAS who are able to sustain attention to structured tabletop work (McCabe et al., 2013). To determine if ReST is a good fit for a child, the authors have created a ReST Readiness Checklist with questions to help identify which children may benefit from this treatment. The URL for the Readiness Checklist can be found in Table 4–4. The online therapy manual provides a flowchart (as shown in Figure 4–15) to guide decisions about where to begin in treatment.

The online therapy manual and other materials and resources are available on the ReST website, and the URLs for those resources are listed in Table 4–4. Some of these resources include a list of polysyllabic words and sentences to use for assessments and/or follow-up probes, sample ReST cards and wordlists, and sample data sheets to transcribe the child's responses and identify if the sounds, beats, and smoothness were correct. When using the word lists from the website, keep in mind that the program is from Australia and, hence, when the

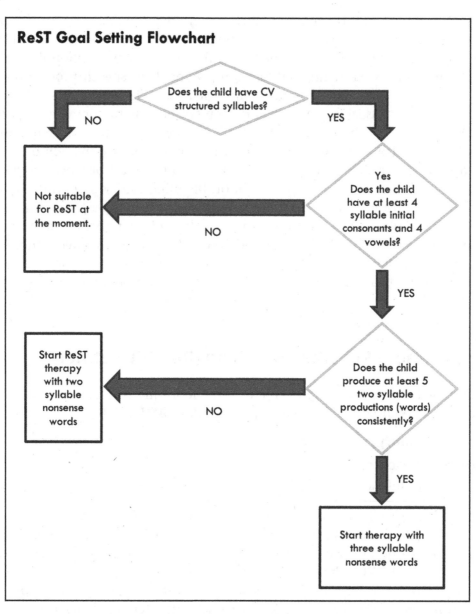

Figure 4–15. ReST goal setting flowchart. ("Clinical Manual for Rapid Syllable Transition Treatment [ReST]," by P. McCabe, E. Murray, D. Thomas, and P. Evans, 2017, p. 9. Reproduced with permission from Patricia McCabe.)

stimuli include vocalic /r/, it is not actually pronounced. For example, the word "farbakee" is actually pronounced as /ˈfɑ.bə.ki/. Instructions are provided on how to make your own stimuli for two- and three-syllable nonsense words. When creating your own nonsense word lists, you are choosing four consonants and three vowels plus a shwa. For two-syllable words, strong-weak and weak-strong (WS) stress patterns are used. For three-syllable words, strong-weak-weak (SWW) and weak-strong-weak (WSW) stress patterns are used. To keep track of the syllable you need to stress, it helps to write your stimuli in International Phonetic Alphabet with the stress marks. It is also helpful to remember that the unstressed syllable in the first or second syllable position will always be a schwa. In Table 4–2, examples of target words are listed for two-syllable nonsense words containing the consonant phonemes /f, d, b, k/ and the vowels /i, ɑ, oʊ, ə/; in Table 4–3, the same consonant and vowel phonemes are used in three-syllable nonsense words.

Various principles of motor learning (described in Chapter 3) guide the design of the ReST treatment protocol (Murray et al., 2012, 2015).

- **pre-practice** to ensure task understanding and allow the learner to experience accurate production of targets
- **practice variability** incorporating phonemes with varied place, manner, and voicing characteristics, as well as varied syllable stress patterns
- **a high number of production trials** completed each session, with the targets practiced in random order
- **feedback** provided as KP in the Pre-practice portion, and KR in the Practice portion of the session

This treatment protocol has shown positive results for supporting improvement in each of ASHA's specified core challenge areas for children with CAS (segmental accuracy/consistency, coarticulation, and prosody). An RCT was conducted comparing ReST and Nuffield Dyspraxia Programme 3rd Edition (NDP3; NDP3 was described earlier). The study found positive efficacy results for both programs (Murray et al., 2015).

The developers of the ReST program have created a clinical manual that can be accessed online (McCabe et al., 2017), as well as a tutorial describing the ReST program (McCabe et al., 2020). These materials provide detailed information about the ReST program, including how to determine if an individual is a good candidate for the program, how to develop treatment materials and target word lists for treatment, and how to track progress.

Table 4–2. Sample ReST Two-Syllable Stimuli

Strong-Weak	Weak-Strong
ˈki.də	kə.ˈdi
ˈboʊ.də	bə.ˈdoʊ
ˈfɑ.bə	fə.ˈbɑ
ˈdoʊ.fə	də.ˈfoʊ
ˈdi.kə	də.ˈki

Table 4–3. Sample ReST Three-Syllable Stimuli

Strong-Weak-Weak	Weak-Strong-Weak
ˈfɑ.bə.kə	fə.ˈbɑ.kə
ˈkɑ.bə.fi	kə.ˈbɑ.fi
ˈdi.fə.bə	də.ˈfi.bə
ˈboʊ.də.fə	bə.ˈdoʊ.fə
ˈkoʊ.fə.bi	kə.ˈfoʊ.bi

Visual Biofeedback

Children with CAS are believed to rely more than children with typical speech development on sensory feedback (the auditory signal following the child's speech production) as a result of poor *feedforward control*. Terband et al. (2009) suggest two possible causes of poor feedforward control: (a) reduced somatosensory awareness and (b) "an increased level of neural noise" (p. 1606).

Because children with CAS often have compromised sensory feedback of their speech production, which can impact knowing where their articulators are in space, it is helpful to augment therapy with visual feedback. Visual biofeedback techniques often utilize technology to provide feedback about accuracy of production of target utterances. A most basic form of visual biofeedback would be the use of a mirror so the child can see if the production is correct (e.g., reducing tongue protruding during production of /l/, facilitating upper teeth contact with the lower lip for /f/). Two types of technology, ultrasound biofeedback and electropalatography, are discussed here.

Ultrasound Biofeedback

Ultrasound biofeedback utilizes ultrasound technology to provide real-time visual feedback of the tongue to facilitate correct production of lingual sounds such as /r, s, l, k, tʃ/. During treatment, an ultrasound probe is placed beneath the chin in one of two directions depending on the view you want to achieve (sagittal or dorsal). The child can view tongue movement on a computer screen in real time during treatment. Descriptions and drawings of the tongue shape and position are provided for comparison of the child's production and the targeted production. For some older children with CAS who have persistent articulation errors, ultrasound biofeedback has been found to be effective in developing increased phoneme accuracy and improved overall speech intelligibility (Preston et al., 2013, 2017). Refer to Figure 4–16A and Figure 4–16B to see sagittal views of correct and incorrect productions of /r/. Figure 4–16C and Figure 4–16D illustrate coronal views of correct and incorrect /s/ production.

It should be noted that the use of visual biofeedback techniques, such as ultrasound biofeedback, should be implemented as part of a motor-based treatment approach when working with children with CAS. Thus, other principles of motor learning would be adhered to during treatment, such as a high number of production trials, careful selection of target utterances to challenge, without overtaxing the motor speech system, and incorporation of pre-practice to shape some accurate productions of the targeted phonemes prior to the practice phase of treatment.

Electropalatography

Electropalatography (EPG) is instrumentation that provides real-time visual feedback of tongue-to-palate contacts and lip closure contacts. An acrylic palate is created from a dental mold of the child's palate. The acrylic palate is covered with over 100 electrodes and is connected to a computer via a USB cable. Both the client and the clinician wear an acrylic palate, and each person's palatal contacts are represented on a split screen on a computer. The client attempts to achieve predetermined placement of the tongue for a specified phoneme by matching the visual display during production of the phoneme in isolation, words, phrases, and sentences. This technology is typically used for children from elementary school through adulthood who

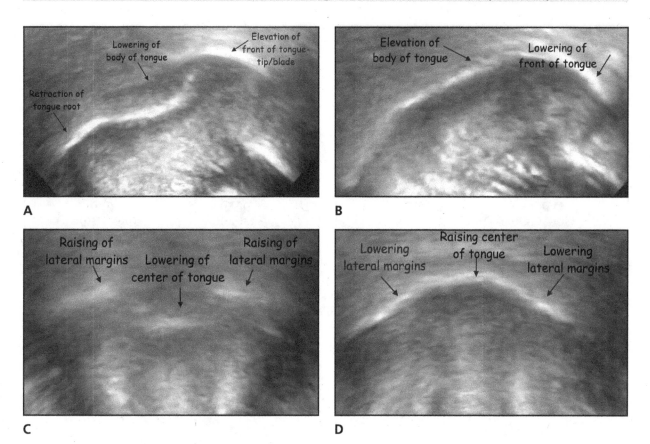

Figure 4–16. A. Ultrasound image sagittal view correct production of /ɚ/. **B.** Ultrasound image sagittal view incorrect production of /ɚ/. **C.** Ultrasound image coronal view correct production of /s/. **D.** Ultrasound image coronal view incorrect production of /s/.

have struggled to achieve certain lingual consonant phonemes or lip-to-lip contact phonemes with the ultimate goal being improvement of speech intelligibility. Lundeborg and McAllister (2007) provided evidence of improvement of articulation of persistent speech sound errors in children with CAS. The most frequently used EPG system on the market currently is the SmartPalate system by CompleteSpeech (more information about the SmartPalate can be found at https://completespeech.com/smartpalate/). Figure 4–17A shows a display of the tongue-to-palate contact for correct production of /ɚ/, whereas Figure 4–17B shows an incorrect production of /ɚ/. Figure 4–18A and 4–18B show displays of tongue-to-palate contact for correct and incorrect production of /k/, respectively. In Figure 4–18C, the child substitutes /t/ for /k/.

Treatments With Preliminary Evidence

Some treatments for CAS have some preliminary evidence of their effectiveness with children with CAS. Two of these programs are discussed next.

Babble Boot Camp

Typically, speech and language therapy is initiated after a child shows signs of a speech and/ or language delay. Children with classic galactosemia (CG) are known to be at high risk of

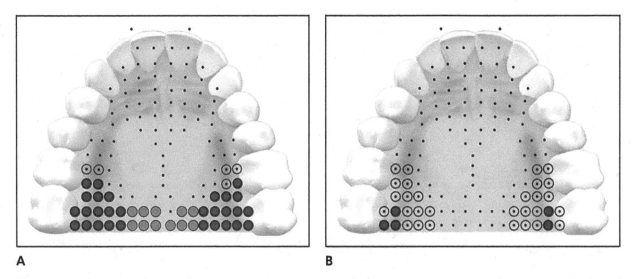

A

B

Figure 4–17. A. EPG display of tongue-to-palate contact for correct /ɑr/ using SmartPalate. **B.** EPG display of tongue-to-palate contact for incorrect /ɑr/ using SmartPalate.

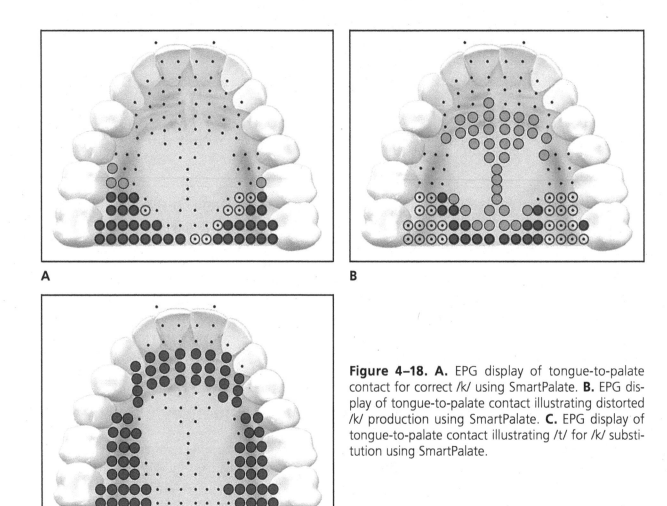

A

B

C

Figure 4–18. A. EPG display of tongue-to-palate contact for correct /k/ using SmartPalate. **B.** EPG display of tongue-to-palate contact illustrating distorted /k/ production using SmartPalate. **C.** EPG display of tongue-to-palate contact illustrating /t/ for /k/ substitution using SmartPalate.

speech and language disorders (Peter et al., 2021). Babble Boot Camp (BBC) was first developed for infants with CG because of their known risk for developing motor speech disorders. Rather than being a reactive treatment, BBC is a proactive intervention model, in which parents are coached via telepractice to implement prespeech, early speech, language stimulation, and language expansion activities in the home (Peter et al., 2021). During the program, parents are trained by an SLP to engage in 17 age-appropriate activities and routines throughout the day that foster communication skills (dyadic interactions, cooing and babbling, use of first words and sentences, vocabulary, and syntax development). These 17 activities and routines are described at the Open Science Framework entry for the BBC (https://osf.io/yzht4/). Examples of activities and routines include responding to baby's coos by imitating what the baby said or saying something back to the baby; showing the baby videos of other babies babbling; stimulating babble by modeling babbling and by gently moving the baby's lips while the baby is vocalizing; pairing gestures and words (e.g., raising arms up for "up" or motioning to "come here"); creating a photo communication book with pictures of important family and friends, favorite foods, and toys, and labeling the pictures in the book as the child looks at the book; and expanding the child's single words with two-word phrases (e.g., baby says, "ball," and parent says, "big ball"). A more detailed description of BBC can be found in Chapter 6.

Kaufman Speech to Language Protocol

The Kaufman Speech to Language Protocol (K-SLP) is a full treatment approach that addresses challenges of children with CAS in the areas of speech, language, and functional communication. K-SLP promotes shaping target words by simplifying motor plans of words/phrases while gradually shaping the child's speech toward accurate productions. The clinician examines the child's production of each target utterance and determines the best approximations to teach to give the child a way to produce the target words in a consistent way as intelligibly as possible. Simplifications of words are chosen based on normal phonological patterns younger children often use when learning speech and are gradually shaped into accurate productions of the target utterances. For example, when teaching the child to say, "bottle," the clinician may initially model "ba" (syllable deletion), then "baba" (reduplication), then "bah doe" (prevocalic voicing and liquid gliding), and eventually, "bottle." Target utterances selection is based on the phonemes and syllable shapes within the child's repertoire, as well as common nouns and functional vocabulary that are meaningful for the child (e.g., favorite foods and toys, names of family members and friends). While working on speech, language is simultaneously being addressed using functional phrases and carrier phrases/pivot phrases to support the child's expressive language development.

When implementing the K-SLP approach, the SLP evaluates where the child is in their motor speech development and figures out the best approximations to teach the child to give them a way to use language and understand the power of language while gradually working toward accurate production of target utterances. The approximations chosen should be the closest approximations of the target utterance the child is able to produce with a high level of accuracy when provided with cueing. Parents and caregivers are provided with coaching to help the child retain their skills in the natural environment and through play. Parents are encouraged to replace the child's typical patterns of communication (e.g., grunts, fussing) with the best possible productions of functional utterances based on common nouns and favorite things and to work on these to perfection. The theoretical underpinnings of K-SLP are based on the principles of applied behavior analysis. The program features the following teaching strategies:

- Define the target speech and language behaviors to be addressed through the process of evaluation.

- Determine target utterances based on assessment and parent/child input.

- Simplify the target utterances based on phonological patterns that would be typical of early speech development and are within the sensorimotor speech capacities of the child.

- Use multisensory cues to establish a high level of accuracy.

- Fade cues gradually to facilitate maintenance and generalization of the targets.

- Use highly preferred items to reinforce and motivate the child.

- Mix and vary the tasks to support generalization.

- Facilitate early language development by incorporating target utterances into functional phrases (I do, me too) and pivot phrases (e.g., put in ____, open ____, I got ___).

Several picture resources are available to support the SLP in the implementation of K-SLP. The K-SLP Treatment Kits include picture cards that are sorted by syllable shape complexity and phonetic features and can be used to provide a visual referent for children to move from imitation to labeling, and ultimately to requesting and commenting in the natural environment. Each picture in the kits has a picture on the front and suggested approximations on the back. The SLP is encouraged to try to facilitate the best production beginning with the correct production and simplifying as needed to reach the closest approximation possible for the child at the point in time. Other books and materials are available to practice functional phrases of increased length and complexity. The Sign to Talk Kits, created by Kasper and Kaufman, are used as resources to implement sign language as a bridge to vocal communication especially for those with autism spectrum disorder (ASD). Figure 4–19 shows examples of K-SLP Treatment Kit materials showing the front and backs of picture cards with the pictures on the front and the target utterances and suggested approximations on the back. The URL for videos and available materials for the K-SLP is found in Table 4–4.

Gomez et al. (2018) collected preliminary evidence on the use of K-SLP with two children and found some evidence for the effectiveness of this approach in children with CAS. Both children in the study improved their percentage phonemes correct on treated words, and the accuracy of these treated words was maintained during the maintenance phase of the study. One of the children in the study showed some generalization of gains to untrained words following the 3 weeks of intensive treatment (four sessions per week). Additional studies of K-SLP are forthcoming.

Online Resources for EBP Programs

A variety of resources can be found online to learn more about the EBP programs described in this chapter or to view the online materials. The URL for each resource is provided in Table 4–4.

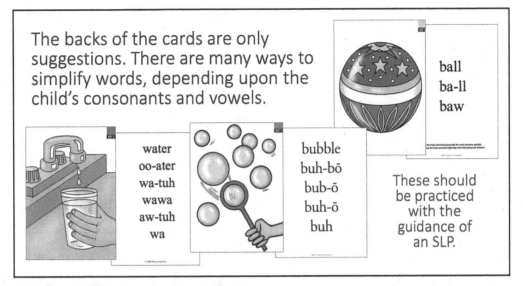

Figure 4–19. Sample K-SLP Treatment Kit 1 pictures. (N. Kaufman, 2013 Used with permission from Nancy Kaufman.)

Table 4–4. Online Resources to Learn More About Evidence-Based Programs for CAS

Program	Type of Resource	Website
Babble Boot Camp (BBC)	Open-source activities and routines of BBC	https://osf.io/sy3en/
BBC	Open-source article	https://pubs.asha.org/doi/full/10.1044/2021_AJSLP-21-00098?af=R
Dynamic Temporal and Tactile Cueing (DTTC)	Online course	https://www.childapraxiatreatment.org/diagnosis-and-treatment-of-cas-online-course/
DTTC	Tutorial article	https://pubs.asha.org/doi/pdf/10.1044/2019_AJSLP-19-0005
Integrated Phonological Awareness (IPA) Program	Manual	https://www.canterbury.ac.nz/media/documents/education-and-health/gail-gillon---phonological-awareness-resources/programmes/preschool/01-Integrated-Phonological-Awareness-Manual-Sept-07.pdf
IPA Program	Additional treatment resources/pictures	https://www.canterbury.ac.nz/education-and-health/research/phonological-awareness-resources/
Nuffield Dyspraxia Programme Third Edition (NDP3)	Website	http://www.ndp3.org

continues

Table 4–4. *continued*

Kaufman Speech to Language Protocol (K-SLP)	Website to locate online materials and webinars	https://www.northernspeech.com/search/author/Nancy_Kaufman/
Rapid Syllable Transition Treatment (ReST)	Program manual	https://rest.sydney.edu.au/wp-content/uploads/2019/07/rest-clinician-manual.pdf
ReST	Additional resources	https://rest.sydney.edu.au/resources/
ReST	Tutorial article	https://pubs.asha.org/doi/full/10.1044/2020_PERSP-19-00165

References

American Speech-Language-Hearing Association. (n.d.). *Key steps in infusing evidence into CE course content: Step 2.* https://www.asha.org/ce/for-providers/ebce step2/

American Speech-Language-Hearing Association. (2007). *Childhood apraxia of speech* [Technical report]. https://www.asha.org/policy/

Baas, B., Strand, E. A., Elmer, L., & Barbaresi, W. (2008). Treatment of severe childhood apraxia of speech in a 12-year-old male with CHARGE association. *Journal of Medical Speech-Language Pathology, 16,* 180–190. https://dx.doi.org/10.1002/14651858.CD006278.pub3

Baker, E., & McLeod, S. (2008, November). *EBP and speech sound disorders: An anthology of 120 peer reviewed studies of phonological intervention 1978–2008* [Paper presentation]. American Speech-Language-Hearing Association Convention, Chicago, IL, United States.

Caruso, A. J., & Strand, E. A. (1999). Motor speech disorders in children: Definitions, background, and a theoretical framework. In A. J. Caruso & E. A. Strand (Eds.), *Clinical management of motor speech disorders in children* (pp. 1–27). Thieme.

Chumpelik, D. A. (1984). The PROMPT system of therapy: Theoretical framework and applications for developmental apraxia of speech. *Seminars in Speech and Language, 5,* 139–155. https://doi.org/10.1055/s-0028-1085172

Dale, P. S., & Hayden, D. A. (2013). Treating speech subsystems in childhood apraxia of speech with tactual input: The PROMPT approach. *American Journal of Speech-Language Pathology, 22,* 644–661. https://doi.org/10.1044/1058-0360(2013/12-0055)

Davis, B. L., Jakielski, K. J., & Marquardt, T. P. (1998). Developmental apraxia of speech: Determiners of differential diagnosis. *Clinical Linguistics & Phonetics, 12,* 25–45. https://doi.org/10.3109/02699209808985211

Edeal, D. M., & Gildersleeve-Neumann, C. E. (2011). The importance of production frequency in therapy for childhood apraxia of speech. *American Journal of Speech-Language Pathology, 20,* 95–110. https://doi.org/10.1044/1058-0360(2011/09-0005)

Gillon, G. T., & McNeill, B. C. (2007). *Integrated phonological awareness: An intervention program for preschool children with speech-language impairment.* College of Education, University of Canterbury, New Zealand. https://www.canterbury.ac.nz/media/documents/education-and-health/gail-gillon---phonological-awareness-resources/programmes/preschool/01-Integrated-Phonological-Awareness-Manual-Sept-07.pdf

Gomez, M., McCabe, P., Jakielski, K., & Purcell, A. (2018). Treating childhood apraxia of speech with the Kaufman Speech to Language Protocol: A phase 1 pilot study. *Language, Speech, and Hearing Services in Schools, 49,* 524–536. https://doi.org/10.1044/2018_LSHSS-17-0100

Hayden, D. A. (2004a). P.R.O.M.P.T.: A tactually grounded treatment approach to speech production disorders. In I. Stockman (Ed.), *Movement and action in learning and development: Clinical implications for pervasive developmental disorders* (pp. 255–297). Elsevier-Academic Press.

Hayden, D. A. (2004b). *P.R.O.M.P.T. Prompts for restructuring oral muscular phonetic targets, introduction to technique: A manual.* PROMPT Institute.

Hayden, D. A. (2006). The PROMPT model: Use and application for children with mixed phonological-motor impairment. *Advances in Speech Pathology, 8,* 265–281. https://doi.org/10.1080/14417040600861094

Hayden, D. A. (2008). *P.R.O.M.P.T. Prompt for restructuring oral muscular phonetic targets, introduction to technique: A manual* (2nd ed.). PROMPT Institute.

Higginbotham, J., & Satchidanand, A. (2019). From triangle to diamond: Recognizing and using data to inform our evidence-based practice. *ASHA Journals Academy.* https://academy.pubs.asha.org/2019/04/from-triangle-to-diamond-recognizing-and-using-data-to-inform-our-evidence-based-practice/

Hume, S. B., Schwarz, I., & Hedrick, M. (2018). Preliminary investigation of the use of phonological awareness paired with production training in children with apraxia of speech. *Perspectives of the ASHA Special Interest Groups SIG 16, 3,* 38–52. https://doi.org/10.1044/persp3.SIG16.38

Kadis, D. S., Goshulak, D., Namasivayam, A., Pukonen, M., Kroll, R., De Nil, L. F., . . . Lerch, J. P. (2014). Cortical thickness in children receiving intensive therapy for idiopathic apraxia of speech. *Brain Topography, 27,* 240–247. https://doi.org/10.1007/s10548-013-0308-8

Kaufman, N. (2013). *Kaufman Speech to Language Protocol Treatment Kits 1 & 2 (Manual).* Nothern Speech Services.

Lim, J., McCabe, P., & Purcell, A. (2019). "Another tool in my toolbox": Training school teaching assistants to use dynamic temporal and tactile cueing with children with childhood apraxia of speech. *Child Language Teaching and Therapy, 3,* 241–256. https://doi.org/10.1177/0265659019874858

Lundeborg, I., & McAllister, A. (2007). Treatment with a combination of intra-oral sensory stimulation and electropalatography in a child with severe developmental dyspraxia. *Logopedics Phoniatrics Vocology, 32,* 71–79. https://doi.org/10.1080/14015430600852035

Maas, E., Butalla, C. E., & Farinella, K. A. (2012). Feedback frequency in treatment for childhood apraxia of speech. *American Journal of Speech-Language Pathology, 21,* 239–257. https://doi.org/10.1044/1058-0360(2012/11-0119)

Maas, E., & Farinella, K. A. (2012). Random versus blocked practice in treatment of childhood apraxia of speech. *Journal of Speech, Language, and Hearing Research, 55,* 561–578. https://doi.org/10.1044/1092-4388(2011/11-0120)

Maas, E., Gildersleeve-Neumann, C., Jakielski, K., Kovacs, N., Stoeckel, R., Vradelis, H., & Welsh, M. (2019). Bang for your buck: A single-case experimental design study of practice amount and distribution in treatment for childhood apraxia of speech.

Journal of Speech, Language, and Hearing Research, 62, 3160–3182. https://doi.org/10.1044/2019_JSLHR-S-18-0212

McCabe, P., Murray, E., Thomas, D. C., Bejjani, L., & Ballard, K. J. (2013, November). *A new evidence-based treatment for childhood apraxia of speech: ReST* [Paper presentation]. American Speech-Language-Hearing Association Annual Convention, Chicago, IL, United States.

McCabe, P., Murray, E., Thomas, D., & Evans, P. (2017). *Clinician manual for rapid syllable transition treatment.* The University of Sydney, Camperdown, Australia.

McCabe, P., Thomas, D. C., & Murray, E. (2020). Rapid syllable transition treatment—A treatment for childhood apraxia of speech and other pediatric motor speech disorders. *Perspectives of the ASHA Special Interest Groups, 5,* 821–830. https://doi.org/10.1044/2020_PERSP-19-00165

McKechnie, J., Ahmed, B., Gutierrez-Osuna, R., Murray, E., McCabe, P., & Ballard, K. J. (2020). The influence of type of feedback during tablet-based delivery of intensive treatment for childhood apraxia of speech. *Journal of Communication Disorders, 87,* 106026. https://doi.org/10.1016/j.jcomdis.2020.106026

McNeill, B. C., & Gillon, G. T. (2021). Integrated phonological awareness intervention. In A. L. Williams, S. McLeod, & R. J. McCauley (Eds.), *Interventions for speech sound disorders in children* (2nd ed.). Paul H. Brookes.

McNeill, B. C., Gillon, G. T., & Dodd. B. (2009). Effectiveness of an integrated phonological awareness approach for children with childhood apraxia of speech (CAS). *Child Language Teaching and Therapy, 25,* 341–366. https://doi.org/10.1177/0265659009339823

Murray, E., McCabe, P., & Ballard, K. J. (2012). A comparison of two treatments for childhood apraxia of speech: Methods and treatment protocol for a parallel group randomised control trial. *BMC Pediatrics, 12.* https://doi.org/10.1186/1471-2431-12-112

Murray, E., McCabe, P., & Ballard, K. J. (2015). A randomized controlled trial for children with childhood apraxia of speech comparing Rapid Syllable Transition Treatment and the Nuffield Dyspraxia Programme (3rd ed.). *Journal of Speech, Language, and Hearing Research.* https://doi.org/10.1044/2015_JSLHR-S-13-0179

Namasivayam, A. K., Huynh, A., Granata, F., Law, V., & van Lieshout, P. (2021). PROMPT intervention for children with severe speech motor delay: A randomized control trial. *Pediatric Research, 89,* 613–621. https://doi.org/10.1038/s41390-020-0924-4

Namasivayam, A. K., Pukonen, M., Goshulak, D., Hard, J., Rudzicz, F., Rietveld, T., . . . van Lieshout, P.

(2015). Treatment intensity and childhood apraxia of speech. *International Journal of Language and Communication Disorders, 50*, 1–18. https://doi.org/10.1111/1460-6984.12154

Olswang, L. B., & Bain, B. (1994). Data collection: Monitoring children's treatment progress. *American Journal of Speech-Language Pathology, 3*, 55–66. https://doi.org/10.1044/1058-0360.0303.55

Peter, B., Davis, J., Cotter, S., Belter, A., Williams, E., Stumpf, M., . . . Potter, N. (2021). Toward preventing speech and language disorders of known genetic origin: First post-intervention results of Babble Boot Camp in children with classic galactosemia. *American Journal of Speech-Language Pathology, 30*, 2616–2634. https://doi.org/10.1044/2021_AJSLP-21-00098

Preston, J. L., Brick, N., & Landi, N. (2013). Ultrasound biofeedback treatment for persisting childhood apraxia of speech. *American Journal of Speech-Language Pathology, 22*, 627–643. https://doi.org/10.1044/1058-0360(2013/12-0139)

Preston, J. L., Leece, M. C., McNamara, K., & Maas, E. (2017). Variable practice to enhance speech learning in ultrasound biofeedback treatment for childhood apraxia of speech: A single case experimental study. *American Journal of Speech-Language Pathology, 26*, 840–852. https://doi.org/10.1044/2017_AJSLP-16-0155

Randazzo, M. (2019). A survey of clinicians with specialization in childhood apraxia of speech. *American Journal of Speech-Language Pathology, 28*, 1659–1672. https://doi.org/10.1044/2019_AJSLP-19-0034

Rosenbek, J. (1985). Treating apraxia of speech. In D. Johns (Ed.), *Clinical management of neurogenic communicative disorders* (pp. 267–312). Little, Brown & Co.

Rosenbek, J., Lemme, M., Ahern, M., Harris, E., & Wertz, T. (1973). A treatment for apraxia of speech in adults. *Journal of Speech and Hearing Research, 26*, 231–249. https://doi.org/10.1044/jshd.3804.462

Strand, E. A. (2020). Dynamic temporal and tactile cueing: A treatment strategy for childhood apraxia of speech. *American Journal of Speech-Language Pathology, 29*, 30–48. https://doi.org/10.1044/2019_AJSLP-19-0005

Strand, E. A., & Debertine, P. (2000). The efficacy of integral stimulation intervention with developmental apraxia of speech. *Journal of Medical Speech-Language Pathology, 8*, 295–300.

Strand, E. A., & Skinder, A. (1999). Treatment of developmental apraxia of speech: Integral stimulation methods. In A. J. Caruso & E. A. Strand (Eds.), *Clinical management of motor speech disorders in children* (pp. 109–148). Thieme.

Strand, E. A., Stoeckel, R., & Baas, B. (2006). Treatment of severe childhood apraxia of speech: A treatment efficacy study. *Journal of Medical Speech-Language Pathology, 14*, 297–307.

Terband, H., Maassen, B., Guenther, F. H., & Brumberg, J. (2009). Computational neural modeling of speech motor control in childhood apraxia of speech (CAS). *Journal of Speech, Language, and Hearing Research, 52*, 1595–1609. https://doi.org/10.1044/1092-4388(2009/07-0283)

Thomas, D. C., McCabe, P., & Ballard, K. J. (2014). Rapid syllable transitions (ReST) treatment for childhood apraxia of speech: The effect of lower-dose frequency. *Journal of Communication Disorders, 51*, 29–42. https://doi.org/10.1016/j.jcomdis.2014.06.004

Williams, A. L., McLeod, S., & McCauley, R. J. (2021). Introduction. In A. L. Williams, S. McLeod, & R. J. McCauley (Eds.), *Interventions for speech sound disorders in children* (pp. 1–22). Paul H. Brookes.

Williams, P., & Stephens, H. (2004). *Nuffield Centre Dyspraxia Programme* (3rd ed.). The Miracle Factory.

World Health Organization. (2007). *International classification of functioning, disability and health: Children and youth version: ICF-CY.*

Establishing Vowel Accuracy and Natural Prosody

Although treatment programs for most children with speech sound disorders typically address improved production of consonant phonemes, most do not address the assessment and treatment of vowel production or prosody. Because challenges with vowels and prosody are features of the speech of children with childhood apraxia of speech (CAS), it is essential that treatment for children with CAS address vowels and prosody as well. These two topics are organized together in this chapter because of the strong interaction between vowels and prosody. Assessment and treatment of both vowels and prosody are discussed in this chapter.

Vowels

Vowels are considered the nucleus of the syllable because, with few exceptions, each syllable contains a vowel. Vowels are different from consonants in their production, as consonants are produced by creating a vocal tract obstruction or constriction (e.g., lip closure for /b/, tongue contacts alveolar ridge for /t/), while vowels are produced with limited vocal tract constriction. They are made distinct from one another by altering the shape of the tongue, which alters the shape of the oral and pharyngeal cavities (Jakielski & Gildersleeve-Neumann, 2018).

Causes and Ramifications of Vowel Challenges in CAS

Vowel errors, including vowel distortions and substitutions and limited vowel inventories are common in children with CAS (Davis et al., 1998; Rosenbek & Wertz, 1972). These errors can have a significant impact on overall speech intelligibility and prosody. Difficulty with *diphthongs* and *rhotic vowels* were consistent findings in children with CAS (Davis et al.,

2005; Pollock & Hall, 1991; Shriberg et al., 1997). Pollock and Hall also noted difficulty with contrasting tense and lax vowels in *neighboring vowel spaces* (vowels that are close to one another on the vowel quadrilateral), such as /i/ and /ɪ/, as well as backing of vowels (e.g., substituting /ɑ/ for /æ/).

What causes children with CAS to exhibit challenges with production of vowels? It is likely that limited vocal tract constriction during vowel production reduces the tactile/kinesthetic feedback the child receives, which contributes to the challenges of many children with CAS in accurate production of vowels. Vowel perception also may contribute to vowel production challenges. Maassen et al. (2003) reported that children with CAS performed more poorly than their same-age peers on tasks of vowel identification and discrimination. Difficulty with discrimination of the duration of vowels as well as the production of duration differences in children with CAS were observed by Ingram et al. (2019).

The ramifications of poor vowel production are significant. Kent and Rountrey (2020) describe how vowels carry acoustical information that provides the listener with a great deal of information about the vowel being produced, the neighboring consonants, age and gender of the speaker, prosodic content of the utterance (e.g., stress, rhythm, intonation), and the mood or intention of the speaker. Vowels also give information about the degree of formality of the speaker, as vowels often are shortened or omitted in less formal connected speech.

It is imperative for clinicians working with children with CAS to understand vowel production, develop strong skills in evaluating vowel accuracy, and learn methods to facilitate accurate production of vowels. This chapter provides an overview of vowel classification and production and addresses assessment and treatment of vowels.

Classification of Vowels

We divide vowels into three basic categories:

- monophthongs
- diphthongs
- rhotic diphthongs and triphthongs

A brief discussion of the phonemes, /w/ and /j/, sometimes referred to as *semivowels* because of their vowel-like quality, also is included in this chapter.

Monophthongs

Monophthongs, sometimes referred to as *pure vowels*, are vowels produced with a single articulatory movement. Figure 5–1 is a visual depiction of a *vowel quadrilateral*. This vowel quadrilateral illustrates both the vertical and horizontal movement of the tongue for production of each monophthong in the American English language. *Tongue height* refers to the vertical dimension or how close the tongue is from the roof of the mouth and is classified as high, mid, or low. *Tongue advancement* refers to the horizontal dimension or how far forward the tongue is positioned in the oral cavity and is classified as front, central, or back.

The phonetic symbols for the vowels on the vowel quadrilateral illustrate the "approximate" location of the tongue during production of each vowel. The positions are considered

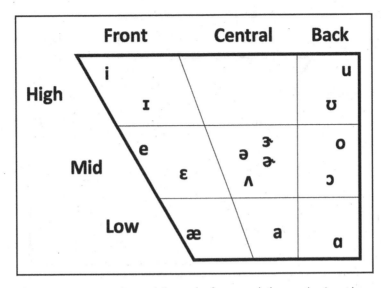

Figure 5–1. Vowel quadrilateral of monophthongs in American English.

approximate because vowel placement is influenced by neighboring consonants, such that a high front vowel is produced more anteriorly following an alveolar phoneme and slightly more posteriorly when it follows a velar phoneme. The highest and most anterior vowel /i/ as in *me, beat, need* is produced with the tongue close to the alveolar ridge. The lowest posterior vowel /ɑ/ as in *hot, mom, stop* is produced with the tongue low and back in the oral cavity. Try alternating between saying /i/ (long "e" sound) and /ɑ/ (short "o" sound) /i, ɑ, i, ɑ, i, ɑ/ several times and notice the movement of the tongue and jaw. Try again without moving the jaw and notice how the tongue retracts and lowers when shifting from /i/ to /ɑ/. These two phonemes are far from one another on the vowel quadrilateral, and the change in articulatory position is quite noticeable. Now try alternating between /i/ and /ɪ/ (short "i" sound as in *hit, sit, sick*) /i, ɪ, i, ɪ, i, ɪ/. Notice how the movement of the tongue is much more subtle, and imagine how making such subtle shifts would be challenging for a child with reduced somatosensory awareness. Keep this in mind later in the chapter when talking about evaluation and treatment of vowel productions.

Vowel Diphthongs

Vowel diphthongs bring two vowels together dynamically by rapidly gliding the tongue and lips from one articulatory position to another. The combining of the two vowels requires the speaker to change the shape of the vocal tract by shifting the position and shape of the tongue and shape of the lips during production quickly and fluidly enough that the production is perceived as a single vowel. There are three vowel diphthongs in the English language including /aɪ/ (b*ye*), /aʊ/ (n*ow*), and /ɔɪ/ (b*oy*). There are also two monophthong vowels, /e/ (h*ay*) and /o/ (n*o*), that sometimes, though not always, are produced as diphthongs /eɪ/ and /oʊ/. Because we recognize the vowels in /ne/ and /neɪ/ and those in /no/ and /noʊ/ as the same vowels, they are considered *allophones* (variations of the same phoneme). The vowel quadrilateral in Figure 5–2 illustrates the articulatory gliding for the diphthongs /aɪ/, /aʊ/, and /ɔɪ/, as well as the /eɪ/ and /oʊ/.

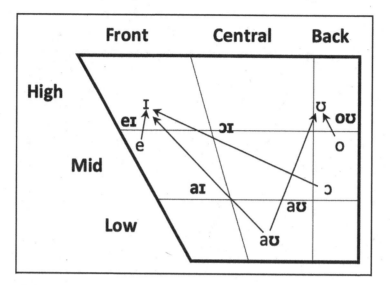

Figure 5–2. Quadrilateral of American English vowel diphthongs.

Rhotic Vowels

Rhotic vowels are vowels in which a rhotic /r/ functions as a vowel. The underlined vowels in the words *her, stir, blurt, butterfly, father,* and *perfect* are rhotic vowels. Rhotics occurring in a stressed syllable are transcribed as /ɝ/ and in an unstressed syllable as /ɚ/. *Rhotic diphthongs* result when a rhotic vowel follows a monophthong /ɪ, ɛ, ʊ, ɔ, ɑ/ to create the diphthongs /ɪɚ, ɛɚ, ʊɚ, ɔɚ, ɑɚ/. *Rhotic triphthongs* result when a rhotic vowel follows a diphthong /aɪ, aʊ, ɔɪ/ to create a triphthong /aɪɚ, aʊɚ, ɔɪɚ/. That is, the symbol /ɑ/, should be changed to /a/.

Phonetic symbols representing each monophthong, diphthong, and rhotic diphthong/triphthong are shown in Table 5–1 along with corresponding words containing each vowel.

Glides

The glides /w/ and /j/ ("y") sometimes are referred to as *semivowels* because they are "vowel-like" and produced in a similar manner to diphthongs or triphthongs. During production of /w/, the lips are rounded, and the tongue is positioned high and back (as in the vowel /ʊ/), then the tongue is quickly glided toward the vowel that follows (e.g., /ʊ/ + /i/ = we; /ʊ/ + /aʊ/ = wow). For /j/, the lips are retracted, and the tongue is positioned high and front (as in the vowel /ɪ/), and then the tongue glides toward the vowel that follows (e.g., /ɪ/ + /ɛs/ = yes; /ɪ/ + /u/ = you). Like diphthongs, there is limited vocal tract obstruction during production of glides. We know that diphthongs can be challenging for many children with CAS, so it follows that glides also would be challenging for some children with CAS.

Development of Vowels

The development of vowels in the first 4 years of life is driven, in part, by anatomy (Kent, 1992). The size and shape of the oral cavity are different in infants and young children than in adults, and these differences impact the attainment of vowels. Kent describes the devel-

Table 5–1. Vowel Classifications and Corresponding Sample Words

Vowel Type With Phonetic Symbol	Sample Words	Vowel Type With Phonetic Symbol	Sample Words
Pure Vowels		**Diphthongs**	
/i/	beet, sea, eat	/aɪ/	right, item, why
/ɪ/	hit, middle, in	/aʊ/	brown, out, now
/e/ or /eɪ/	paint, weigh, ate	/ɔɪ/	boil, enjoy, toys
/ɛ/	penny, went, end	**Rhotic Diphthongs and Triphthongs**	
/æ/	saddle, laugh, and	/ɪɚ/	steered, ear, pier
/u/	cool, losing, new	/ɛɚ/	stairs, air, dare
/ʊ/	shook, would, woman	/ʊɚ/	tour, pure, cure
/o/ or /oʊ/	boat, open, no	/ɔɚ/	forty, or, door
/ɔ/	shawl, lost, raw	/ɑɚ/	party, are, far
/ɑ/	hot, rocket, father	/aɪɚ/	fire, retired, liar
/ʌ/	come, up, above	/aʊɚ/	hour, flower, sour
/ə/	above, banana, zebra	/ɔɪɚ/	foyer, lawyer, employer
/ɝ/	bird, furnace, heard		
/ɚ/	mother, camper, refrigerator		

opment of vowels in children up to 4 years of age. In the first year of life, the most frequent vocalizations are low front, low back, and central vowel-like *vocants*. Though not true vowels, these vocants resemble /ɛ/, /æ/, /ɑ/, /ə/, and /ʌ/. Around age 1 year, children are beginning to produce more adult-like vowels. Stages of mastery of vowels in early development are summarized in Table 5–2. Although there is individual variation of vowel acquisition (Kent & Rountrey, 2020), this table can help guide target utterance selection when addressing vowels in treatment.

Assessment of Vowels

To adequately assess vowels, it is important for clinicians to develop strong skills in their own ability to discriminate vowels and recognize vowel deviations in children with whom they work. Gibbon (2013) describes the importance of strong vowel perception and production skills in clinicians who treat vowel disorders in children, as well as the ability to assess and analyze vowel production and generate appropriate goals and treatment strategies. Because vowel discrimination can be challenging, even for some seasoned clinicians, Strand and McCauley (2019) provide practice in assessment and analysis of vowel accuracy in the online companion videos that accompany the Dynamic Evaluation of Motor Speech Skills (DEMSS).

Table 5–2. Acquisition of Vowel Development in Children

Age	Vowels Acquired
By 1 year	Child produces low front, low back, and central vocants (similar to /ɛ/, /æ/, /ɑ/, /ə/, and /ʌ/)
By 2 years	Child has acquired tense corner vowels /i/, /u/, /ɑ/; tense back vowel /o/; and lax central vowels /ə/ and /ʌ/
By 3 years	Child adds lax mid vowels /ɛ/ and /ɔ/ and diphthongs /aɪ/, /ɔɪ/, and /aʊ/
By 4 years	Child adds lax front vowels /ɪ/ and /æ/, tense front vowel /e/, and lax back vowel /ʊ/
After 4 years	Rhotic vowels /ɝ/ and /ɚ/ emerge

Note. Based on "The Biology of Phonological Development," by R. D. Kent, 1992, in *Phonological development: Models, research, implications*, by C. A. Ferguson, L. Menn, and C. Stoel-Gammon (Ed.), pp. 65–90. Copyright 1992 by York Press.

It is important to assess vowels in a variety of phonetic contexts to capture the child's variability of productions in different contexts. Gibbon (2009) recommends assessing vowels by analyzing productions in a child's speech samples; the findings should be analyzed in several ways, including the following:

- *Independent analysis*—Make a list of each of the vowels the child can produce; this is the child's vowel inventory.

- *Relational analysis*—Identify the vowel errors including substitutions, distortions, and omissions. Describe how the child's vowel productions compare to the expected adult productions; this is the child's vowel error inventory.

- *Variability*—Describe any tendencies for increased errors in utterances of increased length or in more phonetically complex words. Note any token-to-token inconsistency, that is, vowels produced differently in repeated productions of utterances.

- *Facilitating contexts*—Describe "the effect of surrounding consonants on vowel accuracy" (p. 150) (e.g., /i/ may be more accurate if preceded or followed by an alveolar consonant; /u/ may be more accurate if preceded or followed by a velar consonant).

- *Stimulability testing*—Determine which vowels may be potential targets by checking on the vowels for which the child is stimulable.

Although transcription and analysis of vowels in connected speech samples may be ideal, for children who are highly unintelligible it may be difficult to identify the target words the child is saying. In this case, formal tests will be beneficial. Some formal motor speech assessments include analysis of vowel accuracy. Motor speech assessments that examine vowel accuracy are as follows. More detailed information about these tests can be found in Chapter 2.

- Dynamic Evaluation of Motor Speech Skills (DEMSS; 2019)

- Kaufman Speech Praxis Test for Children (KSPT; 1995)

- Verbal Motor Production Assessment for Children, Revised Edition (VMPAC-R; 2021)

Some articulation/phonology assessments also include a vowel examination portion, including Arizona Articulation Proficiency Scale, 4th ed. (AAPS-4; Fudala & Stegall, 2017) and the Diagnostic Evaluation of Articulation and Phonology: Articulation Assessment (DEAP; Dodd et al., 2006). These are described in greater detail in Chapter 2 on assessment.

Facilitating Accurate Production of Vowels

When working with children with CAS, close attention to vowel production is essential. Gibbon and Mackenzie Beck (2002) suggest that to determine the proper approach to treatment of disordered vowels, an identification of the *cause(s)* of the vowel disorder needs to occur. Gibbon and Beck describe three possible factors influencing vowel production errors in children with articulation disorders:

- auditory perceptual challenges (related to hearing loss or significant auditory discrimination difficulties)
- cognitive/linguistic challenges (related to phonological disorders)
- motor/articulatory challenges (related to CAS)

Because CAS implies challenges with motor planning and programming, motor-based treatment approaches would be applicable for addressing the needs of children with distorted vowels and reduced vowel inventories. Motor-based treatment approaches should incorporate multisensory cueing, attention to rate, and careful selection of target utterances. The findings by Maassen et al. (2003) and Ingram et al. (2019) that children with CAS had significantly greater difficulty with vowel identification and discrimination suggest that a combined auditory/motor approach to vowel treatment may be beneficial for at least some children with CAS. Following are suggestions for facilitating accurate vowel production in treatment.

Address Vowels Early in the Process of Treatment

Speech-language pathologists (SLPs) working with children with developmental articulation disorders and phonological disorders are not accustomed to giving much consideration to vowels because the challenges for these children tend to occur in the production of the consonant phonemes. Given the impact of correct vowel production on speech intelligibility, however, it is important to work on accurate vowel production right from the start. For children struggling to connect consonants and vowels to form CV or VC syllables, begin by working on increasing vocalizations and sound play. As children begin to imitate, you can work on meaningful vowels, such as /i, e, a, ɔ, ʌ, o, u, aʊ/ in isolation before moving quickly to CV and VC syllables. Table 5–3 provides recommendations for addressing these isolated vowels in meaningful contexts.

The Nuffield Centre Dyspraxia Programme, Third Edition (NDP3), provides pictures that represent each phoneme, including vowels (Williams & Stephens, 2010). Examples include a monkey for /ʊ/, a fish for /o/, a windy cloud for /u/, and a mouse for /i/. NDP3 provides practice at the isolated phoneme level for children who struggle to combine consonants and vowels before moving to production of alternating sequences such as /i, u, i, u, i, u/ and then to CV and VC words.

Table 5–3. Isolated Vowels Practice Activities

Target Vowel	Recommended Activity

/i/	• Isolated /i/
	  • Child produces the /i/ vowels while singing **E-I-E-I-O** in the Old MacDonald song at a reduced rate.
	  • Produce prolonged /i/ with pitch fluctuations while making emergency vehicle noises during car play activities.
	• Repeated /i i i i/
	  • Produce repeated /i i i i/ while pretending to be a monkey.

/e/	• Produce prolonged /e/ as a sound of cheer during "car race" or other activities. • Produce /e/ to name the letter "a."

/ɑ/	• Isolated /ɑ/
	  • Produce /ɑ/ after giving the dolls drinks of milk.
	  • Produce /ɑ/ while "checking" the puppets during doctor or dentist play activity.
	  • Produce /ɑ/ after smelling the flowers you planted in your pretend garden.
	• Repeated /ɑ ɑ ɑ ɑ ɑ ɑ ɑ ɑ ɑ/
	  • Sing *If All the Raindrops* song

/ɔ/	• Produce prolonged /ɔ/ to denote.
	  • Sympathy for an animal or doll that gets "hurt"
	  • Something is "cute" (e.g., baby animals).
	  • Disappointment about an event (e.g., a car did not make it all the way around a track)

/ʌ/	• Produce /ʌ/ for "uh oh" when crashing cars, pretending toy animals get "hurt," etc. • Produce /ʌ/ while pretending to exert a great deal of effort (e.g., climbing up a mountain, banging a hammer while building a house).
/o/	• Child produces the /o/ vowel while singing E-I-E-I-**O** in the *Old MacDonald* song at a significantly reduced rate. • Child produces /o/ after the therapist produces /ʌ/ for "uh oh" when crashing cars, pretending toy animals get "hurt," etc.
/u/	• Produce prolonged /u/ while pretending to be ghosts. • Produce /u/ to denote something that smells bad (e.g., skunk).
/aʊ/	• Produce /aʊ/ when the toy animals or dolls get "hurt" or as a funny sound when something falls or crashes.

Choose Target Vowels Based on Stimulability and Normal Vowel Development

When making treatment decisions about target utterance selection, consider the child's stimulability for specific vowels, as well as what we know about normal development of vowels (referenced earlier in this chapter in Table 5–2). The vowel /ʌ/ is a good choice for early vowel practice. The vowels /i, u, o, ɑ/ also are early to develop and provide acoustic and motoric contrasts, as well as distinctive lip shapes, making them easier for children to learn. Because the vowels /i, u, o, ɑ/ are tense vowels, they can be taught in both *closed syllables* (those ending in a consonant sound) and *open syllables* (those ending in a vowel sound), so are excellent choices for teaching words with simple CV or CVCV syllable shapes such as *me, do, go, mommy,* and *dada.*

Use Monophthongs to Facilitate Production of Diphthongs and Semivowels (Glides)

Many words common in young children's vocabularies (e.g., hi, my, boy, toy, cow, wow, whee, you) contain diphthongs and glides. Like the early developing vowels described earlier, diphthongs can be produced in closed or open syllables, so target words with diphthongs can be practiced in CV shapes, making them good choices for early target utterances. When a child has learned early vowels, such as /i, ɑ, o, u/, begin working to elicit simple CV words with diphthongs and glides. Model the target words using a slower rate, and exaggerate the gliding manner between the two vowel elements. You can provide multisensory cues by using direct models or simultaneous productions, tactile cueing, phoneme placement cues, and hand gestures to facilitate accurate vowel production. Reduced rate during the early stages of learning also helps increase proprioceptive awareness, making the phonemes more salient for the learner. Once established, move right into functional phrases (e.g., *Hi mom, I do, oh wow, my toy*).

Facilitate Flexibility in Coarticulation Early in Treatment

Children with CAS often demonstrate contextual limitations in phoneme sequencing. A child may be able to produce /o/ but only in a small number of phonetic contexts (e.g., no, go). Therefore, it is important to gradually begin to pair vowels with a wider range of consonants. First choose words with facilitating contexts to reinforce accurate vowel production, then try to increase flexibility by choosing consonants with varied place, manner, and voicing features (e.g., dough, bow, mow, show). Likewise, when a child has achieved production of a specific consonant but only is able to produce the consonant in a small number of vowel contexts (e.g., tea), gradually try to expand the child's flexibility by choosing other vowels with varied tongue height, tongue advancement, and lip shaping (e.g., two, toe, tie, toy).

Picture folders and mini-books are excellent resources for addressing flexible articulatory control of early syllable shapes and can be easily individualized for the needs of specific clients. Velleman (2003) recommends working on CV syllables during warm-up activities to expand coarticulatory flexibility using a "ba-ba" book or flip-book. These resources are described in the following sections.

Picture Folders

Picture folders provide children with opportunities to work on increased coarticulatory flexibility by practicing CV or VC syllables containing varied vowel and consonant phonemes during speech warm-up activities. Figures 5–3 and 5–4 illustrate sample CV picture folders. Picture folders are constructed using a piece of cardboard or a file folder with Velcro buttons to allow for flexibility in selecting and changing the picture targets. Pictures may be sorted in a variety of ways. In

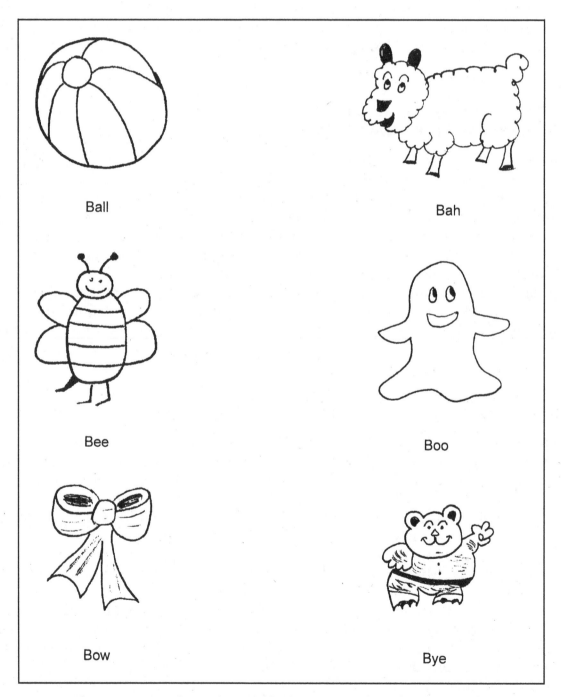

Figure 5–3. Sample CV picture folder for practicing /b/ with varied vowels.

Figure 5–3, the pictures provide repetitive practice of the consonant /b/ with varied vowels. The pictures in Figure 5–4 provide repetitive practice of the /i/ vowel with varied consonants.

Mini Picture Books

Small picture books are another resource for addressing early flexibility in coarticulation of CV or VC words. Separate books can be created for each targeted vowel with varied consonants or

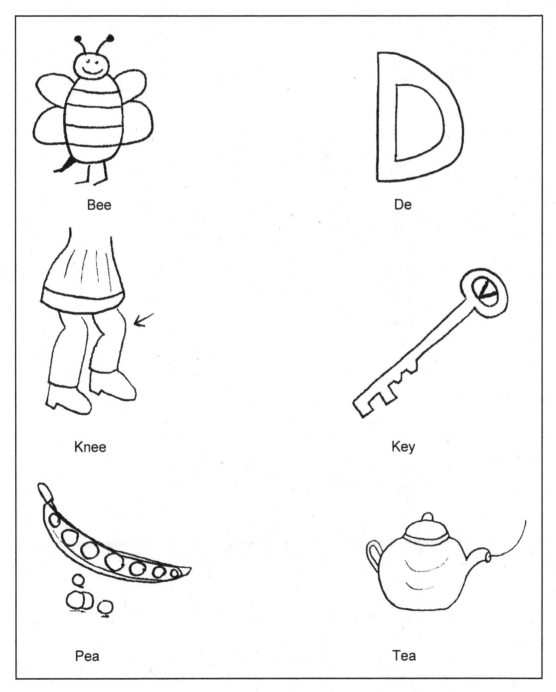

Bee

De

Knee

Key

Pea

Tea

Figure 5–4. Sample CV picture folder for practicing the vowel /i/ with varied consonants.

each targeted consonant with varied vowels. The target words from the books can be practiced during treatment sessions and can be sent home for additional practice. A picture book for the vowel /u/ may include these target words: *Pooh, boo, moo, two, zoo, shoe, who, goo, new,* and *you,* while a picture book for the consonant /m/ may include these target words: *ma, me, moo, mow, more, my, May, aim,* and *em.*

Syllable Flip-Books

Syllable flip-books provide practice in production of CV words. The words are organized in groups of specific consonant phonemes plus a variety of vowels that, when combined, will form picturable words (e.g., bee, bay, ball, bah [sheep], bow [hair bow], boo [ghost], boy, bye, bow [to an audience]). As Figure 5–5 and 5–6 illustrate, multiples of the same pictures are set side by side. In that way, each syllable could be practiced repetitively in two or three picture

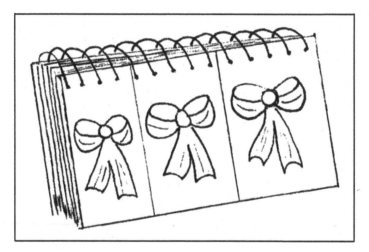

Figure 5–5. Example of repetitive syllable practice using a CV syllable flip-book.

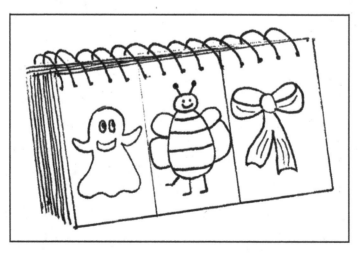

Figure 5–6. Example of varied syllable practice using a CV syllable flip-book.

sets (e.g., *da, da; bah, bah, bah*), or the pages could be flipped so different words could be practiced alternately using the same consonants (e.g., *ma, me; bah, bow, boo*) or varied consonants (e.g., *bah, no, me*). Syllable flip-books can be homemade and sent home with the child for practice. A commercially produced syllable flip-book, Word FLiPS for Learning Intelligible Production of Speech is available through Super Duper Publications.

These types of flip-books provide opportunities to combine syllables for work on CVCV or CVCVCV words by combining pictures to form true words, such as

- reduplicated CVCV (e.g., boo + boo for *boo-boo*)
- consonant harmonized CVCV (e.g., bah + bee for *Bobby*)
- vowel harmonized CVCV (e.g., tea + knee for *teeny*)
- variegated CVCV (e.g., moo + V for *movie*)
- CVCVCV (e.g., toe + May + toe for *tomato*)

To create your own syllable flip-book, use a rectangular spiral blank page notebook approximately 5.5″ × 8.5″, and cut each page so there are three separate flip pages per page. Affix a CV picture to each page, three of the same pictures in a row (e.g., bah, bah, bah; bow, bow, bow; bee, bee, bee). In this way, the child can practice three of the same CV syllables in a row or pages can be flipped to practice varied syllable combinations of either meaningful words (e.g., bow + knee = bony) or nonsense words (e.g., bah + bow + bee). Possible words for the syllable flip-books, picture folders, and mini picture books are listed next.

Word Lists for Picture Folders, Mini Picture Books, and Syllable Flip-Books

Box 5–1 lists sample picturable CV words that can be used when creating picture folders, mini picture books, or flip-books. By combining two CV words, CVCV words and phrases can be created.

Multisensory Cueing and Feedback for Increased Vowel Accuracy

The use of multisensory cues, as described in Chapter 3, is essential for achieving success in CAS treatment. The use of auditory, visual, tactile, and metacognitive cues in treatment of vowels is described next.

Tips for Auditory and Visual Cueing

- *Positioning.* Sit facing the child, so the child has a clear view of your oral-facial structures. Try to position yourself at the same eye level as the child.

- *Rate.* During early practice, model the target utterances using a slower rate and prolong the target vowels to bring the vowels to the attention of the child. Gradually increase the rate to normal as the child's articulatory accuracy increases.

- *Establishing initial articulatory configurations.* Strand (2020) recommends modeling and helping the child assume the initial articulatory configuration (correct lip shaping and jaw height) for the target word with attention to the upcoming vowel. For example, if the target is *me*, the lips would be closed and slightly retracted, and the jaw would be

■ **Box 5–1.** Sample Target Words for Picture Folders, Mini Picture Books, and Syllable Flip-Books

---

CV Words

/b/ bee, bah, boo, bow (for hair or gift), ball (w/out regard to final /l/), bay, bye, bow (to an audience), boy, burr, bear

/p/ pea, pa, Pooh, paw, pay, pie, pow, purr

/m/ me, ma, moo, mow, May, my, meow, more

/w/ whee, wah (crying baby), whoa, way, woo, why, wow, whir

/d/ D, da, dough, day, deer, door

/t/ tea, two, toe, tie, toy

/n/ knee, new, no, neigh, nigh

/l/ la, low, lay

/s/ see, sew, saw, say, sir

/z/ Z, zoo

/f/ fee, fo, foo, fi, fur

/v/ V

/ʃ/ she, shoe, show, shy

/tʃ/ chew, chai, chow

/dʒ/ G, jaw, J

/j/ you, yay, yeah

/r/ rah, row, rye

/k/ key, K, cow, caw, coo

/g/ goo, go, guy, grr (growling bear)

/h/ he, ha, who, hoe, hay, hi, how, her

CVCV Words and Phrases

Words: boo-boo, bye-bye, bah bah, papa, mama, moo moo, dada, tutu, no no, neigh neigh, nigh nigh, la la, ha ha, ho ho, hoo hoo, Bobby, baby, paper, mommy, daddy (da + D), saucer, see-saw genie, kiwi, teeny, teepee, before, below, body, bony, cargo, gopher, hero, honey, lady, lazy, movie, maybe, navy, puma, potty, tiny, today, shiny, wavy, wiper, whiny, zero, cowboy

Phrases: bye bear, bye boy, car key, fee fi, fi fo, guy go, my ma, hi guy, bye guy, see me, my guy, hi boy, hi ma, hi da, hi bear, hi sir, hi cow, bye ma, bye da, bye sir, bye cow, see cow, see ball, my dough, my knee, my ball, my shoe, tie shoe, tie bow, no way, no sir, no bear, no cow, ma go, da go, we go, cow go

---

high. For *boo*, the lips would be closed and rounded, and the jaw would be high. If you are not sure what the initial articulatory configuration would be, simply say the target utterance aloud to yourself while looking at yourself in the mirror or place your fingers near your lips and jaw to see and feel the movement gestures. Notice how the shaping of the lips and the height of the jaw often are more dependent on the shape of the upcoming vowel than the initial consonant phoneme.

- *Natural modeling.* Be sure to model vowels accurately. Say the target words aloud to yourself in a natural way, and determine if any vowels are shortened or produced as a schwa /ə/ (e.g., *believe* would be modeled as [bə.'liv], not [bi.'liv] and *button* would be modeled as ['bʌ.r̩n], with a syllabic /n̩/, not ['bʌ.tɪn]).

- *Stressed syllables in multisyllabic words.* When working on words with two or more syllables, Gibbon and Mackenzie Beck (2002) recommend choosing words in which the target vowel is in a stressed syllable of the word, as the acoustic and proprioceptive information will be stronger. For example, in the words *table*, *mistake*, and *vacation*, the /e/ vowel is in the stressed syllable, whereas the /e/ in *Monday* is in the weak syllable and would be a less desirable target for addressing /e/. As the child's productions improve, targets also can include words with the target vowels in unstressed syllables.

- *Auditory feedback.* Provide auditory feedback by recording and replaying the child's productions so the child can make judgments about accuracy of production. Portable phones and tablet computers offer reasonably good microphones to record and play back the child's productions.

- *Visual feedback.*

  - Use mirrors when facilitating lip rounding or retraction or when helping establish appropriate jaw height.

  - VowelViz and VowelViz Pro are apps by CompleteSpeech (https://completespeech. com/vowelvizpro/) that allow the child to see where their vowel production falls on a vowel quadrilateral. VowelViz ($19.99) provides a basic vowel quadrilateral display, including /ɚ/, and VowelViz Pro ($49.99) comes with pictured flashcards for all monophthongs and rhotic vowels and a variety of background themes (e.g., outer space, flowers, pirates) to sustain the child's interest in the activity.

- *Ultrasound biofeedback.* Ultrasound biofeedback can be particularly useful with rhotic vowels and diphthongs. It is the only technology currently available to SLPs to help the user see the tongue root retraction needed for a good rhotic quality. For diphthongs, the user can observe the gliding of the tongue from one position to another. When working on vowels in neighboring vowel spaces, such as /i/ and /ɪ/, ultrasound biofeedback may not be as useful because the visual difference in tongue position is so subtle. See Chapter 4 for more detailed information regarding using ultrasound biofeedback in therapy for older children.

Tips for Tactile Cueing

Tactile cues can be quite beneficial for helping the child achieve jaw stability, correct jaw height, and appropriate degrees of lip rounding and lip retraction during vowel production.

- *Programs that incorporate tactile cues.* Tactile cues can help the child stabilize the jaw, facilitate grading of jaw height, inhibit jaw sliding, and achieve lip rounding and retraction. Prompts for Restructuring Oral Muscular Phonetic Targets (PROMPT)–trained clinicians are familiar with the use of specific prompts to support correct vowel production and movement between phonemes. Other treatment approaches, including Dynamic Temporal and Tactile Cueing (DTTC) and Motor Speech Treatment

Protocol also incorporate tactile cues into treatment. See Chapter 4 for more detailed information about these treatment programs.

- *Reduce overexaggerated movements.* Keep in mind that children start off using greater jaw excursion than adults. During treatment, you may need to model movements that are more exaggerated than typical adult productions to support the child's ability to recognize differences in lip shaping and vowel height. However, we want to resist training overexaggerated lip and jaw movements for vowels by helping the child achieve more natural degrees of movement necessary for accurate vowel production. Place your fingers under the child's chin to help the child achieve the correct amount of jaw opening for the vowel and to inhibit overexaggerated jaw movements. Place your fingers at the corners of the child's lips to help facilitate just the right amount of lip rounding for /u/, /ʊ/, /o/, and /ɔ/ and lip retraction for /i/, keeping in mind that the accurate amount of jaw lowering and lip rounding/retraction is not static and will vary depending on the surrounding phonemes.

Tips for Metacognitive Cueing

There are many literacy programs that include metacognitive cueing for vowels. The *Lindamood Phoneme Sequencing Program for Reading, Spelling, and Speech* (LiPS; Lindamood & Lindamood, 2011) is an example of one of these programs. When explaining the vowels to the child, they implement a vowel circle that illustrates how the vowels compare to each other in terms of lip retraction and rounding, jaw opening, and tongue position. The child is encouraged to explore the placement of the articulators to figure out where each vowel belongs on a vowel circle (actually a U shape). The order of the vowels is as follows /i, ɪ, ɛ, e, æ, ʌ, ɑ, ɔ, o, ʊ, u/. The vowels are put into three categories, smile vowels /i, ɪ, ɛ, e, æ, ʌ/, open vowels /ɑ, ɔ/, and round vowels /o, ʊ, u/, in which there is a corresponding picture of the mouth for each category. Children are continually encouraged to note the position of their lips, jaw, and tongue as they go through the vowels. Encourage the child to place their fingertip near their teeth for a smile vowel (e.g., /i/) and for a more open vowel (e.g., /æ/) to bring their attention to the contrast in jaw opening between the two vowels. Diphthongs are referred to as "sliders," as the child moves from one position to the next (e.g., /aɪ, aʊ, ɔɪ/). The movement transition can be drawn with the finger on the vowel circle or vowel quadrilateral to go along with the corresponding movement of the articulators. The interactive materials are utilized in a manner for the child to be an interactive problem solver in the process of determining which vowel goes where. Rhotic vowels are referred to as the "r-controlled vowels" /ɝ, ɔ˞, ɑ˞/, and it is explained how the /r/ following the vowel will change the vowel.

Another example of a program that uses metacognitive cueing is Phonic Faces (Norris, 2003). In Phonic Faces, the grapheme is written on a character's face in a manner that shows how the sound is made or provides mnemonic visualization, such as a pair of eyeglasses on the character that represents /aɪ/. In addition, the vowels are presented in tense-lax pairs for each grapheme. Adult characters are used for the long vowels (e.g., /i, e, aɪ, u, o/), and images of babies are used for the short vowels (e.g., /ɛ, æ, ɪ, ɑ/). Figure 5–7 provides an example. In addition, each vowel pair has a story that helps the child remember what the vowel sound is and how it is produced. For example, the character Amy Ann is used for /æ/. She cries a lot using this sound. This helps the child remember that they need to open the mouth a bit more for this sound in a fun interactive way, which is often appealing to younger children.

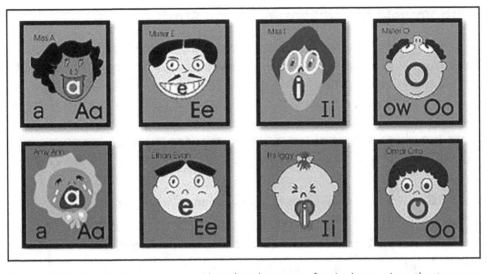

Figure 5–7. Phonic Faces representing the characters for /e, i, aɪ, o/ on the top row and /æ, ɛ, ɪ, ɑ/ on the bottom row. (From Phonic Faces, 2003, by Jan Norris. Used by permission of author.)

Use Minimal Pairs to Establish Vowel Distinctions

Children who struggle with vowel substitutions, such as individuals who substitute the tense vowel /i/ for the lax vowel /ɪ/ (e.g., the child produces "meat" for *mitt*), may benefit from working on *minimal pairs*. When working on minimal pairs, the child needs to change the articulatory movements to make meaningful semantic distinctions. Paired words that compare the target vowel and the contrast vowel are used as stimuli. Before working on production activities, be sure to evaluate the child's ability to discriminate between the target vowel and the contrast vowel and work on auditory discrimination as needed. Box 5–2 provides a few suggestions of minimal pairs activities for addressing vowel accuracy.

■ Box 5–2. Minimal Pairs Activities for Vowels

1. Make two sets of paired pictures/words that vary only by the vowel (e.g., /i/ and /ɪ/—*deep/ dip, feet/fit, green/grin, sheep/ship*; /æ/ and /ɑ/—*ax/ox, black/block, hat/hot, tap/top*; /e/ and /ɛ/—*braid/bread, gate/get, mane/men, rake/wreck*). The child chooses and names a picture, and the partner shows the picture the child said. If the child was correct, the pictures will match; if not, the pictures will not match, and the child will know to change the movement to achieve a more accurate production.

2. Practice minimal pairs by alternating between the paired words (e.g., *meat, mitt, meat, mitt, meat, mitt*) to develop better awareness of auditory and proprioceptive distinctions between the paired words.

3. Practice minimal pairs in triples, with words containing the target vowel in the first and third positions (e.g., *mitt, meat, mitt; bin, bean, bin*).

4. Produce sentences with both words of the minimal pair in the same sentence (e.g., "*I caught the <u>meat</u> with my <u>mitt</u>.*" "*I need a <u>black</u> <u>block</u>.*").

Practice With Vowel-Loaded Sentences and Stories

As a child's accuracy improves, the child can practice target vowels in vowel-loaded sentences, carrier phrases, and stories. In vowel-loaded sentences and carrier phrases, the target vowel will be practiced two or more times within a target utterance, as shown in Box 5–3.

For nonreaders, pictures can be used to address specific vowels in carrier phrases. Figure 5–8 illustrates an example of carrier phrases to work on the /aɪ/ vowel.

Stories that incorporate a set of target words using an "add-on" story technique may be helpful in facilitating the production of target vowels in a connected speech format. Printed

■ Box 5–3. Vowel-Loaded Sentences and Carrier Phrases

Sample Sentences with Two or More Target Vowels

/ʊ/ "He _took_ a _look_ at the _book_."

/ɪ/ "Where _did_ you _put_ _it_?"

/æ/ "The _cat_ is wearing a _hat_."

/o/ "Let's _go_ back _home_."

Target Vowel /ɪ/ With Carrier Phrase—Did you see the ___?

"_Did_ you see the _pig_?"

"_Did_ you see the _hill_?"

"_Did_ you see the _mitten_?"

"_Did_ you see the _zipper_?"

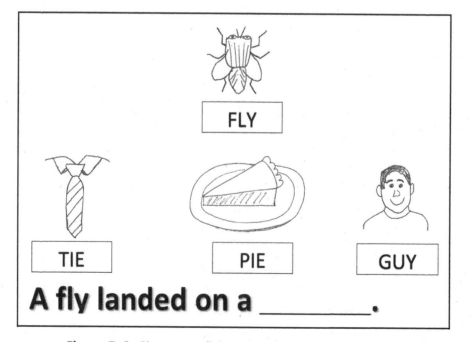

Figure 5–8. Pictures to elicit carrier phrases for /aɪ/ practice.

words or pictures denoting target words are incorporated into a story that is created by the child along with an adult or peer partner. The stories can be silly but should allow for practice of the target vowel in a connected sentence activity.

For the /e/ vowel, a story could be: "A <u>snake</u> woke up one morning and put on his <u>cape</u>. He was almost <u>late</u> for the big <u>game</u>. The <u>snake</u> headed over to the <u>lake</u> to <u>play</u> water polo with <u>Jake</u>. All of the sudden, <u>Jake</u> <u>sprayed</u> water on the <u>snake</u>, and the ref sent <u>Jake</u> to <u>jail</u>."

Most of the words in the sample story and previous sentences are content words. As discussed later in this chapter, content words tend to receive greater relative stress than function words in sentences. Words with greater relative stress may be preferable during initial stages of practice for children with motor speech disorders working on vowels because vowels in stressed syllables are longer in duration relative to surrounding syllables, offering greater auditory and proprioceptive feedback.

Establishing Natural Prosody

Difficulty with prosody is cited frequently as a challenge for children with CAS (Davis et al., 1998; Shriberg et al., 1997). Children with CAS often exhibit excess-equal stress, misplaced stress, syllable segregation, and a slow rate of speech, resulting in monotonous or atypical-sounding speech. Although prosody typically falls under the umbrella of phonology, Gerken and McGregor (1998) suggest that prosody also interacts with and impacts the language systems of syntax and pragmatics. This chapter focuses on understanding these features of prosody and facilitating development of improved prosody in children with CAS:

- **stress:** the relative emphasis given to a certain syllable in a word or a certain word in a phrase or sentence
- **intonation:** variations in pitch that signal the differences between statements and different types of questions; often these pitch changes are used in connection with stress to give emphasis to certain syllables or words in sentences
- **rhythm:** the time intervals between words in connected speech and the timing of stress in sentences
- **chunking:** the grouping of syntactic units between pauses
- **tone of voice:** vocal changes that convey the feelings and mood of the speaker, or denote sarcasm and irony

Features of Prosody

It is important to understand the role of prosody in communication. A child who struggles with prosody will sound unnatural to the listener, even if the segmental and phonotactic features of their speech have improved. The child's speech may have a robotic quality, impacting semantics and syntax. It also may be difficult for the child to match their tone of voice with the mood or feeling they are trying to convey, impacting pragmatic language. Prosodic features are described in greater detail in the following sections. Later in the chapter, suggested treatment strategies to facilitate better prosody in children with CAS are described.

Stress

The use of "inappropriate prosody, especially in the realization of lexical or phrasal stress" (ASHA, 2007, p. 4) is a feature commonly associated with CAS. *Excessive equal stress*, when most or all the syllables in a word or utterance receive pronounced stress, was the most frequently observed prosodic characteristic of children with suspected CAS (Shriberg et al., 1997). Munson et al. (2003) found that children with CAS were able to produce distinctions between stressed and weak syllables, but the distinctions were subtle and were not consistently recognized perceptually by listeners.

The two types of stress discussed in this chapter are *lexical stress* and *sentence stress*. *Lexical stress* refers to word-level stress, in which greater relative stress is placed on a specific syllable or syllables within a word. Words containing more than one syllable, with the exception of some compound words, have both stressed and weak syllables. In the word **mo**mmy, the first syllable is stressed (S), and the second syllable is weak (w) and has a "Sw" stress pattern. In the word *again*, the second syllable has greater relative stress and has a "wS" stress pattern. The pronunciation and stress assignment of some words with identical spellings will change depending on whether the word is a noun or a verb. Consider the words in Table 5–4 and note how the word meaning changes depending on the placement of syllable stress with nouns receiving stress on Syllable 1 and verbs on Syllable 2, illustrating how semantics and syntax influence lexical stress.

Sentence stress refers to both *phrasal stress* and *contrastive stress*. *Phrasal stress* describes the natural stress of a specified language. In English, phrasal stress is marked by applying greater relative stress to content words (nouns, verbs, adjectives, some adverbs) than function words (prepositions, conjunctions, articles, pronouns). In the sentence, "*I was **walk**ing to the **park** with my **BRO**ther on **Sun**day,*" greater relative stress would be applied to the underlined words or syllables, and the strongest stress would occur on the first syllable in the word *brother*. *Contrastive stress* refers to application of stronger stress to a specified word in a sentence and often is used for *clarification* or *emphasis*. Unlike phrasal stress, contrastive stress may be applied to any word in a sentence, not just content words. Consider the use of contrastive stress for clarification in this conversation:

Bob: *"I went to the park with Maya's brother on Sunday."*

Jim: *"Oh, I didn't know you had a brother."*

Bob: *"Not **my** brother; **Maya's** brother."*

Contrastive stress often is used to apply emphasis to certain words in connected speech as in these examples:

*"**MY** turn."*

*"I'm **SO** excited!"*

*"That is **NOT** my ball."*

*"I want the **BLUE** marker."*

Peña-Brooks and Hegde (2007) describe three acoustic features that distinguish stressed syllables from unstressed syllables. These three features—increased loudness, increased duration, and higher pitch—give a stressed syllable greater prominence than the surrounding syllables. The stressed syllables are produced with greater relative vocal intensity (loudness)

Table 5–4. Lexical Stress Contrasts in Noun-Verb Heteronyms

NOUNS	VERBS
conduct	con**duct**
attribute	a**ttri**bute
contest	con**test**
escort	e**scort**
subject	sub**ject**
object	ob**ject**
permit	per**mit**
record	re**cord**

and longer relative duration than the surrounding unstressed syllables. In addition, a stressed syllable often is produced with a higher pitch than the neighboring unstressed syllables. For the speaker to vary the loudness, duration, and pitch of a syllable, motoric adjustments are made in the programming of some spatiotemporal parameters of speech movements, including expelling more air from the lungs, sustaining the duration of the vowel for a longer time frame, and vibrating the vocal folds more rapidly during production of stressed syllables. These subtle motoric variations can be quite challenging for children with CAS.

Intonation

Intonation in English is bound to grammar. Rising and falling pitch patterns are associated with different sentence types. Falling intonation, marked by a fall in pitch at the end of a sentence, is commonly used when producing declarative sentences and "wh" questions. When producing "yes-no" questions or tag questions, rising intonation, where the speaker's pitch rises at the end of the sentence, is used. Consider the dialogue in Box 5–4. The arrows at the end of each sentence indicate falling ↘ or rising ↗ intonation.

■ Box 5–4. Dialogue Illustrating Falling and Rising Intonation

Child: Jenny and I are going to the mall after school. ↘

Parent: You mean after you do your homework, right? ↗

Child: I knew you were going to say that. ↘

Parent: How are you getting there? ↘

Child: We're taking the bus. ↘ Is that okay? ↗

Parent: That's fine. ↘ What time will you be home? ↘

Child: I thought maybe we could eat dinner there? ↗

Parent: That's fine. ↘ Just be sure you're home by 8:00. ↘

Rhythm

The English language is a *stress-timed language*, in which stressed syllables occur at relatively regular intervals regardless of the number of unstressed syllables occurring between each pair of stressed syllables. The unstressed syllables are lengthened or shortened to accommodate these regular intervals of stress. In the first sentence of Table 5–5, stress is placed on the content words (in bold), and the rhythm of the stressed syllables occurs at fairly regular time intervals. Notice that the duration of stressed words/syllables is longer than those not receiving stress. In the second sentence, the words *"to his old"* would be spoken more quickly to maintain the rhythmic interval. Phoneme omissions will help accommodate the more rapid production of that phrase. Children who use excessive equal stress will struggle with the rhythmicity of their language.

 It should be noted that children 5 years of age are still refining this pattern of rhythm in stress-timed languages such as English (Post & Payne, 2018, as cited in Kent & Rountrey, 2020). Thus, addressing the feature of rhythm would not be appropriate in a preschool-age child but would be more appropriate for a school-age or older child.

Chunking

Chunking refers to the grouping of syntactic or semantic units, followed by brief pauses in connected speech. Pauses serve several functions. Pauses are inserted at natural phrase breaks, when naming items in a list, or when trying to establish subtle differences in meaning. Natural phrase breaks are used in longer sentences (e.g., Mommy stopped at the grocery store / to buy some milk / before she took me to school.) We often pause between words in a list as an accommodation to the listener (e.g., I invited Jesse, / Rocky, / Max, / Malcolm, / Hank, / and Sammy to my party.). Pauses also are required to establish meaning differences in sentences. The sentence pairs in Box 5–5 illustrate how important chunking and pausing are to establish differences in meaning.

Tone of Voice

Achieving variations in *tone of voice* requires manipulation of a motoric aspect of speech (vocal quality, rate, pitch, rhythm, intensity) to express different moods or feelings, as well as to denote sarcasm and irony. Struggles with variations in tone of voice will impact children's pragmatic language.

To summarize, the five features of prosody described have their roots in difficulty with motor speech planning and programming. The impacts are widespread across multiple areas of speech and language. Table 5–6 summarizes the underlying deficits and impacts of prosody challenges in children with CAS.

Table 5–5. Rhythm in a Stress Timed Language

The	**boy**	is	**walk**ing	to	**school.**
ðʌ	bɔɪ	ɪz	wɔ.kɪŋ	tu	skul
The	**boy**	is	**walk**ing	to his old	**school.**
ðʌ	bɔɪ	ɪz	wɔ.kɪŋ	tu ɪz ol	skul

Table 5–6. Summarization of the Underlying Deficits and Impacts of Prosody Disturbances

Areas of Challenge	Underlying Planning/Programming and Other Deficits	Impacts on Communication
Stress	DIFFICULTY PLANNING AND PROGRAMMING: **Speech breathing muscles** to achieve variations in loudness and phoneme duration; **laryngeal muscles** to vary vocal pitch	Speech Semantics Syntax Pragmatics
Intonation	DIFFICULTY PLANNING AND PROGRAMMING: **Laryngeal muscles** to vary vocal pitch	Speech
Rhythm	DIFFICULTY PLANNING AND PROGRAMMING: **Laryngeal muscles** to vary vocal pitch; **speech breathing muscles** to achieve variations in vocal loudness and phoneme duration	Speech Pragmatics
Chunking	DIFFICULTY PLANNING AND PROGRAMMING: **Speech breathing muscles** to modulate number of words spoken on a breath and duration of pauses between phrases DIFFICULTY WITH: **Self-monitoring**	Speech Syntax
Tone of voice	DIFFICULTY PLANNING AND PROGRAMMING: **Laryngeal muscles** to modulate voice quality, pitch, and vowel duration; **velopharyngeal muscles** to modulate resonance; **articulatory muscles** to modify rate of speech	Pragmatics

■ Box 5–5. Pauses in Sentences That Clarify Differences in Meaning

> My uncle, / the astronaut, / and my Dad took me to the aquarium.
> My uncle, the astronaut, / and my Dad took me to the aquarium.
>
> I said to him, / "Today we will get it done."
> I said to him today, / "We will get it done."
>
> I want chicken, / soup, / and milk.
> I want chicken soup, / and milk.
>
> And the classic meme
> Let's eat, / Grandma.
> Let's eat Grandma.

Assessment of Prosody

Prosody assessment will depend on the child's age, the nature of the child's prosodic features during spontaneous speech, and the impact of prosody on the child's language (semantics, syntax, pragmatics). Abbiati and Velleman (2021) suggest taking note of the child's use of the features of prosody during spontaneous speech and thinking critically about what you need to assess more specifically. Some formal tests, such as the DEMSS, score prosodic accuracy (word-level stress) for words with two or more syllables. The tasks described in Table 5–7 can be used to informally assess if the child is able to use the various features of prosody.

Table 5–7. Informal Prosody Assessment Tasks

PROSODIC FEATURES	INFORMAL ASSESSMENT TASKS	
Lexical stress *Ask the child to produce these words following a model in single words or in meaningful sentences (e.g., I stepped on a hard **ob**ject. I ob**ject** to these questions.)*	*Can the child accurately apply contrasting lexical stress patterns?*	
	Sample stimuli: **con**trast con**trast** **per**mit per**mit** **ob**ject ob**ject** **pro**gress pro**gress**	ad**dress** **add**ress **con**duct con**duct** **rec**ord re**cord** **en**velope en**vel**ope
Lexical stress *Ask the child to repeat these words following a natural model (without <u>over</u>emphasis on the stressed syllable). If the child's lexical stress is incorrect or if the child produces equal stress, see if more emphatic stress models will facilitate correct stress assignment.*	*Can the child produce lexical stress patterns correctly in two- to four-syllable words?*	
	Sample stimuli: **dad**dy **o**pen **wa**ter a**gain** to**day** be**gin** po**lice** for**got** **rad**io **tri**angle **cer**eal	**news**paper di**rec**tions ba**na**na com**pu**ter re**mem**ber **ex**ercising **tel**evision com**mu**nity in**gre**dients invi**ta**tion Cinde**rel**la
Contrastive stress *This task can be done imitatively or in response to questions (e.g., Who ate the apple? "The **baby** ate the apple." What did the baby eat? "The baby ate the **apple**.") Another option is to model the sentence and then ask a question with a word in error (e.g., Mom got new red shoes. Did **dad** get new red shoes? "No, **mom** got new red shoes.")*	*Can the child shift the relative stress to different words in a sentence?*	
	Sample stimuli: The **baby** ate the apple. The baby ate the **apple**. **Mom** got new red shoes. Mom got **new** red shoes. Mom got new red **shoes**. He **doesn't** like chocolate cake. He doesn't like **chocolate** cake. **He** doesn't like chocolate cake.	
Intonation *Model sentences with either rising or falling intonation at the end. See if the child can repeat the model with the correct intonation.*	*Does the child change pitch to denote different sentence types (e.g., declarative, yes/no and wh- questions)?*	
	Sample stimuli: The baby ate the apple. ↘ Did the baby eat the apple? ↗	

Table 5–7. *continued*

PROSODIC FEATURES	INFORMAL ASSESSMENT TASKS
Intonation *continued*	*Sample stimuli:* continued He found his hat. ↘ Did he find his hat? ↗ What time is dinner? ↘ Is dinner soon? ↗ He can count to 100. ↘ He can count to 100? ↗
Rhythm *Ask the child to repeat sentences and note if the child uses rhythmic stress patterns. Keep in mind that children typically do not stabilize the use of timed stress patterns until approximately 7 years of age.*	*Is the child using a rhythmic stress pattern in sentences with greater stress applied to content words?* *Sample stimuli:* **Mom** is **ma**king a **sal**ad for **din**ner. **When** is **Tom**my **go**ing **home**? He **nev**er **brush**es his **hair**. I **saw** her **dog** be**hind** the **bush**es.
Chunking *If the child's speech intelligibility tends to decline in sentences, see if the child can chunk short phrases from the sentence and pause between these phrases to attain greater intelligibility. Write these sentences on sentence strips with marks to denote where the pause will be inserted and instruct the child to use chunking and pausing to achieve increased intelligibility.*	*Is the child able to chunk phrasal units of a sentence together separated by short pauses?* *Sample stimuli:* She is walking // down the street. She is walking // down the street // to catch the bus. I went to the store // to buy some milk. I went to the store // to buy some milk // for breakfast tomorrow. He plays soccer on Tuesday, // Thursday, // and Saturday. I invited Jose, // his brother Jesse, // and Adam to the party.
Control of tone of voice, loudness, pitch *Provide a list of short sentences and ask the child to produce the sentences with a specified emotion (perhaps explaining the situation), pitch, or loudness. Note if the child can vary these vocal features.*	*Can the child vary vocal quality, pitch, and loudness in sentences?* *Sample stimuli:* I came in second place. (happy/excited) I came in second place. (sad/disappointed) I need to go to bed. (tired) I need to go to bed. (angry) I want more cookies. (childlike voice) I want more cookies. (dad voice) Hi mommy. (whispered) Hi mommy. (loud)

Keep in mind that there can be wide variation in listeners' judgments of children's prosodic control, and listeners often perceive stress and intonation patterns as being inaccurate when they are not, especially when the speaker exhibits substantial speech sound errors (Skinder et al., 1999). Thus, it is imperative to hone your skills in listening to and making judgments about prosody. Audio recording assessments can be beneficial, so you can go back and listen again rather than trying to make judgments on the spot.

Treatment for Prosody

To achieve appropriate prosody requires subtle manipulation of various motor speech variables to vary pitch, loudness, duration, and vocal quality. This can be challenging for children with CAS. Because prosody difficulties are common findings in children with CAS, it is recommended that work on prosody begin early in the treatment process (Strand & Skinder, 1999). There is no need to wait until a child is speaking in sentences before addressing certain elements of prosody, such as intonation, tone of voice, pitch, and loudness. Although SLPs are aware of prosody challenges existing in children with motor speech disorders and autism spectrum disorder, they are less comfortable assessing and treating prosody because they feel they lack knowledge and understanding of proper assessment and treatment techniques (Hawthorne & Fischer, 2020).

The following section offers recommendations for supporting children who struggle with the use of stress, intonation, rhythm, chunking, and tone of voice. In addition to some of the strategies described, there are free and affordable digital tools available, such as the *Waveform, Annotations, Spectrogram & Pitch (WASP)* program (Huckvale, 2021), which can be downloaded or used as a web version (https://www.speechandhearing.net/laboratory/wasp/) and *Voice Analyst: Pitch & Volume*, an app designed for the iPad. WASP allows the speaker to record their or their client's utterance and then see the acoustic correlates of prosody, which are amplitude (loudness), pitch, and duration. When playing the signal back, both the client and SLP can see and hear the production. In addition to being able to better visualize and measure prosodic characteristics, the SLP can also reinforce the concept of smooth coarticulation. The *Voice Analyst: Pitch & Volume* app provides the speaker real-time visual biofeedback of pitch and volume individually or combined on one screen. This is a simpler display than WASP, and you can set parameters for fundamental frequency and decibel level for the client to target or stay within the parameters of. For example, a child who uses a very quiet voice can be given a dB target to hit to be loud enough, and a child who is monotone can be coached to fill in a particular pitch range. See Figures 5–9A and B for further explanation of WASP and Voice Analyst, respectively.

How to Facilitate Appropriate Stress in Treatment

Although most programs that address treatment of speech production typically do not address prosody, there are some programs that specifically address aspects of prosody. Rapid Syllable Transition Treatment (ReST; Murray et al., 2015) specifically addresses syllable stress assign-

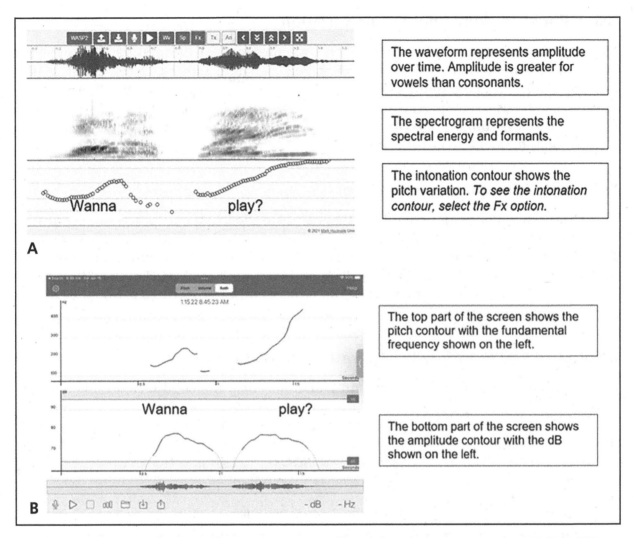

Figure 5–9. A. "*Wanna play?*" waveform, spectrogram, and intonation contour represented on WASP. **B.** "*Wanna play?*" dB and Hz contour on Voice Analyst.

ment and smooth coarticulatory transitions in treatment. DTTC (Strand, 2020) integrates work on variations in loudness, rate, stress, and tone of voice into treatment.

Following are several considerations and activities to support the use of appropriate contrastive and lexical stress for children at various stages of development.

During each of the activities described, appropriate stress should be modeled for the child during treatment, as modeling a staccato pattern of production or placing stress on the wrong syllable may encourage the child to use robotic speech or incorrect lexical stress placement. It can be easy to fall into habits of emphasizing a specific syllable of a word if that is the syllable with which the child is having trouble. For instance, if the target utterance is *Hi mommy*, and the child says, "*Hi mama*," a therapist may be inclined to overemphasize the last syllable and model, "*Hi mommy.*" In this case, it would be more appropriate to use backward chaining, maintaining appropriate syllable stress throughout the process (e.g., Say "me." Now say "**mo**mmy." Now say "Hi **mo**mmy.").

Using Books to Work on Prosodic Variation

Many books for young children provide opportunities to work on prosody (e.g., applying emphatic stress, varying loudness and duration, changing tone of voice). Good choices for early books are those that have few words, so the focus can be on variations in some suprasegmental aspect of speech. The following books offer opportunities to work on prosody. Box 5–6 provides examples of books to work on prosody. They can be worked on during treatment sessions and sent home with children to practice with their families.

Storybooks to Facilitate Emphatic Stress

Classic repetitive line stories often lend themselves to modeling and practicing contrastive stress. Consider the lines, "Somebody's been sitting on *MY* chair" from Goldilocks and the Three Bears; "'Not *I*,' said the cat," from The Little Red Hen; or "I'll huff, and I'll puff, I'll *BLOW* the house down," from The Three Pigs, and "You can't catch *ME* I'm the *GIN*gerbread man." from The Gingerbread Man. These lines all contain words where it would be appropriate to use emphatic stress.

Emphasize Key Words by Incorporating Emphatic Stress

Even very early on in treatment, you can model and help the child increase the duration of vowels and increase vocal intensity in single words and on specific words in phrases and sentences. For younger children, modeling contrastive stress in words and short phrases with high levels of emotional content is beneficial. Some examples include *"OOOH," "AAAH," "WOW," "UH* oh," *"WHEE,"* That's *MINE," "KaBOOM,"* "I *DID* it," "Hoo*RAY*."

■ Box 5–6. Books for Young Children to Address Prosody

Boynton, S. (1984). *Doggies: A counting and barking book.* Little Simon Publishing.

Cook, J. (2014). *Decibella and her 6-inch voice.* Boys Town Press.

Crum, S. (2016). *Uh-oh!* Knopf Books for Young Readers.

Heim, A. (2020). *Quiet down loud town.* Clarion Books.

LaRochelle, D. (2014). *Moo!* Bloomsbury USA.

Munsch, R. (2020). *Up, up, down.* Scholastic Canada.

Patricelli, L. (2003). *Quiet loud.* Candlewick Press.

Patricelli, L. (2003). *Yummy yucky.* Candlewick Press.

Patricelli, L. (2008). *No no yes yes.* Candlewick Press.

Raschka, C. (2007). *Yo! Yes?* HMH Books for Young Readers.

Shannon, D. (1998). *No, David!* Blue Sky Press.

Sullivan, M. (2015). *Ball.* HMH Books for Young Readers.

Tullet, H. (2017). *Say zoop!* Chronicle Books.

Address Contrastive Stress Using Statement Question-Response (SQR)

In the SQR exercise, the child is given a statement and then asked various questions about the statement. The word in the sentence requiring greater relative stress will change depending on the question being asked. For children who can read, an additional cue, such as a chip or block, can be placed on the word of the written sentence that will receive the greatest stress. Examples of SQR are shown in Box 5–7.

 When working to facilitate contrastive stress, multisensory cueing can be quite beneficial. Use accompanying hand gestures and facial expressions when modeling contrastive stress. Talk about how some words or parts of words are louder and longer than other words. Consider incorporating digital materials, such as WASP, into treatment to provide visual representations of the child's production contours. These strategies will help encourage the child to use more robust variations in stress.

In the example in Figure 5–10, WASP is used to provide a visual representation of the contrastive stress in the phrase, "The bird is red." Note the rising contour and bigger sound wave for the words receiving greater relative stress.

Address Contrastive Stress Using a Fix-the-Sentence Exercise

The fix-the-sentence format is similar to the preceding SQR exercise but without questions. The clinician reads a sentence and then repeats it, inserting an incorrect word. The child needs to repeat the original sentence, applying greater stress on the corrected word. Examples of the fix-the-sentence exercise are shown in Box 5–8.

■ Box 5–7. Example of SQR Exercise

Statement: "The bird is red."

   QUESTION: "What *color* is the bird?"

    RESPONSE: "The bird is **RED**."

   QUESTION: "*What* is red?"

    RESPONSE: "The **BIRD** is red."

Statement: "Mom hid the red shoes under the bed."

   QUESTION: "*Who* hid the shoes under the bed?"

    RESPONSE: "**MOM** hid the red shoes under the bed."

   QUESTION: "*Which* shoes did Mom hide under the bed?"

    RESPONSE: "Mom hid the **RED** shoes under the bed."

   QUESTION: "*Where* did Mom hide the red shoes?"

    RESPONSE: "Mom hid the red shoes under the **BED**."

   QUESTION: "*What* did Mom do with the red shoes?"

    RESPONSE: "Mom **HID** the red shoes under the bed."

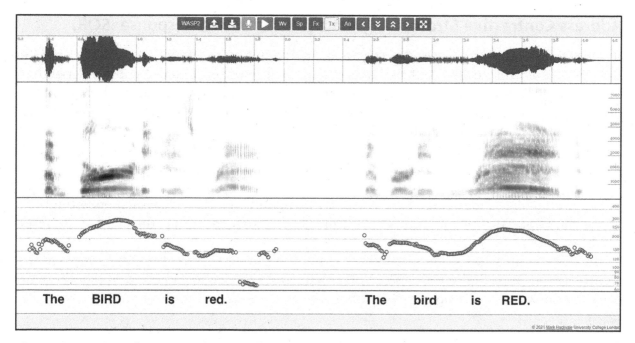

Figure 5–10. View of WASP2 spectrogram illustrating contrastive stress for production of sentences "The BIRD is red." (on left) and "The bird is RED." (on the right).

■ Box 5–8. Example of Fix-the-Sentence Exercise

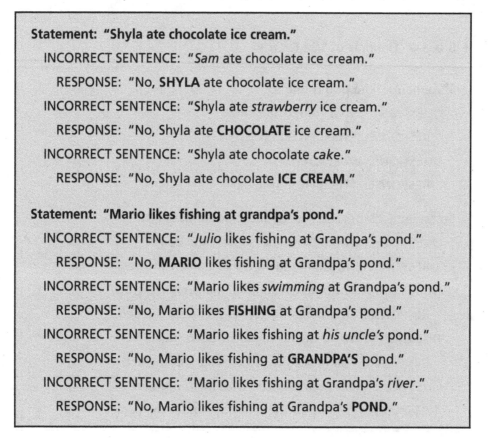

Statement: "Shyla ate chocolate ice cream."

INCORRECT SENTENCE: "*Sam* ate chocolate ice cream."

RESPONSE: "No, **SHYLA** ate chocolate ice cream."

INCORRECT SENTENCE: "Shyla ate *strawberry* ice cream."

RESPONSE: "No, Shyla ate **CHOCOLATE** ice cream."

INCORRECT SENTENCE: "Shyla ate chocolate *cake*."

RESPONSE: "No, Shyla ate chocolate **ICE CREAM**."

Statement: "Mario likes fishing at grandpa's pond."

INCORRECT SENTENCE: "*Julio* likes fishing at Grandpa's pond."

RESPONSE: "No, **MARIO** likes fishing at Grandpa's pond."

INCORRECT SENTENCE: "Mario likes *swimming* at Grandpa's pond."

RESPONSE: "No, Mario likes **FISHING** at Grandpa's pond."

INCORRECT SENTENCE: "Mario likes fishing at *his uncle's* pond."

RESPONSE: "No, Mario likes fishing at **GRANDPA'S** pond."

INCORRECT SENTENCE: "Mario likes fishing at Grandpa's *river*."

RESPONSE: "No, Mario likes fishing at Grandpa's **POND**."

Use Guessing Activities to Support Use of Contrastive Stress

The make-a-guess activities allow for opportunities to practice using contrastive stress. Each participant attempts to guess or make a prediction. Emphatic stress is incorporated into sentences when making a guess and when evaluating the guess or prediction. Following are examples of using contrastive stress during guessing activities.

Example 1. Reading a Flap Book

Activity: While reading a flap book, the student is asked to guess what is hidden behind the flaps.

The guess: "I think it's a **PUPPY**."

If incorrect: "It's **NOT** a puppy. It's a **DUCK**."

If correct: "It **IS** a puppy."

Example 2. Searching for Hidden Objects

The guess: "I think it's under the **TABLE**." The child searches the named location.

If incorrect: "It's **NOT** under the table. Maybe it's under the **CHAIR**." The child searches the new location.

If correct: "It **IS** under the chair."

Example 3. Predicting What Will Happen First

Activity: The child and clinician each guess which of two feathers or balloons will land on the ground first or which race car or wind-up toy will reach the finish line first.

The guess: Child—"I think the **RED** car will win." Clinician—"I think the **BLUE** car will win."

If correct: "I was **RIGHT**. The **RED** car won!"

If incorrect: "**YOU** were right. The **BLUE** car won."

Facilitating Appropriate Lexical Stress

When working with children on improving lexical stress, be sure you are working at the child's optimum challenge point. Gradually increase the level of challenge to encourage success and facilitate generalization. The following sequence is recommended.

1. Identification of lexical stress
2. Production of single words with correct stress assignment
   a. imitatively
   b. spontaneously
3. Production of correct stress assignment in phrases and sentences
   a. imitatively
   b. spontaneously
4. Production of varied lexical stress patterns in conversational and connected speech activities

To work on identifying lexical stress, begin with two-syllable words and determine if the child can identify which syllable has greater stress (which syllable was longer and/or louder). Initially, you may need to exaggerate the stressed syllable to demonstrate greater contrast between the stressed and weak syllable. As the child's ability to identify stressed syllables improves, you will reduce the exaggeration of the syllable stress. Negative practice also can help children identify lexical stress. Have the child produce a word, first placing stress on one syllable and then on the other syllable (or listen to you produce a word with stress on opposing syllables) and see if the child recognizes which one sounds correct. Some children will continue to struggle with identification of syllable stress, even when they are beginning to produce syllable stress correctly, so there's no need to wait for lexical stress identification to emerge before moving on to production.

During production activities, begin by modeling correct lexical stress. The verbal models can be accompanied by a variety of other cues, for example, you can model the word while using hand gestures (e.g., mimicking stretching of dough). Blocks can be used to denote stressed and weak syllables with large blocks for stressed syllables/small blocks for weak syllables. If the child can read, you can use graphic cues, such as denoting the stressed syllable with larger letters than the weak syllables, placing a chip above the stressed syllable, or using a highlighter to bring the child's attention to the stressed syllable. Examples of visual cues are illustrated in Figure 5–11.

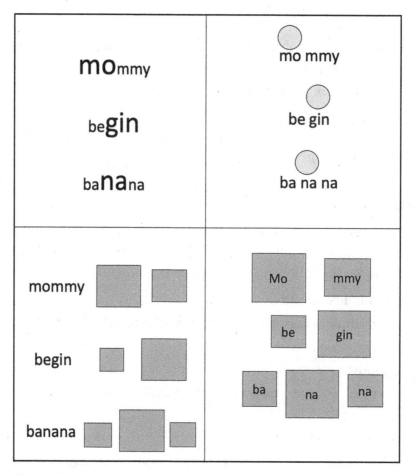

Figure 5–11. Examples of visual cueing for addressing lexical stress assignment.

Visual biofeedback tools, like WASP and Voice Analyst, can be used to provide explicit instruction when working on lexical and sentential stress. In Figure 5–12, observe the difference in amplitude and pitch when the child produces the word *contrast* with stress on the second syllable (on the left) versus the first syllable (on the right).

When choosing target utterances containing two or more syllables for treatment, begin by choosing words with *trochaic* stress patterns, in which a strong syllable is followed by a weak syllable (e.g., edit, bottom, separate, exercising). Words with *iambic* stress patterns, in which a weak syllable is followed by a stressed syllable or other nontrochaic stress patterns (e.g., surprise, believe, volunteer, community), can be targeted later in treatment. Careful selection of carrier phrases also influences the ease with which a child may be able to produce a target word in a phrase or sentence. When choosing carrier phrases, consider incorporating trochaic words into carrier phrases that follow a trochaic stress pattern and iambic words into phrases with iambic stress patterns (Bowen, 2009). Examples of trochaic and iambic words and carrier phrases are shown in Box 5–9.

Lexical stress should always be addressed within the context of sentences, rather than stopping at the single-word level, to support flexibility and generalization of prosody within the context of connected speech. Worksheets can be found in the online materials along with practice word lists as exercises for developing more accurate lexical stress starting with syllable stress identification and moving through use of appropriate lexical stress within sentence contexts.

Facilitating Appropriate Intonation

Within the context of speech production activities, you can incorporate work on using rising and falling intonation patterns. A variety of activities can be used to help children use appropriate and more varied intonation in their speech.

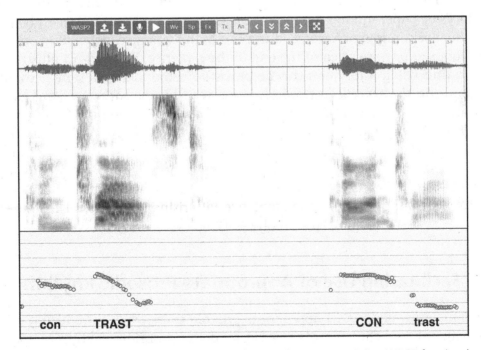

Figure 5–12. Lexical stress variations in the word "contrast" using WASP for visual biofeedback.

■ Box 5–9. Examples of Trochaic and Iambic Words and Carrier Phrases

Trochaic words and carrier phrases

I can *eat* the (<u>ap</u>ple/<u>car</u>rot/<u>coo</u>kie/<u>pea</u>nut <u>but</u>ter).

Do you *have* the (<u>pup</u>py/<u>but</u>ton/<u>hel</u>icopter/<u>tel</u>evision)?

Put the (<u>bas</u>ket/<u>can</u>dle/<u>pen</u>ny) *on* the *ta*ble.

Iambic words and carrier phrases

I *bought* a *big* (gi<u>raffe</u>/bal<u>loon</u>/a<u>quar</u>ium).

I *know* you *won't* (a<u>gree</u>/be<u>lieve</u>/par<u>tic</u>ipate).

He *wants* to *play* (cro<u>quet</u>/to<u>day</u>/Mo<u>nop</u>oly).

Count Items Using Falling Intonation

Counting is an activity that facilitates use of a falling intonation pattern at the end of the sequence. When counting objects with a child, an exaggerated intonation pattern should be modeled, with the final number accentuated and prolonged, and an obvious change in pitch. This type of exaggerated intonation during counting can be accompanied by hand gestures that match the intonations used (falling) to provide an accompanying visual cue.

Differentiate Sentence Types Using Falling and Rising Intonation

Children with CAS may benefit from opportunities to practice using falling and rising intonation to differentiate between different types of sentences. The use of falling and rising hand gestures to accompany the intonation pattern provides a beneficial visual cue for some children. Blocks or paper squares used to denote each word of a sentence can be placed on a table, with the blocks raised or lowered at the end of the sentence, depending on whether the child needs to lower or raise pitch at the end of the sentence. Figure 5–13 illustrates how the use of falling and rising intonation can be practiced using identical sentences, alternating between producing the sentence as a declarative with falling inflection and as a question with rising inflection, as well as inflection changes between yes-no questions and declarative sentences. Children can be taught to identify yes-no questions words at the start of a sentence (e.g., is, are, can, does, do, will) that would trigger the use of rising intonation and then practice varying pitch to express rising and falling intonation in production practice.

In Figure 5–14, the first two sentences from Figure 5–13 were recorded using WASP2, the first sentence with falling and the second sentence with rising intonation. The figure illustrates the sentence, "Bob ate 12 apples." and "Bob ate 12 apples?"

Facilitating Use of Appropriate Prosodic Rhythm

Just as the clinician would model appropriate syllable stress when introducing multisyllabic words in treatment, the clinician also would model appropriate rhythm of speech during sentence-level productions. Bringing a child's attention and awareness to the rhythm of

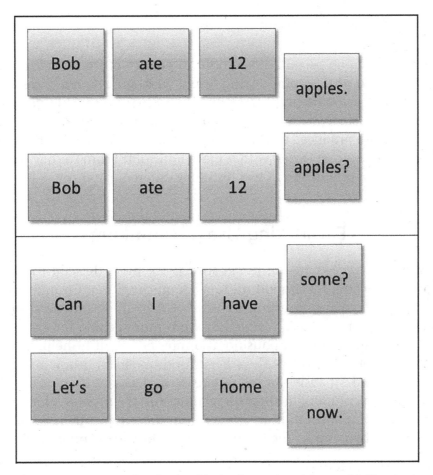

Figure 5–13. Example of using blocks for cueing rising and falling intonation patterns.

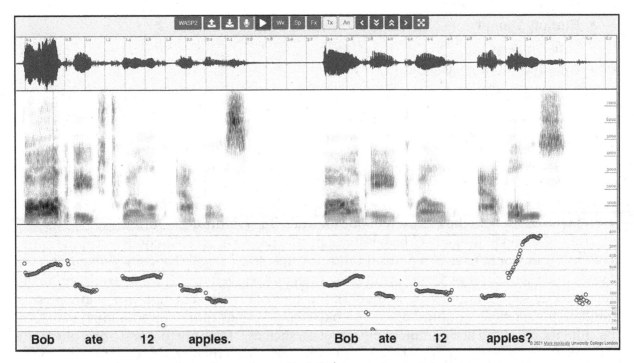

Figure 5–14. Identical sentences with falling intonation and then rising intonation.

237

language can be challenging because it is a natural pattern of stress and rhythm. Nevertheless, the use of modeling with accompanying visual cues, such as hand gestures that follow the rise and fall of stress in a sentence, can be useful. It also may be useful to contrast different ways of producing a sentence, such as contrasting a sentence produced with a robotic stress pattern versus a sentence produced with rhythmic application of stress. Children can practice saying the sentence "like a robot" and with a more natural rhythm so they can begin to hear and feel the difference in production of two distinctly different rhythmic patterns.

Facilitating Use of Chunking

For children whose sentences and connected speech are more difficult to understand than their single-word production, it is important to work on chunking. Chunking of phrases into smaller clusters and practicing inserting pauses between these phrase chunks may make the motor plan for longer sentence production more manageable for children with motor planning difficulties. Chunking and pausing also may be useful in helping children gain a greater consideration for the needs of the listener and understand how things they do with their speech can help make it easier for the listener to understand them.

One way to work on chunking is through reciting nursery rhymes. Nursery rhymes often utilize short phrases with pauses that are longer than those typically used in conversational speech. These nursery rhymes may facilitate the use of chunking and pausing:

- Eeny, Meeny, Miny, Moe
- Georgie Porgie
- Hey Diddle Diddle
- Hickory Dickory Dock
- Humpty Dumpty
- Little Bo Peep
- One, Two, Buckle My Shoe
- Pat-a-Cake, Pat-a-Cake, Baker's Man
- Rain, Rain, Go Away
- Star Light, Star Bright

Another way of introducing more natural sounding chunking and pausing in treatment is reciting the alphabet. There are natural pauses between letter chunks in alphabet recitation, and children can learn to tune into where these pauses occur and attempt to produce this well-rehearsed list with the insertion of pauses where they naturally would occur.

Teach children to recognize where natural phrase breaks occur in language, first in shorter sentences that would have two phrasal units and one pause (e.g., "They are walking / to the store,") and then in longer phrases with more than one pause (e.g., "They are walking / to the store / to buy some cookies.") To accomplish this type of activity, children can read sentences and determine where a natural phrase break(s) would occur. In sentence-building activities, the child produces the first portion of the sentence, such as, "Mommy took me," and gradually expands the sentence, "Mommy took me / to the park," and then "Mommy took me / to the park / on Saturday morning." Another activity could involve creation of silly sentences, in which the child chooses phrases from two or more piles that could be connected to form a longer sentence (e.g., The purple dinosaur / ate four cookies / at the rodeo).

Children can practice using juncture by reciting lists. As a listener, it is easier to make sense of lists of items if the speaker produces the lists with a slight pause between the items on the list. Practice inserting pauses between words in well-rehearsed lists, such as counting from one to 10, listing the months of the year, or reciting the colors of the rainbow in the correct order. From there, children can begin to work on using pauses when producing novel lists, such as items on a birthday wish list, their favorite superheroes, or items on a shopping list.

Facilitating the Use of Varied Tones of Voice

Varying tone of voice can begin quite early in treatment, but activities appropriate for older children can be introduced in treatment as well.

Introduce Exaggerated Tone of Voice Early in Treatment

When working with very young children or older children with minimal expressive language, exclamations can be taught by modeling exaggerated tones of voice. Table 5–8 provides examples of words or phrases that may be introduced early in treatment to facilitate the use of exaggerated intonation patterns.

Recognize Different Tones of Voice

Children can be taught to recognize that different vocal tones can be associated with different emotions and different speakers. Treatment activities may involve contrasting different vocal tones and asking the child to determine what emotion is being expressed (e.g., sad, happy, angry, tired). Pictures of faces that match various emotions may be beneficial during this

Table 5–8. Eliciting Varied Intonation Patterns Through Use of Exclamations

Word/Phrase Exclamations	Contexts for Teaching Exclamations
"Whee!"	Sending cars, toy animals, or toy people down a slide
"Wow!"	Observing results from playdough machine
"Ready, set, *go*!"	Going on a swing, slide, or toy car
"Yikes!"	Toy vehicles crashing together
"*Uh* oh!"	Object falling to the ground
"Ka . . . *boom*!"	Block tower falling or being pushed over
"Mmm" or "Yuck"	Feeding food to dolls or puppets
"Oh, *no*!"	Toy animal or doll getting "hurt"
"Ta *da*!"	Completing a puzzle or other building toy
"Yahoo!"	Child accomplishing a challenging task

activity. Helping children recognize differences in pitch and vocal quality also can be addressed using characters from books or television programs or from play characters (mommy, daddy, baby). Producing sentences using different character voices and asking a child to guess who was speaking (e.g., Cookie Monster versus Elmo) can help children recognize these differences in vocal tone and quality. Older children may be asked to distinguish between spoken sentences that sound sincere versus those that are spoken with a sarcastic tone of voice.

Produce Different Tones of Voice

From very early on in treatment, children can be encouraged to practice using different tones of voice. They can pretend to "Say it like Cookie Monster" and then "Say it again like Elmo." Children can help read along with familiar books that emphasize contrasts in vocal tone. An example would be *The Three Bears*. The child would be asked to say the lines the way the papa bear, the mama bear, and the baby bear would say them. Another activity would be to have the children choose an emotion card and produce a target utterance using a tone of voice that matches the emotion on their card. The same target utterances could be used, but the child practices manipulating various suprasegmental components such as pitch, loudness, vocal quality, and rate.

For older children, using variations in vocal tone can be practiced while reading books or comic strips. Choose books that contain lots of dialogue and a wide variety of characters with different personality traits. Comic strips are an excellent choice because they are loaded with dialogue and typically incorporate characters with very transparent personality characteristics. Help the child understand and use variations in pitch, rate, and vocal quality to achieve distinctions in tone of voice.

In summary, working on vowels and prosody is incredibly important and rewarding when supporting children with CAS. By working on these two areas in treatment, you are helping facilitate increased intelligibility, as well as helping the children's speech sound more natural.

References

Abbiati, C., & Velleman, S. (2021, July 8–10). *Prosody!? Reducing the stress of assessment and intervention* [Paper presentation]. Apraxia-Kids National Conference, Plano, TX, United States.

American Speech-Language-Hearing Association. (2007). *Childhood apraxia of speech* [Technical report]. http://www.asha.org/policy

Bowen, C. (2009). *Children's speech sound disorders*. Wiley-Blackwell.

Davis, B. L., Jacks, A., & Marquardt, T. P. (2005). Vowel patterns in developmental apraxia of speech: Three longitudinal case studies. *Clinical Linguistics and Phonetics, 19*, 249–274. https://doi.org/10.1080/02699200410001695367

Davis, B. L., Jakielski, K. J., & Marquardt, T. M. (1998). Developmental apraxia of speech: Determiners of dif- ferential diagnosis. *Clinical Linguistics & Phonetics, 12*, 25–45. https://doi.org/10.3109/02699209808985211

Dodd, B., Hua, Z., Crosbie, S., Holm, A., & Ozanne, A. (2006). *Diagnostic Evaluation of Articulation and Phonology (DEAP)*. Pearson Assessment.

Fudala, J. B., & Stegall, S. (2017). *Arizona Articulation and Phonology Scale, Fourth Revision (Arizona-4)*. Western Psychological Services.

Gerken, L., & McGregor, K. (1998). An overview of prosody and its role in normal and disordered child language. *American Journal of Speech-Language Pathology, 7*, 38–48. https://doi.org/10.1044/1058-0360.0702.38

Gibbon, F. E. (2009). Vowel errors in children with speech disorders. In C. Bowen (Ed.), *Children's speech sound disorders* (pp. 147–151). Wiley-Blackwell.

Gibbon, F. E. (2013). Therapy for abnormal vowels in children with speech disorders. In M. J. Ball & F. E. Gibbon (Eds.), *Handbook of vowels and vowel disorders* (pp. 429–446). Psychology Press.

Gibbon, F. E., & Mackenzie Beck, J. (2002). Therapy for abnormal vowels in children with phonological impairment. In M. Ball & F. Gibbon (Eds.), *Vowel disorders* (pp. 217–248). Butterworth-Heinemann.

Hawthorne, K., & Fischer, S. (2020). Speech-language pathologists and prosody: Clinical practices and barriers. *Journal of Communication Disorders, 87,* 106024. https://doi.org/10.1016/j.jcomdis.2020.106024

Huckvale, M. (2021). *Waveform, Annotations, Spectrogram & Pitch (WASP)* (Version 2.1) [Mobile app]. https://www.speechandhearing.net/laboratory/wasp/

Ingram, S. B., Reed, V. A., & Powell, T. W. (2019). Vowel duration discrimination of children with childhood apraxia of speech: A preliminary study. *American Journal of Speech-Language Pathology, 28,* 857–874. https://doi.org/10.1044/2019_AJSLP-MSC18-18-0113

Jakielski, K. J., & Gildersleeve-Neumann, C. E. (2018). *Phonetic science for clinical practice.* Plural Publishing.

Kent, R. D. (1992). The biology of phonological development. In C. A. Ferguson, L. Menn, & C. Stoel-Gammon (Ed.), *Phonological development: Models, research, implications* (pp. 65–90). York Press.

Kent, R. D., & Rountrey, C. (2020). What acoustic studies tell us about vowels in developing and disordered speech. *American Journal of Speech-Language Pathology, 29,* 1749–1778. https://doi.org/10.1044/2020_AJSLP-19-00178

Lindamood, P. C., & Lindamood, P. D. (2011). The *Lindamood Phoneme Sequencing Program for Reading, Spelling, and Speech* (LiPS; 4th ed.). Pro-Ed.

Maassen, B., Groenen, P., & Crul, T. (2003). Auditory and phonetic perception of vowels in children with apraxic speech disorders. *Clinical Linguistics and Phonetics, 17,* 447–467. https://doi.org/10.1080/026992 0031000070821

Munson, B., Bjorum, E. M., & Windsor, J. (2003). Acoustic and perceptual correlates of stress in nonwords produced by children with suspected developmental apraxia of speech and children with phonological disorder. *Journal of Speech, Language, and Hearing Research, 46,* 189–202. https://doi.org/10.1044/1092-4388(2003/015)

Murray, E., McCabe, P., & Ballard, K. J. (2015). A randomized controlled trial for children with apraxia of speech comparing Rapid Syllable Transition Treatment and the Nuffield Dyspraxia Programme (3rd ed.). *Journal of Speech, Language, and Hearing Research, 58,* 669–686. https://doi.org/10.1044/2015_JSLHR-S-13-0179

Norris, J. (2003). *Phonic Faces* (2nd ed.). EleMentory.

Peña-Brooks, A., & Hegde, M. N. (2007). *Assessment and treatment of articulation and phonological disorders in children* (2nd ed.). Pro-Ed.

Pollock, K. E., & Hall, P. E. (1991). An analysis of the vowel misarticulations of five children with developmental apraxia of speech. *Clinical Linguistics and Phonetics, 5,* 207–224. https://doi.org/10.3109/02699 209108986112

Post, B., & Payne, E. (2018). Speech rhythm in development: What is the child acquiring? In N. Esteve-Gibert & P. Prieto (Eds.), *Prosodic development in first language acquisition* (pp. 125–144). John Benjamins. https://doi.org/10.1075/tilar.23.07pos

Rosenbek, J., & Wertz, R. (1972). A review of fifty cases of developmental apraxia of speech. *Language, Speech, and Hearing Services in Schools, 3,* 23–33. https://doi.org/10.1044/0161-1461.0301.23

Shriberg, L. D., Aram, D. M., & Kwiatkowski, J. (1997). Developmental apraxia of speech: II. Toward a diagnostic marker. *Journal of Speech, Language, and Hearing Research, 40,* 286–312. https://doi.org/10.1044/jslhr.4002.286

Skinder, A., Strand, E. A., & Mignerey, M. (1999). Perceptual and acoustic analysis of lexical and sentential stress in children with developmental apraxia of speech. *Journal of Medical Speech-Language Pathology, 7,* 133–144.

Strand, E. A. (2020). Dynamic temporal and tactile cueing: A treatment strategy for childhood apraxia of speech. *American Journal of Speech-Language Pathology, 29,* 30–48. https://doi.org/10.1044/2019_AJSLP-19-0005

Strand, E. A., & McCauley, R. J. (2019). *Dynamic Evaluation of Motor Speech Skill (DEMSS).* Paul H. Brookes.

Strand, E. A., & Skinder, A. (1999). Treatment of developmental apraxia of speech: Integral stimulation methods. In A. Caruso & E. Strand (Eds.), *Clinical management of motor speech disorders in children* (pp. 109–148). Thieme.

Velleman, S. L. (2003). *Childhood apraxia of speech resource guide.* Delmar Learning.

Williams, P., & Stephens, H. (2010). The Nuffield Centre Dyspraxia Programme. In L. Williams, S. McLeod, & R. McCauley (Eds.), *Interventions for speech sound disorders in children* (pp. 159–177). Brookes.

Facilitating Speech and Language in Minimally Verbal Children

The suggestions provided in earlier chapters describe methods to shape increasingly accurate and flexible speech production in children with childhood apraxia of speech (CAS). For children to increase the complexity of word shapes and precision of articulation, however, they need to have some volitional control over the movement and timing of the speech mechanism. They need to be able to imitate with some degree of reliability. What about very young children who are at risk for sensorimotor speech and language impairment (e.g., children with a known etiology associated with sensorimotor speech impairment) and children who are not yet reliably able to coordinate the movement and timing of respiration, phonation, resonance, and articulation? This chapter focuses on ways to facilitate speech and language development in infants and toddlers at risk for speech and language delays, to motivate young children and children who are reluctant to attempt speech, and to facilitate vocal and verbal development in young children with suspected CAS or older children with very severe CAS who do not yet readily imitate. It also addresses development of early expressive language skills in children with CAS and the use of augmentative and alternative modes of communication (AAC).

Some of the strategies described in this chapter are beneficial in treatment of nonverbal or minimally verbal children despite their etiology. It is important to keep in mind, however, that a child's absence of verbal language and lack of verbal imitation skills can be attributed to etiologies unrelated to sensorimotor speech planning deficits. For example, a child with a severe cognitive impairment may not have some of the underlying cognitive/linguistic capacities required to develop verbal communication skills. A child with autism spectrum disorder may have weak communicative intent that will lead to delayed use of expressive language. A thorough discussion of differential diagnosis can be found in Chapter 2.

Infant Vocal Development

The vocal development of very young children is an evolving process. Although there is a general sequence from very early *reflexive* and vegetative *sounds* beginning at birth to production of *jargon* by the middle of the second year of life, there is overlap among the stages in the vocal development process. Nathani et al. (2012) describe the stages of vocal development in children from birth to 18 months. Box 6–1 summarizes these stages. Note how there is overlap between the stages. For example, a child will continue producing *quasi-resonant nuclei* even as they enter the stage where they begin to produce some fully resonant vowel-like sounds. When working with children who are not yet producing true words, you can chart their stage of vocal development and begin to build upon what they do have to move them closer to true canonical babbling, which is a precursor to use of true words.

Programs for Establishing Early Sensorimotor Speech Development and Expressive Language Skills in Infants and Toddlers at Risk for Sensorimotor Speech Disorders

A number of programs have been used to facilitate speech and language in very young children with delayed speech and language development or who are at risk for communication challenges. Three of these programs are described here.

Babble Boot Camp

An exciting new area of research pertaining to early intervention is showing us how children at risk for speech and language disorders can benefit from a proactive therapy approach starting with infants as young as 2 months old. The therapy program is called Babble Boot

■ Box 6–1. Summary of Vocal Development From Birth to 18 Months

0–2 months: Child produces reflexive sounds; vegetative sounds (burps, sneezes); crying and fussing; quasi-resonant nuclei (e.g., grunt-like sounds that lack full resonance)

1–4 months: Child produces clicks and raspberry noises; laughter; CV-like syllables without true vowels; vowel-like sounds that are fully resonant but not able to be transcribed

3–8 months: Child produces fully resonant vowels and sequences of vowels; squeals; marginal babbling

5–10 months: Child produces true CV syllables; repeated CV syllables

9–18 months: Child produces complex syllables beyond CV syllables (e.g., VC, CCV, CCVC); two-syllable sequences (e.g., VCV, VCVC); diphthongs; jargon (i.e., series of syllables with varied prosodic patterns)

Based on Nathani, Ertmer, & Stark (2006).

Camp (BBC). BBC is implemented through parent training by a speech-language pathologist (SLP) who specializes in early child development. Beate Peter, PhD, and her research team from Arizona State University, Washington State University, University of Washington, University of Minnesota, and Saint Louis University have been studying the effect of BBC on children with classic galactosemia (CG) ages 8 to 24 months. CG is a genetic disorder where the child is unable to metabolize galactose and often results in sensorimotor speech disorders and language impairment. Babies are universally screened for CG; thus, parents know immediately if their child has it. The high incidence of speech and language disorders and the early diagnosis make this the ideal population to study the impact of proactive intervention in the first 2 years of life. Preliminary results are very promising (Peter et al., 2019, 2021). Previous research indicates that 24% to 63% of children with CG have CAS, and 50% to 78% have a developmental language disorder (Peter et al., 2021). However, results from their 2021 study showed that after participation in BBC, all 12 children in the study receiving treatment had typical language scores, and 11 of the 12 had typical articulation scores. In the control group, one of the three untreated children had low articulation and expressive language scores. Hence, the evidence strongly supports this proactive method. With the increase in genetic testing and knowledge of which genes lead to disruption in neural development, the likelihood of other populations benefiting from this approach is high. It is also important to point out that BBC is taking place via telepractice. Given the increase in telepractice since COVID-19, this turned out to be fortuitous (for detailed instructions on BBC, go to https://osf.io/sy3en/). Following is a brief summary of the program.

Parents are first educated on typical communication milestones, as well as red flags for delays. Parents are then introduced to a progression of activities and routines that support typical development, and are coached in strategies to elicit specific communicative behaviors. Table 6–1 provides a summary of the activities and routines associated with BBC. An expected age of achievement for each activity/routine is provided; however, each child progresses through the program at their own rate, regardless of their chronological age. Parents are provided with a pamphlet that explains each activity and how often to engage in the activity. The activities are to occur at least 5 minutes a day (5+) or as part of the daily routine.

Although many of these activities may seem like they would naturally occur between a caregiver and their child, parent-child interactions tend to wain when a baby lacks vocalizations and babbling, as there is little initiation from the baby or reinforcement to the parent when the baby does not babble in response to the parent's vocalizations. Activities 7 and 8 could be extremely beneficial in assisting the parent during this important stage of development. Babbling is crucial to the child's speech development, as this is when "the infant is learning the mapping between acoustic-phonetic targets and the movement of their articulators to achieve those targets" (Rvachew & Brosseau-Lapré, 2021, p. 207). Using videos of babies babbling is consistent with research on the benefits of video modeling (Beating & Maas, 2021). Research from Franklin et al. (2014) further supports the benefits of parental interaction on the development of infant vocalizations and *volubility* and suggested that their TD participants learned that their vocalization had social value for parental interactions by 6 months of age.

There are potential effects on the child's skill development when treatment is provided proactively in children at risk for significant communication disorders. Early eye contact and talking to the baby set the stage for coupling of visual and auditory signals, while expressing emotion through our tone of voice and facial expression helps the child develop increased

Table 6–1. Progression of Activities and Routines for Infants and Toddlers Based on Babble Boot Camp Research

Expected Age of Acquisition in Typically Developing Children	Progression of Activities and Routines
Birth to 24 months	1. Make regular eye contact with the baby to establish and maintain bonding.
Birth to 4 months	2. Talk to the baby and imitate the child's nonreflexive sounds to establish turn taking.
Birth to 8 months	3. Use facial expressions to show emotions to establish and maintain bonding.
2–8 months	4. Reinforce vocalizations by activating a light-up toy in response to volitional sound production.
2–8 months	5. Imitate or respond to the child's cooing to reinforce vocalizations.
4–8 months	6. Reinforce dyadic exchanges by making silly faces and playing Peek-a-Boo.
6–12 months	7. Model babbling and gently move the child's lips while the child is vocalizing to stimulate babbling.
6–10 months	8. Increase quantity and quality of babbling by visiting with other babies or showing the child videos of other babies babbling.
6–12 months	9. Model and shape greetings (such as waving, saying "Hi") to increase social interaction skills.
6–12 months	10. Facilitate increased receptive vocabulary by pairing verbal cues with nonverbal cues.
6–24 months	11. Read books together to support increased receptive and expressive vocabulary.
8–18 months	12. Create a photo book to show the child pictures of important people, places, and objects in the family to increase receptive and expressive vocabulary.
8–24 months	13. Sing songs and pair the speech rhythm with the music rhythm to build rhythmic, phonemic, and rhyme awareness.
8–24 months	14. Label the people and objects to which the baby points to build receptive and expressive vocabulary.
10–24 months	15. Make comments about things that are happening using simple sentences to build language comprehension.
12–18 months	16. Use expansion by producing simple phrases/sentences in response to the child's single-word utterances to build expressive syntax.
14–24 months	17. Expand the child's short utterances by repeating them in longer sentences to build expressive syntax.

Note. Adapted from B. Peter (2020). Babble Boot Camp Activities and Routines.

awareness of pragmatic communication. When the parent responds to the child's vocalizations and models and responds to babbling, the child begins to associate the auditory and motor behaviors for vocalizations and speech-like sounds and increase their phonetic inventory. Further improvements in phonemic inventory and articulation skills are enhanced when the parent labels objects in the environment and models words. The use of *expansion* will support an increase in the complexity of the syntax of the child's language.

Given the success of BBC for children with CG, the research has expanded to children with Down syndrome and children who were born prematurely.

Wee Words

There are other programs that support children ages 2 years and above with suspected speech and language disorders. One such structured treatment program for children of at least 2 years of age is the Wee Words program. The Wee Words program (Kiesewalter et al., 2017) was designed for children ages 2:0 to 3:6 with suspected speech sensorimotor planning difficulties. Wee Words is a parent-child group-based program that focuses on facilitating development of children's imitation skills, speech sound repertoires, intelligibility, and expressive vocabulary development. Wee Words combines principles of motor learning using a variety of multisensory strategies to facilitate imitation skills, increase complexity of syllable shapes, increase phoneme repertoire, and increase expressive language skills. During an initial parent training session, parents are provided with information about typical speech sound development, principles of motor learning, and strategies to elicit communication and imitation skills (e.g., cueing, imitating the child, encouraging the child to watch their face while modeling, providing specific feedback).

Treatment occurred in groups, with five parent-child dyads, along with an SLP and a communicative disorders assistant who led group activities (e.g., songs, book reading). In addition, they provided coaching for each individual parent-child dyad. Each parent-child dyad would be provided with a specific set of toys and suggestions for how to facilitate production of target utterances, target phonemes, and selected syllable shapes during the activities. In a clinical report of pre- and posttreatment measures, Kiesewalter and colleagues reported that the children who received treatment showed improvement in expressive vocabulary, imitation skills, and increased their consonant phoneme repertoire and variety of word shapes.

Let's Start Talking

The Let's Start Talking (LST) program (Hodge & Gaines, 2017) provides support for preschool-age children of approximately 3.0 to 3.5 years of age with normal receptive language and severely delayed expressive speech and language by "helping children to learn to produce intelligible one- and two-syllable words with simple word shapes, using their existing phonetic inventory, in addition to systematically building their inventory (including vowels)" (p. 37). LST follows and builds upon Dynamic Temporal and Tactile Cueing (DTTC) and the PROMPT Motor Speech Hierarchy (see Chapter 4). Ten parent-child dyads received 8 weeks of twice-weekly individual treatment. Following treatment, significant increases were observed in several areas of speech development, including number of consonant types produced, syllable shape and consonant accuracy, use of recognizable speech sounds, number of intelligible words, and number of intelligible word types.

Facilitating Vocal and Verbal Development in Minimally Verbal Children

When children are able to imitate at least some speech sounds, their productions can be shaped into intelligible words. For children who do not imitate speech reliably, however, other treatment strategies must be utilized. DeThorne et al. (2009) described six evidence-based treatment strategies for facilitating speech development in young children who are not yet readily imitating speech sounds. The six strategies are as follows:

- **Minimize the pressure on the child to speak** because pressure to speak may increase frustration and anxiety related to communication.

- **Imitate the child's actions and sounds** to facilitate the child's own imitation skills.

- **Utilize exaggerated intonation** and slowed tempo when speaking to the child so the child develops a greater awareness of the salient aspects of the sounds and words you are attempting to elicit.

- **Provide salient auditory, visual, tactile, and proprioceptive feedback** so the child's ability to process information related to articulatory movement is maximized.

- **Provide access to AAC,** even while working on sensorimotor speech planning, to support the child's social and linguistic skill development.

- **Avoid emphasis on nonspeech oral motor exercises (NSOMEs),** as these have not been shown in peer-reviewed research to facilitate speech production.

These and other strategies are described in the following section in further detail.

Minimizing Pressure on the Child to Speak

When a child is reluctant to attempt verbal imitation, DeThorne et al. (2009) recommend reducing use of commands to speak or requiring the child to say a word before receiving a desired outcome (e.g., If you want the ball, tell me "ball."). Instead, they suggest using these tactics:

- Follow the child's lead during play, commenting on what the child is interested in.

- Use puppets as interactive partners. The child can interact vocally, verbally, and gesturally with the puppet, observe the clinician interacting with the puppet, and direct the puppet to do and say things (e.g., when playing doctor, direct the puppet to say, "ah").

- Incorporate familiar routines and interactions in naturalistic settings (e.g., giving baby a bath, feeding baby, and putting baby to bed).

- Avoid "test questions" that put the child on the spot (e.g., Tell us who you saw at the playground today. What did you eat for lunch?) and requests for direct imitation (e.g., "Say hi").

- Reduce time pressure to communicate.

Certainly, the child can be encouraged to communicate verbally, just not pressured to do so. When the child does vocalize, the clinician can assign meaning to the child's vocalization. If the child says "baba" while babbling, the clinician can bring out the bubbles, saying, "*I've got bubbles right here. Bubbles!*" If the child is pointing to a ball and says "da," the clinician can recognize "da" as a communicative request, give the child the ball, and tell the child how much you love their sounds and words (e.g., *"Oh, you want the ball. I love when you use your words to tell me what you want!"*). When the child makes babbling sounds, encourage the caregivers to express joy and excitement about how much they love the child's sounds and guide them in ways to make those sounds meaningful.

Build anticipatory vocal and verbal routines into play with the child. Games like *peekaboo* or verbal routines like *"ready, set, go"* provide the child with anticipation of what word is going to come next. If the child is engaged in a game of peekaboo and wants to keep going, you can pause right before saying "boo" and see if the child responds. Sometimes children will not speak the word but may close and round their lips as if they are getting ready to say the word. Reinforce the child's movement gestures by saying, *"Your mouth was ready to say 'boo!' Great job moving your lips!"* Building anticipatory routines is gradual and can take time for children with severe sensorimotor planning challenges. Box 6–2 provides an example of a routine that encourages both gestural and vocal responses.

■ Box 6–2. Building and Shaping Anticipatory Responses

The child and adult are playing on the floor. The child is feeding a baby doll and pretending to drink from a cup. The child offers a cup to the adult.

Adult: (Making drinking noises while pretending to drink from the cup with one hand and pointing to the approximate place of constriction for /g/ near the throat with the other) "guh guh guh guh guh guh guh, ah"

Child: (Giggles)

Adult: (Pretends to drink from the cup again) "guh guh guh guh guh guh guh, ah"

Child: (Giggles)

Adult: (Pretends to drink from the cup again) "guh guh guh guh guh guh guh, ah"

Child: (Giggles even more loudly)

Adult: (Holds the cup up, but does not pretend to drink; pauses and waits for a response from the child)

Child: (Pushes the cup toward the adult's mouth and smiles up at the adult expectantly)

Adult: (Pretends to drink from the cup) "guh guh guh guh guh guh guh, ah"

Child: (Giggles loudly)

Adult: (Sets the cup down)

Child: (Picks up the cup and hands it to the adult, then moves the cup toward the adult's mouth)

Adult: (Tips the cup, as if drinking, but does not make the associated drinking noises)

Child: (Says [dʌ] while looking up at the adult)

Adult: (Continues to "drink" from the cup) "guh guh guh guh guh guh guh, ah"

Child: (Smiles and giggles)

Imitate the Child's Movements and Sounds

For children who have not yet begun to imitate reliably, the clinicians and caregivers can begin imitating what the child is doing. When the child makes raspberry sounds or bangs their hands on the highchair tray, the adult can do what the child does in a joyful and animated way. If the child enjoys the adult reaction, they will want to keep this activity going by repeating the same action, or the child may do something new and see what type of reaction the child receives. This turn-taking routine, when solidly established, can be shifted from child-led to adult-led, so the child and adult are mirroring one another. DeThorne et al. (2009) described research by Snow (1989) that showed positive associations when adults increased their imitation of the child and an increase in the child's use of imitation.

When a child begins to vocalize and verbalize, it is beneficial to talk with the child about what the child is doing and how the child is doing it. If the child is producing /ba.ba.ba/, tell the child that their lips are opening and closing. The child who is making raspberry sounds can be told that their lips are vibrating or that the child sounds like a motorboat. These descriptions may lay a foundation for the child to understand their movements and can be used as reminders later for how to produce specific target sounds and words.

Model Using Exaggerated Intonations and Slowed Tempo

DeThorne et al. (2009) recommend using more exaggerated intonation patterns and speaking at a slower rate of speech when providing models for minimally verbal children. They suggest the "primary rationale for this strategy is that neural mechanisms involved in singing can be used to 'bootstrap' speech production due to partially distinct but also overlapping neural networks" (DeThorne et al., 2009, p. 138). The enhanced melodic nature of speech when we model with an exaggerated intonation pattern is similar to singing or chanting. Introducing melody and slower speaking rates enhances the speech model for the child. Exaggerated prosody can be combined with *Focused Stimulation* (Ellis Weismer & Robertson, 2006). Focused stimulation is used to heighten the child's awareness of specific phonemes or phoneme combinations. Target utterances can be emphasized by using these strategies:

- **Pausing** just before the target word is produced (e.g., *"Look, I found a . . . ball. Oh, here's another . . . ball."*).

- **Producing target words more slowly** and more frequently (e.g., *"Duck's going uuuup the ladder. Here he goes—uuuup, uuuup, uuuup. Duck's going uuuup."*).

- **Securing the child's visual attention** toward your mouth by pointing to your mouth, using gestural cues, or holding desired items near your mouth while you produce the target words.

- **Using greater vocal intonation** when modeling the target word. You can make your voice slightly louder and incorporate more dramatic vocal intonation and prosody when producing the target word.

By combining pausing, slower productions, visual attention, and vocal inflection when modeling target words, these keywords become more salient for the child, increasing the likelihood that the child will attempt to imitate them.

Singing provides a natural way of incorporating exaggerated prosodic patterns, vowel prolongation, and repeated modeling of target utterances. In addition to singing familiar children's songs, you can sing while modeling target utterances and create personal tunes that incorporate the child's target utterances. For example, for a child working on the phrase, "*Let me do it*" or the word "do," the clinician could sing "*Let me do it*" to the melody of *Frere Jacques* repeating the target multiple times, pausing where appropriate to allow the child to fill in some of the words:

Let me do it, let me do it.

Let me do it! Let me do it!

Let me let me do it. Let me let me do it.

Let me do it! Let me do it!

Chanting provides a fun way of using a call-out and response-style melody during therapy. Chants can incorporate functional words and phrases that are child specific:

Clinician: My name is Aaron. My name is . . .

Child: Aaron

Clinician: Yeah my name is Aaron. My name is . . .

Child: Aaron

Clinician: People call me Aaron. People call me . . .

Child: Aaron

Clinician: Yeah people call me Aaron. People call me . . .

Child: Aaron

Table 6–2 provides a list of several songs for young children that are useful for facilitating sound effects, simple word production, vowel variety, vocal imitation, and nonvocal imitation.

Provide Salient Auditory, Visual, Tactile, and Proprioceptive Feedback

Children with CAS may have reduced somatosensory awareness and respond less favorably to sensory feedback in natural circumstances. Thus, providing more salient sensory feedback is recommended. DeThorne et al. (2009) recommend using amplification (e.g., speaking through an Echo-microphone—available at some toy stores, party stores, or online; a Toobaloo—small U-shaped toy that can be held up to the ear and mouth; paper towel or wrapping paper rolls; or a piece of PVC pipe) to provide altered and enhanced auditory feedback.

Cueing can be enhanced using mirrors and puppets with movable mouths or placing a wide tube around the clinician's mouth so the child can focus on the clinician's mouth movements with reduced distractions.

Many children with apraxia demonstrate reduced tactile and proprioceptive processing (Ayres, 2005). By adding tactile and proprioceptive cues, we increase the child's ability to process information related to the motion, direction, force, and timing of the articulators. For example, when modeling the word *moo*, the clinician could press their fingers against the child's lips and hold for a second for /m/ before transitioning to the vowel. Shaping the child's lips in a rounded formation for the /u/ vowel in *moo* also offers increased tactile/proprioceptive saliency for the child. These cues provide a child with a sense of what it should feel like to say the target words, thus helping the child associate the feeling of the movement gesture with the sound of the utterance.

Table 6–2. Popular Children's Songs and Chants to Promote Early Speech Skills in Children

Song Titles	Speech and Language Skills Facilitated
Apples and Bananas	Vowel variety
Baby Bumblebee	Animal sounds; simple word production
BINGO	Vowel /o/
Down by the Bay	Rhyming; simple word production; vowel variety
Eentsy Weentsy Spider	Simple word production through sentence completion
Five Little Ducks	Counting; simple word production through sentence completion
Five Little Monkeys Jumping on the Bed	Counting; simple word production through sentence completion
Head, Shoulders, Knees, and Toes	Simple word production; vowel variety
I Love You (The Barney Song)	Simple word production
I Caught a Fish Alive	Counting; simple word production through sentence completion
If You're Happy and You Know It	Vocal and nonvocal imitation
John Jacob Jingleheimer Schmidt	Complex word production
London Bridge Is Falling Down	Simple word production through sentence completion
Old Macdonald Had a Farm	Animal sounds and vowel variety
One, Two, Buckle My Shoe	Simple word production; counting
Pat-a-Cake	Simple word production (especially bilabials)
Pop Goes the Weasel	Simple word production; nonvocal imitation
Ring Around the Rosy	Simple word production
Row, Row, Row Your Boat	Simple word production; early developing vowels /i, o/
The Alphabet Song	Vowel variety; production of CV and VC combinations
The Wheels on the Bus	Simple word production
This Is the Way . . .	Vocal and nonvocal imitation; simple word production
This Old Man	Simple word production
Twinkle, Twinkle Little Star	Simple word production
Wibbely Wobbely Woo	Complex word production

Embed AAC Into Treatment

According to ASHA (n.d.), "Augmentative and alternative communication (AAC) describes multiple ways to communicate that can supplement or compensate (either temporarily or permanently) for the impairment and disability patterns of individuals with severe expressive communication disorders." AAC does not imply a specific mode of communication but, rather, a wide array of communication methods that can be used in combination. Communication modes typically are divided into two types: aided and unaided communication. *Unaided communication* is any type of communication that relies only on the person's body to convey the message (e.g., speech, gestures), whereas *aided communication* requires the use of an external tool to convey the message. The range of aided communication options is broad and may include low-tech options such as writing or picture boards, as well as high-tech options such as voice output communication aids (VOCAs). Figure 6–1 provides a diagram of various communication systems sorted between aided and unaided modes. These modes of communication can be used in combination; therefore, it is highly unusual for an individual to rely solely on one mode to meet all communication needs. In fact, multimodal communication should be encouraged.

Benefits of AAC

AAC can be particularly beneficial for children with severe sensorimotor speech disorders who have limited expressive speech or reduced speech intelligibility. A child with very limited speech may rely on AAC as the primary means of communication. For a child who produces speech, but whose speech intelligibility is limited, AAC can be a way to augment existing speech.

Whether AAC is used regularly or intermittently, temporarily, or long term, children with CAS may receive several benefits from its use:

- increased efficiency of communication
- increased effectiveness of communication
- increased quantity and quality of the child's language
- increased opportunities for social interaction across a wider range of settings, with a wider variety of individuals, and for a wider range of communicative functions
- decreased reliance on familiar adults to serve as interpreters
- decreased communicative passivity
- reduced challenging behaviors caused by limited ability to express ideas

Considerations in Use of AAC in Treatment

A number of dilemmas face SLPs with regard to the use of augmentative communication as part of treatment programs for children with apraxia of speech. Questions may surface concerning when the right time would be to introduce AAC into treatment, how much time to spend teaching the child to use the augmentative system when a significant amount of time is needed to address speech itself, which augmentative system is most appropriate for a given child at a given age, what vocabulary to select for a communication device, and how to

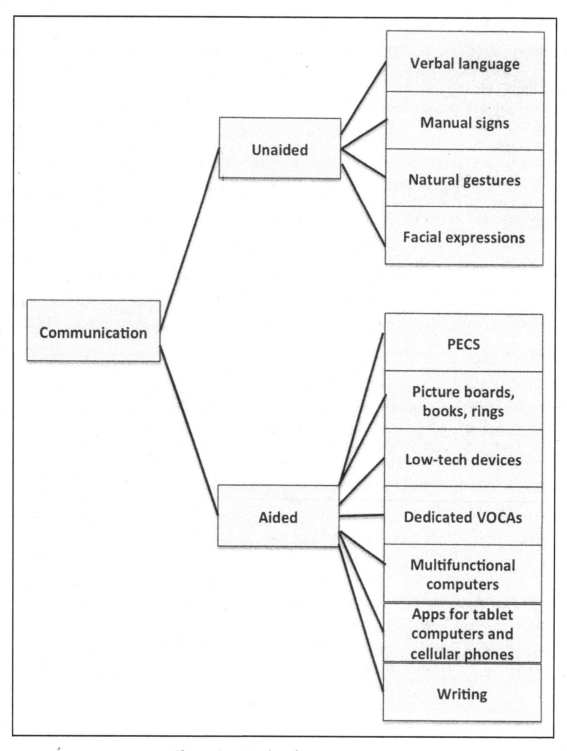

Figure 6–1. Modes of communication.

introduce the topic of AAC with parents. When AAC looks like it may be used as more than a temporary incorporation of some manual signs or use of a limited selection of pictures to use when verbal communication is breaking down, it will be important to complete a multi-disciplinary AAC evaluation where a team of professionals assesses cognitive function, motor accessibility, visual acuity and hearing status, and speech and language skills. This will help guide the team toward selecting the most appropriate AAC system for the child. Kuhlmeier (2021) recommends applications like AAC Genie (https://humpsoftware.com/aacgenie.html), the Communication Matrix (https://www.communicationmatrix.org/), and the Student, Environment, Task, and Tools (SETT) framework (Zabala, 2005) as frameworks for selection of AAC systems.

When Should AAC Be Introduced Into Treatment?

Basic manual signs and communication boards can be introduced right from the start of treatment, even for very young children with CAS. There is no need to wait for extended periods of time before introducing signs, gestures, or picture selection strategies into treatment. If AAC is provided only as a last resort and only after all attempts to elicit speech have been tried, the child will have missed months or years of opportunities to establish intentional, symbolic communication, and to become an active participant in the communication process. The child can be taught manual signs and natural gestures for high-frequency words (more, mine, all done, yes, no) while simultaneously working on verbal production of these same words. Picture boards and books can be provided, and the child can be taught to use these pictures to make choices or comments during various routines (play, mealtime, bath). After adequate verbal production has been attained for the target word, the use of signs or picture selection strategies will be extinguished naturally.

How Much Time Should Be Devoted to Use of AAC?

Intensive work to address the child's speech production should be at the forefront of the treatment program for a child with CAS. To support the child's expressive language and social communication, however, a multimodal program of communication should be integrated into the child's treatment. Cumley and Jones (1992) recommend facilitating the use of gestures, manual signs, and picture symbols as adjuncts to speech therapy in young children with CAS. Finding the right balance of intensive practice in speech praxis and continuing to enhance expressive language using an augmentative system of communication is challenging, but necessary, for some children with CAS. When AAC is introduced, parents should be taught how to incorporate it into the child's daily routines. If children have opportunities to practice communicative interaction using AAC in a wider range of settings, it allows the SLP to spend a greater portion of time addressing prevocal and vocal communication goals during the treatment sessions.

What Type(s) of AAC Systems Are Most Beneficial for Children With CAS?

The types of communication modes that would be most beneficial would depend on the individual needs and abilities of each child. To determine which type(s) of AAC to introduce to a child, consider the following factors:

- **Portability.** How easy is it for the child to transport the system?
- **Readability.** Can the communicative partners easily interpret the child's message?
- **Cost.** What is the cost of the system, including programming and repairs?

- **Flexibility and efficiency.** How much flexibility does the system offer to formulate any possible message, and how quickly and efficiently can the child formulate a message?
- **Motor requirements.** Does the child have the sensorimotor skills and coordination necessary to use the system effectively?

Selecting Vocabulary for Communication Boards

When selecting vocabulary for communication boards (picture boards, low- and high-tech systems), be sure to choose appropriate vocabulary. Consider the following:

- Choose vocabulary that will facilitate a wide range of communicative functions (e.g., greeting, requesting, rejecting, protesting, describing, commenting, providing information, expressing feelings, joking).
- Vocabulary should be appropriate for the child's age and cognitive functioning.
- Incorporate vocabulary that is specific to the child's environments and interests (home, school, community).
- Select vocabulary that represents a wide range of linguistic categories to allow for opportunities to combine words into phrases and sentences (e.g., names, nouns, verbs, descriptors, interjections, conjunctions).
- Vocabulary should provide opportunities for the child to participate more fully in imaginative play.
- Select vocabulary that helps facilitate greater participation in the classroom and other group activities (circle-time, curriculum units, games).
- Change vocabulary as needed to facilitate linguistic growth.

Cumley and Jones (1992) recommend the use of miniboards for children who are mobile to reduce the challenges of portability. Miniboards, described by Beukelman and Mirenda (1992), are single topic boards that are placed in specific locations (e.g., bathtub area, kitchen table, the child's play area, reading corner in the classroom), so they are available readily without having to be transported from place to place. Miniboards can be created to facilitate communication related to specific books the child is reading, specific thematic units in school, and special activities or events (holidays, birthday parties, field trips). Portability also can be achieved by using communication wallets that can be placed in a pocket or picture rings that can be attached to a belt or backpack. These may be handy to use in the community (e.g., ordering food at a restaurant) or for quick access to frequently used phrases across multiple environments.

Addressing Parent Concerns About AAC

Parents often express serious concerns regarding the introduction of augmentative communication into treatment. Understandably, they worry about whether their child may lose the desire or motivation to work on verbal communication if the child is provided with an easier way to express ideas. Take time to educate parents about the complex nature of communication and how all areas of communication—receptive and express language, social language, and articulation—need to grow together in unison. If speech is very slow in coming and the child has no other ways to reliably communicate, the child's expressive language development and social language functioning will be compromised. It can be helpful to share with parents that speech development is facilitated when AAC is incorporated into communication programs (Millar et al., 2006; Zangari & Kangas, 1997).

Avoid Emphasis on NSOMEs

There has been a great deal of controversy regarding the use of NSOMEs in speech therapy. No study has been published to date in peer-reviewed journals showing NSOMEs facilitating any significant changes in speech production of a child with CAS. That said, it may be appropriate to work on some functional, nonspeech skills—such as blowing, kissing, licking lips, and so forth—that may have social implications for a child with oral apraxia. It may also be appropriate to *shape* the movement required for accurate production of a specific phoneme using a nonspeech activity. A child struggling to achieve lip rounding for /u/ and /o/ may benefit from rounding lips around a lollipop or straw to achieve lip rounding while being asked to vocalize the vowel. Tongue clicks may help shape production of alveolar phonemes, and coughing may be beneficial for shaping velar phonemes. A note of caution here is that intensive, repetitive production of NSOMEs to build muscle strength is not appropriate for treating children with CAS, as children with CAS need to work on volitional speech productions to build muscle memory, not on strength building.

Facilitate More Robust Imitation

Treatment of CAS requires the child to watch the clinician and try to imitate what the clinician says. Young and minimally verbal children may struggle with imitation, so imitation will need to be taught. Begin by determining what types of movements (gross motor, fine motor, oral-facial, vocalizations, speech) the child is able to imitate, and progress from there. The following is a general guide to facilitating motor imitation skills in children who do not readily imitate speech. Although this list is a progression from simple to more challenging motor movements, these stages overlap, so it should be considered a rough guide:

- large motor movements (e.g., clapping hands, banging on a table, stomping feet)
- actions with objects (e.g., banging a stick on a table like a drum, banging two blocks together)
- more subtle movements, gestures, and signs (e.g., wiggling fingers, shaking head, producing simple manual signs such as *more*, *eat*, or *cookie*)
- oral-facial movements (e.g., clicking and protruding tongue, licking lips, blowing kisses, smacking lips)
- vocal play (e.g., raspberries, gurgling)
- vocal imitation (e.g., "baba," "puhpuhpuh," "mmmm," "uh oh")

Encourage the child to make silly noises and produce environmental sounds. Sounds such as animal and vehicle noises often develop prior to the production of true words. Examples of toys that may elicit these early sounds include the following:

- toy animals (growling bear, panting, or barking dog, meowing cat, braying horse, snorting pig, chattering monkey, buzzing bee)
- toy vehicles (beeping truck horn, helicopter propeller, zooming motorcycle, screeching car brakes, steam engine noise, train horn noise)

- food-related toys (popcorn popping, fry pan sizzling, water faucet noise, gulping drinks, "ah" after a thirst-quenching drink, noisy chewing, yummy "mmmmm" food, microwave beeping)
- dolls and other people toys (hiccups, coughing, sneezing, burping, startle "ah," noisy yawn)

Many books for young children encourage the production of sound effects. The books in Box 6–3 offer opportunities to facilitate sound effects such as animal noises and environmental sounds.

■ Box 6–3. Books to Elicit Environmental Sounds

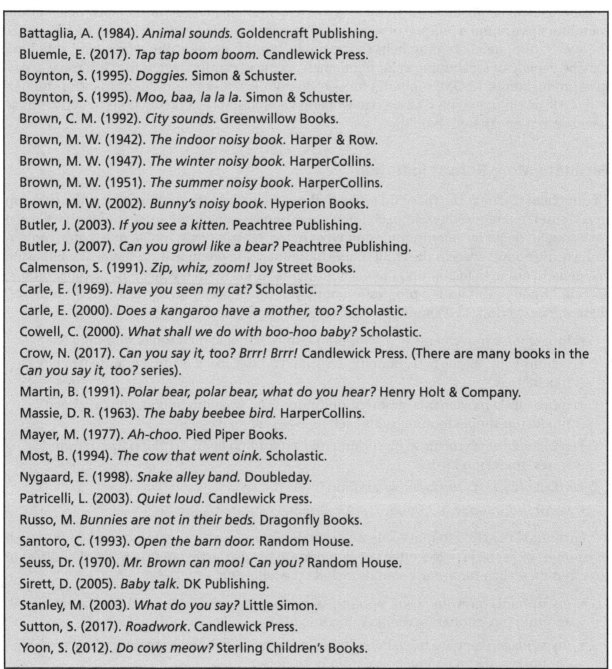

Battaglia, A. (1984). *Animal sounds.* Goldencraft Publishing.

Bluemle, E. (2017). *Tap tap boom boom.* Candlewick Press.

Boynton, S. (1995). *Doggies.* Simon & Schuster.

Boynton, S. (1995). *Moo, baa, la la la.* Simon & Schuster.

Brown, C. M. (1992). *City sounds.* Greenwillow Books.

Brown, M. W. (1942). *The indoor noisy book.* Harper & Row.

Brown, M. W. (1947). *The winter noisy book.* HarperCollins.

Brown, M. W. (1951). *The summer noisy book.* HarperCollins.

Brown, M. W. (2002). *Bunny's noisy book.* Hyperion Books.

Butler, J. (2003). *If you see a kitten.* Peachtree Publishing.

Butler, J. (2007). *Can you growl like a bear?* Peachtree Publishing.

Calmenson, S. (1991). *Zip, whiz, zoom!* Joy Street Books.

Carle, E. (1969). *Have you seen my cat?* Scholastic.

Carle, E. (2000). *Does a kangaroo have a mother, too?* Scholastic.

Cowell, C. (2000). *What shall we do with boo-hoo baby?* Scholastic.

Crow, N. (2017). *Can you say it, too? Brrr! Brrr!* Candlewick Press. (There are many books in the *Can you say it, too?* series).

Martin, B. (1991). *Polar bear, polar bear, what do you hear?* Henry Holt & Company.

Massie, D. R. (1963). *The baby beebee bird.* HarperCollins.

Mayer, M. (1977). *Ah-choo.* Pied Piper Books.

Most, B. (1994). *The cow that went oink.* Scholastic.

Nygaard, E. (1998). *Snake alley band.* Doubleday.

Patricelli, L. (2003). *Quiet loud.* Candlewick Press.

Russo, M. *Bunnies are not in their beds.* Dragonfly Books.

Santoro, C. (1993). *Open the barn door.* Random House.

Seuss, Dr. (1970). *Mr. Brown can moo! Can you?* Random House.

Sirett, D. (2005). *Baby talk.* DK Publishing.

Stanley, M. (2003). *What do you say?* Little Simon.

Sutton, S. (2017). *Roadwork.* Candlewick Press.

Yoon, S. (2012). *Do cows meow?* Sterling Children's Books.

Limit the Number of Target Stimuli

For children who are minimally verbal, the number of target utterances introduced during a session should be limited to just a few (Strand, 2020). Follow a blocked practice schedule when introducing new targets by repeating the same target many times in a row before moving on to a different stimulus item. By limiting the number of stimulus items per session, the child has the opportunity to practice a small set multiple times to begin to establish volitional control and develop sensorimotor plans for producing those words. If five or six target utterances are chosen for a session, one or two specific utterances can be incorporated into each practice activity so as not to overwhelm the child by trying to practice too many new movement plans at once.

Using Scaffolding and Shaping

Scaffolding and shaping are extremely beneficial during the treatment process, even with minimally verbal children. As a child gains sensorimotor control over a simplified production of a target utterance, the complexity of the target gradually can be increased. The sample script in Box 6–4 offers an example of using scaffolding to facilitate production of a CV word with a child who is minimally verbal.

■ Box 6–4. Using Scaffolding From Isolated Vowel to Elicit CV Production

Clinician: Whose turn is it to blow the bubbles?

Child: (points to Mom)

Clinician: Okay, Mommy's blowing bubbles! (Mom blows bubbles and child pops them) Who popped all those bubbles?

Child: (points to self) "eeee" [i]

Clinician: Wow! You popped a lot of bubbles. I like how you pointed to yourself and said, "Me." Let's practice the word "me" again. Close your lips and say, "me."

Child: [i]

Clinician: Great smiley lips, but we need to use the humming sound, "mmm." Let's do it together. Close your humming lips and say "me."

Clinician and Child together: Clinician–"me," Child—[i]

Clinician: You're trying hard. We'll practice our humming lips again. Time to blow more bubbles. (child blows bubbles) Who blows bubbles now?

Child: (points to self) "eeee" [i]

Clinician: Let's practice "me" again. We'll just say the last part, "ee."

Clinician and child together: [i]

Clinician: Great, let's do a few more—"ee."

Child: [i, i, i, i]

continues

■ Box 6–4. *continued*

Clinician: You did it just like me. Now let's try a new way. Close your lips. Let's see your humming lips.

Child: (closes lips)

Clinician: Yay, your lips are ready to go. Say [mi] (the /m/ model is prolonged).

Clinician and Child together: [mi] (Clinician applies a tactile cue to facilitate production of /m/)

Clinician: Yes! You made your humming sound—"me" (/m/ is prolonged; bubbles are offered for the Child to blow). Whoo hoo! So many bubbles that time! Now who gets to blow the bubbles?

Child: (points to self) [i]

Clinician: Woops. Let's find that humming sound. (pretends to look around for the sound) Oh, there it is. Right on your lips! "Me." (/m/ is prolonged)

Clinician and Child together: [mi, mi, mi] (using tactile cue)

Clinician: Fabulous humming lips! Time to blow some bubbles. Whoa! Who made all those big bubbles? Let's make our humming lips together. . . .

Clinician and Child together: [mi] (no tactile cue, just simultaneous production)

Clinician: Great humming! Four more. (Clinician holds up four fingers)

Clinician and Child together: [mi mi]

Child alone: [mi mi] (Clinician miming)

Clinician: That was terrific. So many humming sounds. You can blow bubbles two times for all those great humming sounds!

Addressing Language Goals in Treatment

Children with CAS frequently demonstrate significant expressive language challenges including limitations in the areas of syntax and morphology (Ekelman & Aram, 1983). Ekelman and Aram's findings suggest that the mean length of utterance (MLU) of children with CAS was not a good indicator of the integrity of the syntactic or grammatical abilities of the children. Children with CAS exhibited omissions or incorrect productions of grammatical elements and pronouns that could not be attributed to limitations in sensorimotor speech planning or phonology. Lewis et al. (2004) found that many children with CAS exhibited significant receptive as well as expressive language deficits, although expressive language typically lagged behind receptive language. An important role of the SLP is to assess, identify, and prioritize all the child's communicative needs and determine how and when to address each deficit area.

Expand Vocabulary Variety to Facilitate Phrase Production

A careful analysis of a child's expressive vocabulary will help provide ideas of ways that early phrases can be facilitated. It also may uncover holes in the child's vocabulary that reduce the opportunities for combining words to form phrases. For instance, a child whose vocabulary consists primarily of object labels will have difficulty formulating meaningful phrases. Some ready-made picture sets for apraxia and articulation will hinder the expansion of vocabulary from a wider range of parts of speech. Vocabulary will need to be expanded beyond labels to include pronouns, verbs, adjectives, adverbs, prepositions, conjunctions, articles, and interjections.

Use Carrier Phrases to Expand Utterances

The use of *carrier phrases* is a common treatment strategy in apraxia intervention (Velleman, 2003). When teaching carrier phrases, the phrase shell remains the same, with the exception of the target word(s), which changes. Considerations when choosing carrier phrases include the following:

- Initially the stable portion of the carrier phrase should be relatively easy for the child to produce (e.g., *"Hi ___;" "more ___;" "no ___;" "___ in"*) so that the child is not challenged on the target word and the carrier phrase simultaneously.
- The carrier phrase should be functional so there are opportunities to practice the phrase in a variety of settings and within the context of a variety of activities.
- As children advance, the complexity of the carrier phrase can be more challenging:
  - *Target phoneme /s/. "Sit on a _____."* (seat, sock, seven, circle)
  - *Target phoneme /dʒ/. "I jumped over a _____."* (jet, jelly bean, giant, giraffe)

Table 6–3 lists several sample carrier phrases with play activities that could be used to practice these phrases and short sentences in a session.

Facilitate Early Semantic Relations

An additional benefit of moving quickly into production of phrases and sentences is that it enables the child to begin to develop more complex syntactic structures. Developing more complex syntax is essential because the clarity of a speaker's message is not based solely on the integrity of the articulation but also on the complexity of the language. For instance, a child may produce the word "ball." Out of context, it is difficult for the listener to interpret the meaning of the message. The child may be trying to request a ball, show someone a ball, indicate that Dad possesses a ball, or request assistance in finding a ball that has been lost. Unless more linguistic information is provided, the interpretation of the message can be understood only in context.

Children combine words in a variety of ways that Brown (1973) described as "minimal two-term relations" (p. 173) that are prevalent in Stage I (MLU <1.75), and our target utterance selection should reflect that variety. The semantic relations described by Brown include the following:

- Agent and action—*"Daddy go."*
- Action and object—*"drink juice"*
- Agent and object—*"Daddy juice"*
- Action and location—*"go home"*
- Entity and location—*"book car"*

Table 6–3. Carrier Phrases with Corresponding Language Activities

Two-Word Carrier Phrases	Corresponding Language Activities
Hi _____.	Greeting toy characters: "Hi, Mommy."
Bye-bye _____.	Putting toys away: "Bye-bye, bunny."
(subject word) _____ go	Animals, characters, or toy people going down slide: "Boy go"
(subject word) _____ in/on/up	Animal characters going on a school bus: "Cow in"
	Toy characters climb up a mountain: "Pooh up"
More _____	Blowing bubbles: "More blow"
No _____	Reading "Where's Spot?" book: "No puppy"
(number word) _____	Reading counting books: "one sheep, two sheep, three sheep"
(color word) _____	Making a potato head toy or a jack-o-lantern picture: "blue eyes" "red mouth"
My _____	Choosing food for cooking activity: "My apple"
Three-Plus Word Carrier Phrases	**Corresponding Language Activities**
It's a _____.	Using feely box—place hand inside box, feel what's inside, and tell what it is: "It's a spider."
I got a _____.	Playing Go Fish game or Memory game—tell what you got when you turned over a picture: "I got a duck."
I found a _____.	I Spy game—using a flashlight, find "hidden" toys: "I found a ring"
I have (a) _____ _____. You have (a) _____.	Describing clothing or physical characteristics of self and other person: "I have blue socks." "You have no socks."
I want (a) _____. I want (a) _____ _____.	Telling what piece you need to complete a sticker picture or block structure: "I want a red block."
Do you have a _____?	Playing Go Fish game: "Do you have a big house?"

- Possessor and possession—"*mama shoe*"
- Entity and attributive—"*big book*"
- Demonstrative and entity—"*there ball*"

In addition, Brown describes other two-term semantic relations cited in research literature, including the following:

- Nominative—"*that ball*"
- Recurrence—"*more dog*"
- Nonexistence—"*no hat*"

Brown described four common three-term relations observed at Stage I:

- Agent, action, and object—"*Doggy eat bone.*"
- Agent, action, and location—"*Daddy go home.*"
- Agent, object, and location—"*Mommy hat chair*"
- Action, object, and location—"*roll ball hole*"

Combining Word Shape Goals and Grammar Goals

Facilitating production of morphological markers (e.g., present progressive "-ing," first person singular "s," plural "s" and "es," past tense "ed," possessive "s") can be accomplished within the context of speech praxis treatment. When choosing targets, consider the word shape complexity required for incorporating various morphological markers into language. A word shape goal can be combined with a grammar goal, allowing the child to upgrade sensorimotor speech planning while simultaneously developing more complex grammar skills. Table 6–4 provides sample lists demonstrating how word shape goals and grammar goals can be combined within the context of treatment along with sample words for each goal area.

When introducing morphological markers, Velleman (2003) puts forth a suggested order when working with children with CAS. One of her recommendations is to choose targets in which the addition of a *bound morpheme*, such as plural "s" or past tense "ed," does not require the child to produce a final cluster. It likely would be easier for a child to produce plural "s" in words like "eyes," "bows," and "toys," than in words like "hats," "ducks," and "cups," just as it would be easier for a child to produce past tense "ed" in words like "cried," "mowed," and "dried," than in words like "hopped," "brushed," and "opened."

Another way to introduce morphological markers is to practice groups of words that have like endings. Table 6–5 shows how words with similar movement patterns can be grouped to help establish motor patterns that may make the targets easier to produce. Picture cues for the present progressing "ing" endings or plural, third person singular, and possessive "s" endings can provide an additional cue to remind the child of the insertion of the morphological marker, as shown in Figure 6–2.

Incorporate Repetitive Line Books and Counting Books Into Treatment

Repetitive line books provide another way of facilitating repeated productions of target words and phrases in treatment in a more naturalistic manner. Books can be read verbatim or modified to encourage production of specific targets. Lederer and Arnston (2008) and Ellis Weismer and Robertson (2006) recommend using books that offer multiple opportunities for the target to be modeled using a focused stimulation approach when working with children with early language delay and expressive language disorders. For instance, a children's book such as *Where's Spot?* (Hill, 1980) offers multiple opportunities to practice words such as "open," "no," and "door." Sample repetitive line books are listed in Box 6–5.

Counting books also are useful in treatment, as there are multiple opportunities to practice the target utterances in a natural language activity. Rather than counting "1, 2, 3, 4 . . . ," the pictures are used to prompt production of target utterances each time they appear.

Table 6–4. Addressing Syllable/Word Shape Goals and Grammar Goals Simultaneously

WORD SHAPE GOAL: IMPROVE PRODUCTION OF CVC SHAPE	
Grammar Goals: Increase Production of . . .	**Sample Words**
Third person singular 's' marker	goes, buys
Plural 's' marker	toys, bees
Possessive 's' marker	guy's, cow's
Regular past tense verbs	rowed, mowed
Contractions	he's, she's

WORD SHAPE GOAL: IMPROVE PRODUCTION OF VCC SHAPE	
Grammar Goals: Increase Production of . . .	**Sample Words**
Third person singular 's' marker	eats, aims
Plural 's' marker	eggs, apes
Possessive 's' marker	Ed's, Ann's
Regular past tense verbs	aimed, owned
Contractions	it's, aren't

WORD SHAPE GOAL: IMPROVE PRODUCTION OF CVCC SHAPE	
Grammar Goals: Increase Production of . . .	**Sample Words**
Third person singular 's' marker	gets, hops
Plural 's' marker	hats, bones
Possessive 's' marker	dog's, dad's
Regular past tense verbs	pushed, moved
Contractions	don't, that's

WORD SHAPE GOAL: IMPROVE PRODUCTION OF CV.CVC SHAPE	
Grammar Goals: Increase Production of . . .	**Sample Words**
Present progressive '-ing'	baking, digging
Regular past tense verbs	waited, needed
Third person singular 'es' marker	buzzes, loses
Plural 'es' marker	buses, noses
Possessive 's' marker	Liz's, goose's
Contractions	should've, could've

WORD SHAPE GOAL: IMPROVE PRODUCTION OF CVC.CVC SHAPE	
Grammar Goals: Increase Production of . . .	**Sample Words**
Present progressive '-ing'	painting, bending
Regular past tense verbs	wanted, painted
Third person singular 'es' marker	rinses, dances
Plural 'es' marker	benches, fences

Table 6–5. Grouping Words With Similar Motor Patterns to Facilitate Production of Grammatical Morphemes

Present Progressive '-ing'	
[-kɪŋ]	walking, taking, making, working
[-dɪŋ]	hiding, riding, feeding, kidding
[-sɪŋ]	crossing, dressing, passing, missing
[-mɪŋ]	drumming, humming, swimming, coming
[pkɪŋ]	hopping, hoping, wiping, keeping
[-wɪŋ]	sewing, mowing, doing, rowing
[-tʃɪŋ]	marching, teaching, reaching, catching
Regular Past Tense	
[-ɑpt]	stopped, popped, dropped, hopped
[-ɪpt]	slipped, tripped, dipped, tipped
[-ɛrd]	shared, cared, stared, dared
[-eɪd]	played, neighed, paid, weighed
Irregular Past Tense	
[-ɔt]	bought, fought, caught, taught
[-ɛpt]	wept, kept, slept, leapt
[-ʌŋ]	hung, sung, wrung, flung
/-u/	drew, flew, grew, knew
Plural 's'	
/æts/	hats, cats, bats, mats
/ɑɪz/	eyes, ties, flies, guys
/æps/	maps, caps, laps, naps
Third Person Singular 's'	
/ɑɪz/	flies, buys, tries, dries
/ɪts/	sits, fits, hits, knits
/ɑps/	hops, drops, pops, stops

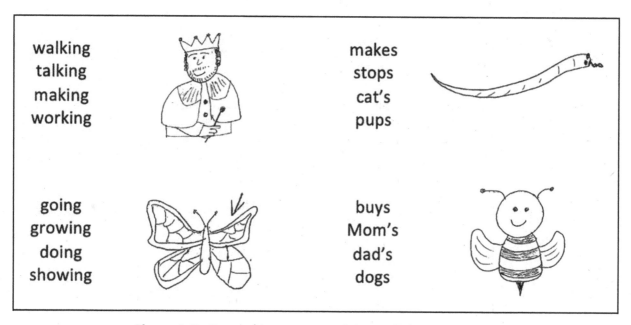

walking
talking
making
working

makes
stops
cat's
pups

going
growing
doing
showing

buys
Mom's
dad's
dogs

Figure 6–2. Sample picture cues to elicit morphological markers.

■ Box 6–5. Repetitive Line Books

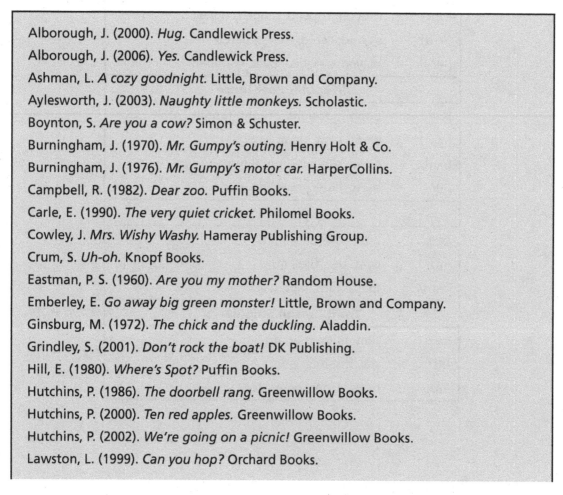

Alborough, J. (2000). *Hug.* Candlewick Press.

Alborough, J. (2006). *Yes.* Candlewick Press.

Ashman, L. *A cozy goodnight.* Little, Brown and Company.

Aylesworth, J. (2003). *Naughty little monkeys.* Scholastic.

Boynton, S. *Are you a cow?* Simon & Schuster.

Burningham, J. (1970). *Mr. Gumpy's outing.* Henry Holt & Co.

Burningham, J. (1976). *Mr. Gumpy's motor car.* HarperCollins.

Campbell, R. (1982). *Dear zoo.* Puffin Books.

Carle, E. (1990). *The very quiet cricket.* Philomel Books.

Cowley, J. *Mrs. Wishy Washy.* Hameray Publishing Group.

Crum, S. *Uh-oh.* Knopf Books.

Eastman, P. S. (1960). *Are you my mother?* Random House.

Emberley, E. *Go away big green monster!* Little, Brown and Company.

Ginsburg, M. (1972). *The chick and the duckling.* Aladdin.

Grindley, S. (2001). *Don't rock the boat!* DK Publishing.

Hill, E. (1980). *Where's Spot?* Puffin Books.

Hutchins, P. (1986). *The doorbell rang.* Greenwillow Books.

Hutchins, P. (2000). *Ten red apples.* Greenwillow Books.

Hutchins, P. (2002). *We're going on a picnic!* Greenwillow Books.

Lawston, L. (1999). *Can you hop?* Orchard Books.

■ **Box 6–5.** *continued*

Litman, E. *Groovy Joe: Disco party bow wow.* Scholastic.

Litman, E. *Groovy Joe: Ice cream and dinosaurs.* Scholastic.

Marshall, J. (1989). *The three little pigs.* Scholastic.

Mayer, M. (1983). *I was so mad.* Golden Books.

Mayer, M. (1983). *Me, too.* Golden Books.

Mericle Harper, C. *Go! Go! Go! Stop!* Knopf Books.

Patricelli, L. *Yummy yucky.* Candlewick Press.

Seuss, Dr. (1960). *Green eggs and ham.* Random House.

Shannon, D. *Duck on a bike.* Blue Sky Press.

Shaw, C. (1947; 1988). *It looked like spilt milk.* HarperCollins.

Waddell, M. (1992). *Owl babies.* Candlewick Press.

Watts, F. (2010). *That's not my _____* [collection of books]. Usborne.

West, C. (1997). *"Buzz, buzz, buzz," went Bumblebee.* Candlewick Press.

West, C. (1997). *"I don't care!" said the bear.* Candlewick Press.

Wilburn, K. (1984). *The gingerbread boy.* Grosset & Dunlap.

Williams, L. (1986). *The little old lady who was not afraid of anything.* HarperCollins.

Williams, S. (1989). *I went walking.* Harcourt Brace Jovanovich.

Wilson, K. *Bear feels scared.* Margaret K. McElderry Books.

Wood, A. (1984). *The napping house.* Harcourt Brace.

Wood, A. (1985). *King Bidgood's in the bathtub.* Harcourt Brace.

Wren, R. *Yum, yum, baby!* Cottage Door Press.

Zimmermann, H. W. (1989). *Henny Penny.* Scholastic.

Consider making your own counting books and fill them with pictures representing the targets your client is working on. Figure 6–3 provides an example of a counting book for a child working on functional words and phrases. Those that require fewer repetitions are placed on the first pages, and words requiring more practice are on subsequent pages.

Modification of Target Utterances

When functional target utterances are challenging for children, consider ways to make the target stimuli more manageable. This can help the child gain linguistic control of functional words and phrases, enhance motivation to speak, and increase overall volubility of speech. Three specific ways in which target utterances can be modified to build success are described. Each of these modification strategies provides children with a different way of producing the target utterance *for now*. As children's sensorimotor skills improve, there also would be an

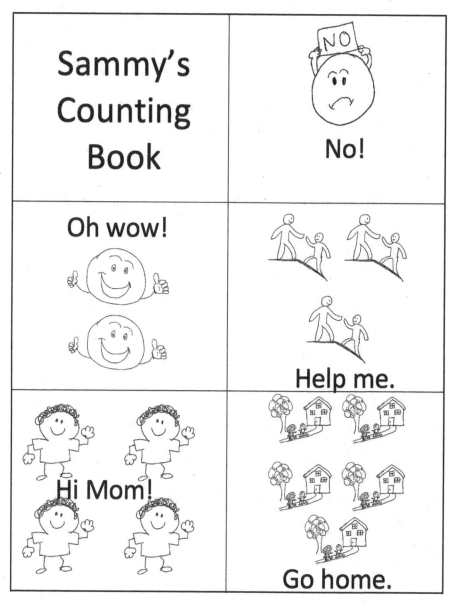

Figure 6–3. Counting book to address functional words/phrases.

expectation that the complexity of the target utterance would shift from the simplified production toward the correct adult form of the utterance.

When choosing a simplification of a target word for a child, it is important to keep other people with whom the child interacts regularly apprised of the acceptable modifications. This may include parents, grandparents, siblings, teachers, and other clinicians. In this way, the child's best speech attempts can be validated and reinforced. The following strategies for modifying target stimuli are described in the next sections:

- choose alternate target vocabulary
- teach successive approximations
- allow for nonstandard articulatory placement

Alternate Target Vocabulary

When a specific target word is too challenging for a child, another word that is synonymous with the target word can be used in its place. Table 6–6 provides suggestions for choosing alternate targets when the child's sensorimotor skills do not support the production of the adult form of the target. One example listed in Table 6–6 is substituting "Uh uh" for "No." Not having a way to express opposition, refusal, or rejection can be frustrating for children and their families. Providing a child with the means to express feelings of opposition by offering a substitute word can be very empowering and help reduce frustration.

Successive Approximations

Successive approximations, based on the concept of shaping from behavioral psychology theory, are commonly used for treatment of articulation disorders (Bankson & Bernthal, 2004; Secord et al., 2007). When using successive approximations, you allow the learner to produce target utterances that are phonetically modified to make them more manageable. In articulation treatment, successive approximation moves the client gradually closer to the desired target phoneme through a series of progressive steps. A systematic approach using successive approximation for treatment of CAS was developed and described by Kaufman (1998), who describes her Kaufman Speech to Language Protocol (K-SLP) as "the employment of phonological processes to simplify words so the child can then learn successive approximations toward target words to achieve a 'functional' vocabulary" (p. 1). Target utterances are taught through a series of small steps that move the learner gradually closer to the desired behavior: the correct adult form of the utterance. A more detailed description of K-SLP can be found in Chapter 4.

Nonstandard Articulatory Placement

Occasionally compensatory placements for phonemes are beneficial when working with children with CAS. For instance, if a child struggles with production of alveolar phonemes

Table 6–6. Suggested Alternate Targets

Target Utterance	Suggested Alternate Target
Cow	"Moo moo"
Sheep	"Bah bah"
Grandma	"Nana"
Grandpa	"Papa"
Yes	"Uh huh," "Yeah," or "Mm hmm"
No	"Uh uh"
Refrigerator	"Fridge"
Ghost	"Boo"
Train	"Choo choo"
Be quiet	"Shh"

such as /t, d, n, l/, they may be achieved by teaching a slight dental production, thus providing greater tactile feedback to the speaker. As the child gains more motor control and gradation of movement, they will be able to shift to a more traditional placement of the target phoneme.

It can be quite challenging to work with minimally verbal children who do not readily imitate speech. Meeting them where they are in their development and using evidence-based treatment strategies to support their speech and language development can help them become more competent communicators.

References

American Speech-Language-Hearing Association. (n.d.). *Augmentative and alternative communication* [Practice portal]. https://www.asha.org/Practice-Portal/Profes sional-Issues/Augmentative-and-Alternative-Com munication/

Ayres, A. J. (2005). *Sensory integration and the child: Understanding hidden sensory challenges*. Western Psychological Services.

Bankson, J. E., & Bernthal, N. W. (2004). Treatment approaches. In N. W. Bernthal & J. E. Bankson (Eds.), *Articulation and phonological disorders* (5th ed.). Allyn & Bacon.

Beating, M., & Maas, E. (2021). Autism-centered therapy for childhood apraxia of speech (ACT4CAS): A single-case experimental design study. *American Journal of Speech-Language Pathology, 30*, 1525–1541. https://doi.org/10.1044/2020_AJSLP-20-00131

Beukelman, D. R., & Mirenda, P. (1992). Serving young children with AAC needs. In D. Beukelman & P. Mirenda (Eds.), *Augmentative and alternative communication: Management of severe communication disorders in children and adults* (pp. 175–202). Paul H. Brookes.

Brown, R. (1973). *A first language: The early stages*. Harvard University Press.

Cumley, G., & Jones, R. (1992). Persons with primary speech, language, and motor impairments. In D. Beukelman & P. Mirenda (Eds.), *Augmentative and alternative communication: Management of severe communication disorders in children and adults* (pp. 229–251). Paul H. Brookes.

DeThorne, L. S., Johnson, C. J., Walder, M. A., & Mahurin-Smith, J. (2009). When "Simon says" doesn't work: Alternatives to imitation for facilitating early speech. *American Journal of Speech-Language Pathology, 18*, 133–145. https://doi.org/10.1044/1058-0360 (2008/07-0090)

Ekelman, B. L., & Aram, D. M. (1983). Syntactic findings in developmental verbal apraxia. *Journal of Communication Disorders, 16*, 237–250. https://doi .org/10.1016/0021-9924(83)90008-4

Ellis Weismer, S., & Robertson, S. (2006). Focused stimulation approach to language intervention. In R. McCauley & M. Fey (Eds.), *Treatment of language disorders in children* (pp. 175–201). Paul H. Brookes.

Franklin, B., Warlaumont, A. S., Messinger, D., Bene, E., Iyer, S. N., Lee, C. C., . . . Oller, D. K. (2014). Effects of parental interaction on infant vocalization rate, variability and vocal type. *Language Learning and Development, 10*(3), 279–296. https://doi.org/10.10 80/15475441.2013.849176

Hill, E. (1980). *Where's Spot?* Penguin Books.

Hodge, M., & Gaines, R. (2017). Pilot implementation of an alternate service delivery model for young children with severe speech and expressive language delay. *Canadian Journal of Speech-Language Pathology and Audiology, 41*, 34–57.

Kaufman, N. R. (1998). *Kaufman Speech Praxis Treatment Kit For Children*. Northern Speech Services.

Kiesewalter, J., Vincent, V. A., & Lefebvre, P. (2017). Wee words: A parent-focused group program for young children with suspected motor speech difficulties. *Canadian Journal of Speech-Language Pathology and Audiology, 41*, 58–70.

Kuhlmeier, A. (2021). *AAC evaluations: Criteria and considerations for a successful outcome* [Paper presentation]. Virtual Apraxia-Kids 2021 National Conference on Childhood Apraxia of Speech.

Lederer, S., & Arnston, R. (2008). *Beyond Brown Bear: First words, focused stimulation, storybooks & songs* [Paper presentation]. 2008 ASHA Conference, Chicago, IL, United States.

Lewis, B. A., Freebairn, L. A., Hansen, A. J., Iyengar, S. K., & Taylor, H. G. (2004). School-age follow-up of children with childhood apraxia of speech. *Language, Speech, and Hearing Services in Schools, 35*, 122–140. https://doi.org/10.1044/0161-1461(2004/014)

Millar, D., Light, J. C., & Schlosser, R. W. (2006). The impact of augmentative and alternative communication intervention on the speech production of individuals with developmental disabilities: A research review. *Journal of Speech, Language, and Hearing Research, 49*, 248–264. https://doi.org/10.1044/1092-4388(2006/021)

Nathani, S., Ertmer, D. J., & Stark, R. E. (2006). Assessing vocal development in infants and toddlers. *Clinical Linguistics & Phonetics, 20*, 351–369. https://doi.org/10.1080/02699200500211451

Peter, B. (2020). *Babble Boot Camp activities and routines.* https://osf.io/sy3en/

Peter, B., Davis, J., Cotter, S., Belter, A., Williams, E., Stumpf, M., . . . Potter, N. (2021). Toward preventing speech and language disorders of known genetic origin: First post-intervention results of Bubble Boot Camp in children with classic galactosemia. *American Journal of Speech Language Pathology, 30*, 2616–2634. https://doi.org/10.1044/2021_AJSLP-21-00098

Peter, B., Potter, N., Davis, J., Donenfeld-Peled, I., Finestack, L., Stoel-Gammon, C., . . . VanDam, M. (2019). Toward a paradigm shift from deficit-based to proactive speech and language treatment: Randomized pilot trial of the Babble Boot Camp in infants with classic galactosemia. *F1000Research, 8*, 271. https://doi.org/10.12688/f1000research.18062.5

Rvachew, S., & Brosseau-Lapré, F. (2021). Speech perception intervention. In A. L. Williams, S. McLeod, & R. J. McCauley (Eds.), *Interventions for speech sound disorders in children* (pp. 201–224). Paul H. Brookes.

Secord, W. A., Boyce, S. E., Donohue, J. S., Fox, R. A., & Shine, R. E. (2007). *Eliciting sounds: Techniques and strategies for clinicians* (2nd ed.). Thomson Delmar Learning.

Snow, C. E. (1989). Imitativeness: A trait or a skill? In G. E. Speidel & K. E. Nelson (Eds.), *The many faces of imitation in language learning* (pp. 73–90). Springer-Verlag.

Strand, E. A. (2020). Dynamic temporal and tactile cueing: A treatment strategy for childhood apraxia of speech. *American Journal of Speech-Language Pathology, 29*, 30–48. https://doi.org/10.1044/2019_AJSLP-19-0005

Strand, E. A., & Skinder, A. (1999). Treatment of developmental apraxia of speech: Integrated stimulation methods. In A. J. Caruso & E. A. Strand (Eds.), *Clinical management of motor speech disorders in children* (pp. 109–148). Thieme.

Velleman, S. L. (2003). *Childhood apraxia of speech resource guide.* Delmar Learning.

Zabala, J. (2005). Ready, SETT, go! Getting started with the SETT framework. *Closing the Gap: Computer Technology in Special Education and Rehabilitation, 23*(6), 1–3.

Zangari, C., & Kangas, K. (1997). Intervention principles and procedures. In L. Lloyd, D. Fuller, & H. Arvidson (Eds.), *Augmentative and alternative communication* (pp. 235–253). Allyn & Bacon.

CHAPTER

Addressing Early Literacy Concerns in Children With Childhood Apraxia of Speech

The Relationship Between Speech and Literacy

Parents of children with severe speech sound disorders frequently express concern about what impact their child's speech impairment may have on later literacy development. They may question whether a child who is unable to say words accurately also may have difficulty reading and spelling those words. Research has demonstrated that *phonological awareness* is known to be a critical factor in literacy success (Catts & Kamhi, 2005). *Phonological awareness* is defined as "the ability to reflect on and manipulate the *structure* of an utterance (e.g., into words, syllables, or sounds) as distinct from its meaning" (Stackhouse, 1997, p. 157). It involves the awareness that words can be broken down into smaller segments such as the individual syllables of a multisyllabic word (e.g., ba + na + na = "banana"), onset and rime (e.g., m + ap = "map"), or individual sounds (e.g., /k/ + /o/ + /t/ = "coat").

A study by Bird and colleagues (1995) found that children with speech sound disorders (SSDs) performed more poorly on phonological awareness tasks than their peers, even if they did not have accompanying expressive language problems. This was confirmed by Anthony et al. (2011), who found that children with SSDs demonstrated poorer performance on phonological awareness tasks than language-matched peers without SSDs. They also found that weak underlying *phonological representations* may contribute to poor performance on phonological awareness and reading tasks. Preston and Edwards (2010) observed that preschoolers with SSDs (not specifically childhood apraxia of speech [CAS]) who exhibited atypical sound errors (e.g., intervocalic consonant deletion; additions of syllables, vowels, and consonants; backing of front consonants; replacement of stops with fricatives; prevocalic devoicing) performed more poorly on phonological awareness tasks than children with more typical sound errors or

273

distortion errors. McNeill and colleagues (2008) reported that children between the ages of 4 and 7 years with CAS performed more poorly on phonological awareness tasks than children with typical speech-language development and children with inconsistent speech disorder. Challenges in phonological awareness, reading, and spelling in children with CAS have been cited by many researchers (e.g., Lefebvre et al., 2017; Lewis et al., 2004; Marion et al., 1993; Miller et al., 2019). Not all children who have a history of speech and/or language challenges will have later challenges with literacy; however, when significant speech difficulties persist past 5 years of age, the risk for literacy difficulties increases (Stackhouse, 1997). If we know that children with CAS are at much greater risk for literacy challenges than their typically developing peers, it behooves speech-language pathologists (SLPs) to integrate phonological awareness intervention in conjunction with motor speech intervention to strengthen phonological awareness development and early reading skills (Gillon & Moriarty, 2007).

A wide range of skills and knowledge bases come together to support literacy development. Some of these include vocabulary development, morphological knowledge, language comprehension, prior background knowledge, strength of phonological representations, exposure to print, letter recognition, phonological awareness, sound-letter knowledge, and orthographic knowledge. The SLP plays a crucial role in assessing (or being sure someone on the child's team is assessing) the child's skill development in all of these areas and addressing those areas of need that may contribute to the child's literacy success (Schuele & Boudreau, 2008). For a review of the roles and responsibilities of SLPs with respect to reading and writing, refer to the American Speech-Language-Hearing Association (ASHA) guidelines (2001).

Supporting Literacy Development in Children With Severe SSDs

A question that comes to mind is how the SLP can support a child's development across multiple areas in an effective and efficient way. Anthony et al. (2011) suggest "that the most efficient forms of therapy for children with SSDs may be those that comprehensively integrate training in speech perception, expressive phonology, speech motor coordination, phonological awareness, and phonics rather than . . . treatment approaches with a more narrow focus" (p. 157). Many of the skills that underlie literacy can be addressed in the context of speech praxis treatment without compromising the goal of improving speech intelligibility. In a study by Gillon (2005), children as young as 3 and 4 years of age with moderate to severe SSDs (not specifically CAS)—who received intervention targeting improving speech intelligibility, facilitating phoneme-level phonological awareness skills, learning sound-letter names, and developing sound-letter correspondence—made remarkable gains in all targeted areas of treatment. Further, children who received this combined intervention demonstrated greater reading and spelling success in early elementary grades than children whose intervention only addressed speech intelligibility. It should be noted that the combined intervention program did not compromise children's progress in speech development. Studies by McNeill, Gillon, and Dodd (2009, 2013) utilized an integrated phonological awareness program to facilitate speech and phonological awareness development in children with CAS. The majority of children in the study demonstrated gains in speech, phoneme awareness, and letter-sound knowledge, suggesting that integrated phonological awareness intervention facilitates improved phonological awareness and speech development in some children with CAS. Their follow-up study (2013) indicated that although the participants improved in these areas immediately following intervention, their rate of growth in these skills did not continue post intervention, suggesting that children with CAS will need ongoing support with written language skills.

A variety of tips and activities for supporting phonological awareness, letter knowledge, and sound-letter association are described in this chapter. The following activities are not intended to be an exhaustive list or a complete phonological awareness program, but rather suggestions for efficient ways to incorporate phonological awareness, in particular, *phoneme awareness*, into the context of apraxia treatment. Phoneme awareness relates to "conscious awareness that words are made up of individual sounds" (Gillon, 2005, p. 309).

When Introducing Letters and Sound-Letter Correspondence, Draw the Child's Attention to the Look and Feel of the Sound

Lease (2014) recommends taking opportunities during articulation therapy to talk with the child about what is happening motorically when producing various sounds. This may include information like whether the primary movement is occurring in the lips or the tongue, the shape of the lips, if airflow is prominent, if the sound is quick or prolonged, or if the voice is turned on or off. Multisensory cueing like this is a key component of literacy programs and tools that are available, for example, *Lindamood Phoneme Sequencing Program for Reading, Spelling, and Speech (LiPS)* (Lindamood & Lindamood, 2011), the *Orton-Gillingham Program Approach* https://www.ortonacademy.org/), the *Barton Reading & Spelling System* (https://bartonreading.com/), *Lively Letters* (https://www.readingwithtlc.com/), and *Phonic Faces* (https://www.elementory.com/).

Use Written Letters as Cues When Working on Specific Phonemes

The letter(s) representing the speech sound the child is working on can be written on an index card, on each practice picture, or on the board (Figure 7–1). A game board, with a game path in the shape of the letter representing a specific target phoneme, can be used in treatment to bring the child's attention to the letter-sound association for the practice sounds.

Visually Supported Alphabets

Many children struggle to understand how the graphemic representation of a letter makes a sound. This could partly be due to how letter sounds are often taught. For example, the instructor may say "A is for apple" and "B is for banana." A child will only be successful with knowing the first letter represents the sound if they are capable of segmenting the sounds of the word and isolating the first sound. Phonological awareness tasks such as this can be difficult for some children with CAS (Gillon & Moriarty, 2007). When this is the case, consider tools that provide additional cues to help the child conceptualize the sound the letter is making. *Lively Letters* (https://www.readingwithtlc.com/) is a program that provides an embedded image in the letter and uses mouth, hand, and body cues, in addition to musical animations, and mnemonic stories, that make learning the letter sounds more engaging and salient. Their materials can be found on the readingwithtlc.com website. Similarly, *Phonic Faces* (Norris, 2003) also uses multisensory cues and graphics to teach letter sounds. Imagery is incorporated by embedding the letter(s) representing the phoneme on a character's face in the place and/ or manner that the sound is produced. For example, the /p/ is taught as a sound Peter Pops

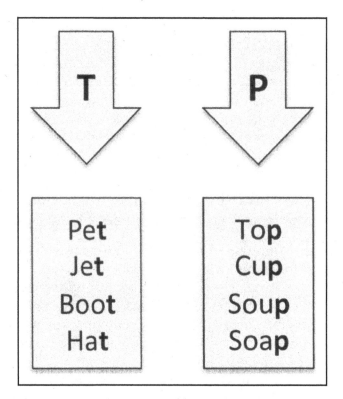

Figure 7–1. Facilitating sound-letter association in speech therapy.

produces with the letter "p" coming off the lips and a puff of air. Figure 7–2 provides examples of the graphemic images used for phonemes /p, t, k, ʃ/ and /r/. (*Phonic Faces* was discussed in Chapter 5 for teaching vowels.) The *Phonic Faces* program also uses mnemonic stories, handwriting methods, and multiple activities, which are available on their website (elementory. com) and in their manual for teaching letter-sound correspondence, blending sounds into words, spelling words, and understanding phonics principles.

Tools such as *Lively Letters* and *Phonic Faces* are particularly useful with children in preschool through second grade and children with intellectual and developmental disabilities. These visually supported alphabets, which include multisensory cuing (e.g., tactile, kinesthetic, visual, and auditory cues), can help the child with both perception of the sound and production of the letter sound. The visual supported alphabet will then need to be faded to transfer these skills to traditional grapheme identification (i.e., letters). This, in turn, should result in stronger letter-sound correspondence skills, which is a crucial building block in the development of early literacy skills (Schuele & Boudreau, 2008).

Write the Target Words on Practice Word Cards

When the target words are written on each practice picture (Figure 7–3), the SLP can draw the child's attention to various aspects of the written words.

A specific letter or letters can be highlighted with a marker to make an orthographic element(s) more salient. Target sound letters can be written larger than the other letters or in a different color than other letters. Specific syllables in multisyllabic words can be highlighted,

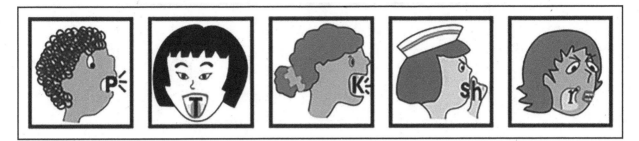

Figure 7–2. Phonic faces representing the letters for /p, t, k, ʃ/ and /r/. (*Phonic Faces* reprinted with permission from Janet Norris.)

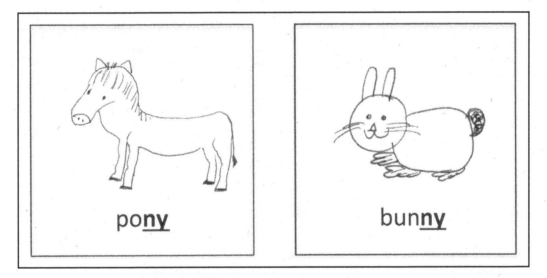

Figure 7–3. Speech picture cards with attention to sound-letter association.

written with a space between them, or written in different colors. These visual cues can be used to help children recognize the following:

- Specific sounds generally correspond with specific alphabetic letters.
- Words that begin or end with the same sound often are written with the same letter(s).
- Different letters may correspond to the same sound (e.g., F = /f/; PH = /f/; GH = /f/).
- Longer words (typically) have more letters than shorter words.
- Words that rhyme often are written with the same ending letters (e.g., *at* in cat, hat, rat, bat).
- Syllables in multisyllabic words can be separated and counted.
- Sounds in words can be separated (segmented) and put back together (blended).

Use Blocks or Another Visual Cue System to Support Syllable Blending and Sound Blending

Using blocks that represent syllables or individual sounds (Figure 7–4) may help children develop improved syllable-level and phoneme-level awareness.

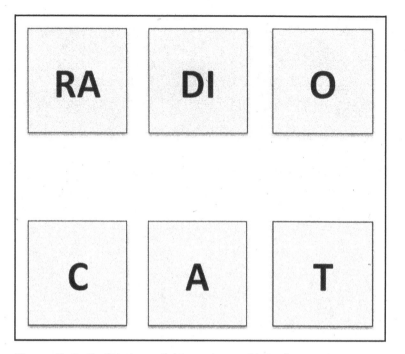

Figure 7–4. Facilitating syllable and sound blending and segmenting in context of speech praxis treatment.

It may be necessary to introduce blending in an order from syllable blending (e.g., "I'm going to say a word in a funny way. Try to guess what word I'm saying: *pea . . . nut.*"), to onset and rime blending ("*m . . . at*"), and then phoneme blending ("*f . . . a . . . n*"). Working on phoneme blending is important because phoneme-level awareness was strongly predictive of later reading skills (Hulme et al., 2002). Blending and segmenting tasks involving individual phonemes and letters should be introduced as early as children are able to manage work at this level.

To make blending tasks more manageable, early on the child can be asked to identify the blended word from a set of picture choices (e.g., "Look. There are three pictures here. I'll name each picture in a funny way, and I want you to find the picture I am naming. Find *b . . . u . . . s*"). When appropriate, integrate the child's target stimuli for speech practice into this and other phonological awareness activities.

Create New Words Using Phoneme Replacement Activities

When helping children establish production of CVC, CVCC, and CCVC word shapes, the clinician can use words with the same rime pattern (e.g., *at* "cat," "bat," "hat," "sat," "mat") and change the onset portion of the word to create different words. Provide a card for the rime portion of the word (e.g., "at") and change the onset portion of the word by adding different letters (as shown in Figure 7–5). Developing flexibility in both speech and the corresponding phoneme-level awareness associated with those phonemes can be beneficial for children. Phoneme manipulation tasks initially involving changing one letter of VC (it, in, if), CV (no, go, so), or CVC (top, hop, mop, pop; bet, bed, beg, Ben) words can help strengthen children's phoneme awareness (e.g., "This word says *at*. If we want to change *at* to *am*, what letter would

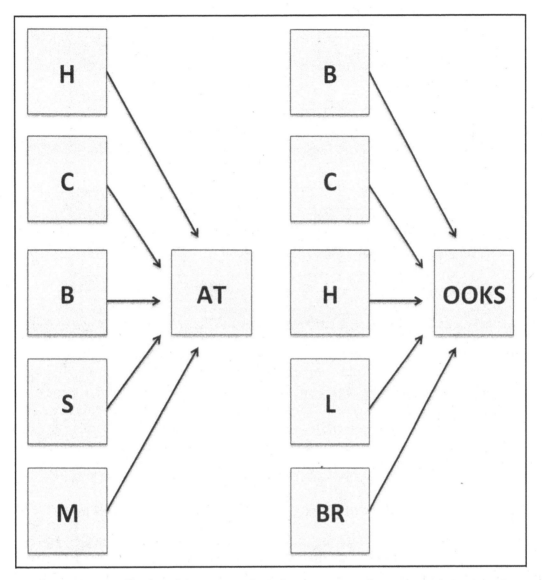

Figure 7–5. Facilitating phoneme manipulation in context of speech praxis treatment.

we need to put in the place of 't'?"). Introducing phonemes that are easy for the child to identify and to discriminate (e.g., /m/ versus /t/) would be introduced first.

Assist the Child in Sorting the Target Words or Picture Cards in Various Ways

The child's target words and picture cards can be sorted in a variety of ways, as shown in Boxes 7–1 and 7–2, to help children recognize common features. They can be sorted by beginning sound, ending sound, number of syllables, ending syllable, or vowel. For example, a child working on two-syllable words with varied consonants and vowels may sort the words ending with the same final syllable. A child working on differentiating sibilant sounds may sort words beginning with the /s/ sound versus /ʃ/ sound. Discussion related to different ways the /s/ and /ʃ/ sounds can be spelled also would support literacy.

■ BOX 7–1. Examples of Sorting Targets by Same Second Syllable

bunny, funny, honey, pony, penny

waited, stated, hated, rated

walking, raking, talking, making

busy, dizzy, fuzzy, crazy, lazy

■ BOX 7–2. Examples of Sorting Targets by Same Initial Consonant

sick, cell, circus, sign

shell, shock, chef, Chicago

Incorporate Books Containing Rhyming and Alliteration Into Treatment

Books that reinforce rhyme patterns in words containing word shapes or phonemes the clinician is addressing in treatment can be incorporated into therapy sessions. The use of rhyming books and books with *alliteration* (many words beginning with the same phoneme) is an efficient way to address target phonemes in treatment, while reinforcing preliteracy skills. Many of the Dr. Seuss books incorporate rhyme and alliteration patterns. Usborne Books (http://www.usborneonline.com/speech.htm) offers a collection of rhyming stories for children ages 3 years and up.

Incorporate Songs, Finger Plays, Poems, and Nursery Rhymes Into Treatment

Rhyme is a feature of phonological awareness that can be incorporated easily into treatment using songs, poetry, and children's nursery rhymes. Drawing children's attention to word endings based on common sound patterns supports both speech practice and phonological awareness. Lists of nursery rhymes and songs appropriate for young children can be found in Chapter 6.

Group Instruction

Often the research gives SLPs and parents the impression that children with CAS are best served in a one-on-one therapy session. Although this may be true for obtaining multiple repetitions for the purpose of improving sensorimotor planning skills, it is not always the case for working on language and literacy skills. Many of the techniques discussed up to this point can be worked on in a group setting. It is estimated that between 20% and 30% of children in the early grades struggle with learning how to read (IRIS Center, n.d.). Hence, addressing early literacy skills is crucial for a population much larger than just our children with CAS. Children with reading disabilities typically need explicit phonological awareness instruction. "The more sensitive that children are to the sound structure of spoken words, the more likely that they will become strong readers irrespective of educational measures, such as socioeconomic status, intelligence, and receptive vocabulary" (Carson et al., 2013, pp. 147–148). Research has clearly shown the benefits of addressing phonological awareness in the classroom, starting as young as preschool, for children with and without SSDs (e.g., Carson et al, 2013; Ehri et al., 2001; Gillon et al., 2020).

As alluded to earlier, the SLPs' background knowledge in phonological awareness can be a critical asset to the educational team (Schuele & Boudreau, 2008). It behooves the school SLP, early educators, and reading specialists to work as a team to ensure the children at risk for reading disabilities are being identified early and are receiving evidence-based phonological awareness instruction. In addition, the SLP could assist the teacher and reading specialist in differentiating early literacy instruction and understanding the unique needs of children with CAS so that each child is being challenged at the appropriate level. The SLP may also provide small-group intervention, allowing for further scaffolding supports for children with greater needs. Addressing the child's early literacy needs in small groups and in the classroom will allow the SLP more time to integrate phonological awareness into their speech practice during their individual sessions.

References

American Speech-Language-Hearing Association. (2001). *Roles and responsibilities of speech-language pathologists with respect to reading and writing in children and adolescents* [Guidelines]. https://www.asha.org/policy.

Anthony, J. A., Greenblatt Aghara, R., Dunkelberger, M. J., Anthony, T. I., Williams, J. M., & Zhang, Z. (2011). What factors place children with speech sound disorders at risk for reading problems? *American Journal of Speech-Language Pathology, 20*, 146–160. https://doi.org/10.1044/1058-0360(2011/10-0053)

Bird, J., Bishop, D. V. M., & Freeman, N. H. (1995). Phonological awareness and literacy development in children with expressive phonological impairments. *Journal of Speech and Hearing Research, 38*, 446–462. https://doi.org/10.1044/jshr.3802.446

Carson, K., Gillon, G., & Boustead, T. (2013). Classroom phonological awareness instruction and literacy outcomes in the first year of school. *Language, Speech, and Hearing Services in Schools, 44*, 147–160. https://doi.org/10.1044/0161-1461(2012/11-0061)

Catts, H., & Kamhi, A. (2005). Defining reading disabilities. In H. Catts & A. Kamhi (Eds.), *Language and reading disabilities* (2nd ed., pp. 50–71). Pearson Education.

Ehri, L. C., Nunes, S. R., Willows, D. M., Schuster, B. V., Yaghoub-Zadeh, Z., & Shanahan, T. (2001). Phonemic awareness instruction helps children learn to read: Evidence from the National Reading Panel's meta-analysis. *Reading Research Quarterly, 36*(3), 250–287. https://doi.org/10.1598/RRQ.36.3.2

Gillon, G. (2005). Facilitating phoneme awareness in 3- and 4-year-old children with speech impairment. *Language, Speech, and Hearing Services in Schools, 36*, 308–324. https://doi.org/10.1044/0161-1461(2005/031)

Gillon, G., McNeill, B., Denton, A., Scott, A., & Macfarlane, A. (2020). Evidence-based class literacy instruction for children with speech and language difficulties. *Topics in Language Disorders, 40*(4), 357–374. https://doi.org/10.1097/TLD.0000000000000233

Gillon, G., & Moriarty, B. (2007). Childhood apraxia of speech: Children at risk for persistent reading and spelling disorder. *Seminars in Speech and Language, 28*(1), 48–57. https://doi.org/10.1055/s-2007-967929

Hulme, C., Hatcher, P. J., Nation, K., Brown, A., Adams, J., & Stuart, G. (2002). Phoneme awareness is a better predictor of early reading skill than onset-rime awareness. *Journal of Experimental Child Psychology, 82*, 2–28. https://doi.org/10.1006/jecp.2002.2670

IRIS Center. (n.d.). *What approaches are available to schools to help struggling readers and to efficiently identify students who need special education services?* https://iris.peabody.vanderbilt.edu/module/rti01/cresource/q1/p01/#:~:text=On%20average%2C%2025%25%20(typically, of%20instruction%20in%20each%20school

Lease, S. (2014). Beyond articulation. *ASHA Leader Live.* http://blog.asha.org/2014/09/23/beyond-articulation-dont-forget-reading/

Lefebvre, P., Gaines, R., Staniforth, L., & Chiasson, V. (2017). Emergent literacy skills in English-speaking preschoolers with suspected childhood apraxia of speech: A pilot study. *Canadian Journal of Speech-Language Pathology, 41*(1), 128–142.

Lewis, B. A., Freebairn, L. A., Hansen, A. J., Iyengar, S. K., & Taylor, H. G. (2004). School-age follow-up of children with childhood apraxia of speech. *Language, Speech, and Hearing Services in Schools, 35*, 122–140. https://doi.org/10.1044/0161-1461(2004/014)

Lindamood, C., & Lindamood, P. (2011). *Lindamood Phoneme Sequencing Program for Reading, Spelling, and Speech* (4th ed.). Pro-Ed.

Marion, M. J., Sussman, H. M., & Marquardt, T. P. (1993). The perception and production of rhyme in normal and developmentally apraxic children. *Journal of Communication Disorders, 26*, 129–160. https://doi.org/10.1016/0021-9924(93)90005-U

McNeill, B. C., Gillon, G. T., & Dodd, B. (2008). Phonological awareness and early reading development in childhood apraxia of speech (CAS). *International Journal of Language & Communication Disorders, 44*, 175–192. https://doi.org/10.1080/13682820801997353

McNeill, B. C., Gillon, G. T., & Dodd, B. (2009). Effectiveness of an integrated phonological awareness approach for children with childhood apraxia of speech (CAS). *Child Language Teaching and Therapy, 25*, 341–366. https://doi.org/10.1177/0265659009339823

McNeill, B., Gillon, G., & Dodd, B. (2013). The longer term effects of an integrated phonological awareness intervention for children with childhood apraxia of speech. *Asia Pacific Journal of Speech, Language and Hearing, 13*, 145–161. https://doi.org/10.1179/136132810805335074

Miller, G. J., Lewis, B., Benchek, P., Freebairn, L., Tag, J., Budge, K., . . . Stein, C. (2019). Reading outcomes for individuals with histories of suspected childhood apraxia of speech. *American Journal of Speech-Language Pathology, 28*(4), 1432–1447. https://doi.org/10.1044/2019_AJSLP-18-0132

Norris, J. (2003). *Phonic Faces* (2nd ed.). EleMentory.com

Preston, J., & Edwards, M. L. (2010). Phonological awareness and types of sound errors in preschoolers with speech sound disorders. *Journal of Speech, Language, and Hearing Research, 53*, 44–60. https://doi.org/10.1044/1092-4388(2009/09-0021)

Schuele, C. M., & Boudreau, D. (2008). Phonological awareness intervention: Beyond the basics. *Language, Speech, and Hearing Services in Schools, 38*, 3–20. https://doi.org/10.1044/0161-1461(2008/002)

Stackhouse, J. (1997). Phonological awareness: Connecting speech and literacy problems. In B. Hodson & M. Edwards (Eds.), *Perspectives in applied phonology* (pp. 157–196). Aspen.

CHAPTER

Supporting the Needs of Older Children With Ongoing Communicative Challenges

As children with a history of childhood apraxia of speech (CAS) reach elementary school age and beyond, they often have ongoing communicative challenges. These challenges may be mild in nature, as in a child whose sensorimotor speech challenges appear to be resolved with the exception of attainment of some later developing phonemes. Some children may continue to exhibit substantial speech, language, and/or social communication challenges even after years of intensive speech therapy. This chapter describes how to address some of the ongoing speech, language, and social communication challenges of children elementary school age and older with CAS, as well as ways to enhance motivation and support generalization.

Ongoing Communication Challenges Impacting Older Children With CAS

Some elementary school–age children make dramatic improvement in their sensorimotor planning skills by the time they reach grade school but may exhibit residual articulation errors or phonological patterns that are unresolved. Other children may continue to exhibit more severe and widespread challenges resulting from CAS. Some comorbid challenges in speech and language may also be observed in elementary school–age and older children with CAS, including any of the following:

- *residual articulation errors*, particularly on later developing phonemes (e.g., /θ, ð, ʃ, tʃ, dʒ, l, r/), as well as poor stability of production of earlier developing phonemes (e.g., /k, g, f, v, s, z/)

283

- unresolved phonological patterns
- challenges with complex phoneme sequences in single words, phrases, and sentences including the following;
  - initial, medial, and final consonant clusters of two and three phonemes, including words with more than one cluster in the word
  - weak syllable deletion in multisyllabic words
  - words or sentences containing both a challenge phoneme and the substitution phoneme
  - omission of unstressed words in sentences (e.g., articles, prepositions)
- voicing errors, the most common of which is voicing of initial voiceless stops (e.g., bot for pot; do for two; gat for cat)
- vowel distortions, the most prevalent of which are on rhotic vowels, diphthongs, lax front and back vowels /ɪ, ɛ, æ, ʊ/, and the tense front vowel /e/
- difficulties with the suprasegmental features of speech (e.g., syllable segmentation, excessive equal stress, difficulty varying intonation)
- reduced overall *comprehensibility*
- limited generalization of speech skills
- language challenges affecting syntax, morphology, and attainment of higher-level vocabulary
- social communication challenges
- difficulty with literacy skill development in reading, writing, and spelling

Each of the areas of challenge listed is described in greater detail.

Residual Articulation Errors and Ongoing Errors on Earlier Developing Phonemes

Although a child may have demonstrated dramatic improvement in sensorimotor speech planning, the child may be delayed in acquiring one or more of these later developing phonemes. Treatment may shift to a more traditional articulation approach to address the phoneme or phonemes in error.

When addressing articulation errors in children with a history of CAS, it is important to recognize that dynamic, motor-based treatment principles still need to be incorporated into treatment (e.g., carefully assessing facilitative contexts to support stimulability; using dynamic cueing strategies to encourage high levels of accuracy).

Specific methods for treating eight later developing phonemes, including /θ, ð, s, z, l, r, ʃ, tʃ /, are described by Bleile (2018). For each of the eight phonemes, Bleile suggests *key phonetic environments* and describes useful *metaphors*, *touch cues*, *phonetic placement methods*, and *shaping techniques*. Secord et al. (2007) describe popular methods for eliciting each phoneme of the English language, including vowels. These include *imitation*, identification of *facilitating contexts*, *phonetic placement*, the *motokinesthetic method*, and *sound approximation*. Visual biofeedback tools, such as ultrasound biofeedback (Preston et al., 2013) and electropalatography (EPG; Lundeborg & McAllister, 2007), have been found to be useful for older children with ongoing articulation errors. Ultrasound and EPG are described in greater detail in Chapter 4.

Many children's books provide multiple opportunities to practice specific phonemes. For example, the /s/ phoneme can be practiced several times while reading the book, *Dear Zoo* by Rod Campbell. It contains the repetitive lines, "So they sent me a ___" and "I sent him back." A list of other books to reinforce specific phonemes is available in the online materials.

Several other digital visual biofeedback applications are available to support acquisition of phonemes. Though not an exhaustive list, a few of these applications are described in Box 8–1.

Persistence of Phonological Patterns

Phonological patterns may persist after a child has made substantial gains in the control of their sensorimotor speech skills. Although a child's sensorimotor planning and programming have improved, they may continue to exhibit difficulty learning the sound distinctions or phonemic rules of language. This results in specific patterns of errors (e.g., fronting of velar phonemes, stopping of continuant phonemes). For a child whose residual errors tend to be more representative of a developmental phonological disorder, the treatment protocol may shift to one of the phonological approaches to treatment.

■ Box 8–1. Digital Visual Biofeedback Tools to Support Phoneme Acquisition

Seeing Speech is an online resource that allows you to view video-animated images, as well as ultrasound and magnetic resonance images of the movements of the vocal tract for many phonemes in the International Phonetic Alphabet.

Speech Racer is an iOS app that provides visual biofeedback for /r/, /r/ clusters, and vocalic /r/. The visual biofeedback is provided in game format, allowing the learner to produce /r/ in words and isolation and determine if their production was accurate.

Vowel Viz is an app available for iOS that provides visual biofeedback to analyze accuracy of English vowel production. The speech-language pathologist (SLP) chooses among a variety of visual feedback tools, so the learner can see if their vowel production in isolation or words was accurate. Monophthongs, diphthongs, and rhotic vowels are included.

Windows Tool for Speech Analysis (WASP) is a free program for analyzing the acoustic qualities of speech. With WASP, you can record speech, then replay and view waveforms, spectrograms, and pitch-tracking of the speech signal. The spectrograph is especially helpful for illustrating the formant transitions for liquids /r/ and /l/, glides /w/ and /j/, and diphthongs. The example in Figure 8–1 shows how the formants change when the diphthong is produced correctly versus staying flat when it is reduced in the word "bike." When a child produces steady-state formants, you can encourage them to experiment with the sound and see if they can make the lines move. They do not need to take a course in speech and hearing sciences to understand that when the tongue moves, the formants change. They are also able to play back their speech to see if it matched the model the clinician provided. The WASP tool can be found at https://www.speechandhearing.net/laboratory/wasp/

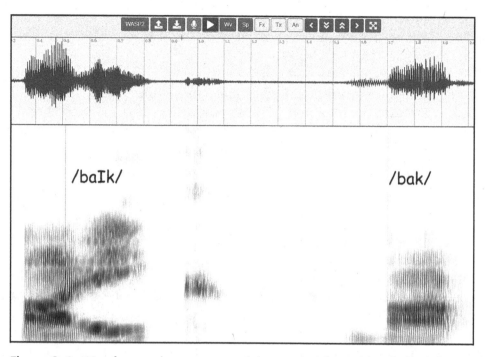

Figure 8–1. Waveform and spectrogram of the word "*bike*" said with the full diphthong on the left / bɑɪk/ and reduced diphthong on the right /bɑk/.

Keep in mind, however, that children with a history of CAS may need a more scaffolded approach to treatment of phonological patterns. Careful attention to facilitative contexts and use of shaping strategies will be critical for success when addressing phonological error patterns. There are many approaches commonly used in treatment of phonological patterns, a few of which include Minimal Pairs Intervention (Baker, 2021); Multiple Oppositions Intervention (Williams & Sugden, 2021); the Cycles Approach (Perzas et al., 2021); and Integrated Phonological Awareness Intervention (McNeill & Gillon, 2021). A thorough description of these and other approaches to treatment of phonological impairments is beyond the scope of this book, but resources regarding treatments are widely available. Baker et al. (2018) provide a thorough analysis of elements comprising phonological intervention and is an excellent resource for understanding what various approaches and interventions offer so you can more easily match the treatment to the child's specific profile.

Difficulty With Complex Phoneme Sequences

- Challenges with complex phoneme sequences in single words, phrases, and sentences including the following:
  - initial, medial, and final consonant clusters of two and three phonemes, including words with more than one cluster in the word
  - weak syllable deletion in multisyllabic words
  - words or sentences containing both a challenge phoneme and the substitution phoneme
  - omission of unstressed words in sentences (e.g., articles, prepositions)

Some older children with CAS continue to demonstrate challenges producing complex phonemic sequences. We observe **cluster reduction, weak syllable deletion, phoneme omissions, unstressed word omission,** and **phoneme confusion.** These errors may be prevalent at the single-word level or may be observed only in longer utterances or during a child's connected speech. Each of these errors is described as follows.

Cluster reduction can have a significant impact on intelligibility. Many therapy resources are designed to facilitate only acquisition of two-element clusters in the initial position of words; however, clusters are more varied and include

- clusters in the medial and final positions of words (e.g., accomplish, conclusion, difference)

- triple consonant clusters (e.g., **strong, camped, asked**)

- targets containing more than one consonant cluster within the same word (e.g., **president, congratulations, demonstrates**)

Weak syllable deletion occurs when a child deletes or omits the unstressed or weak syllable of a multisyllabic word (e.g., /bʌ.flaɪ/ for butterfly; /mɛɚ.ə.kə/ for America).

Phoneme omissions and **substitutions** and errors of **phoneme confusion** resulting in **assimilation** (a phoneme changes to become more similar to a nearby phoneme, as in /ʃʌn.ʃaɪn/ for sunshine) also are prevalent in older children with CAS. In addition, errors of **omission of unstressed words and syllables in sentences** and connected speech are commonly observed (e.g., "Guess what, our substitute teacher is not giving us any homework tonight" produced as /dɛs wʌt aʊ sʌtut titʃʊ nat dɪbiŋ ʌs ɛji homwʊk tənaɪt/). Of course, omission of unstressed words in sentences may be tied to underlying expressive language issues, as well as sensorimotor speech challenges.

Assimilation often is observed when a phoneme that previously was in error and appears to have been mastered (e.g., /r/) occurs in a word or phrase with the old substitution phoneme (e.g., /w/), as when a word like *worry* is produced as /wʊ.wi/, or the sentence *Are we going the right way?* is produced as /aɚ wi goɪŋ ðə raɪt reɪ/. The frequency of these types of errors increases dramatically during connected speech, when the child's rate of speech increases, and when the linguistic load of the child's speech is greater. Examples of the types of errors that may be observed during production of complex, multisyllabic words can be seen in Table 8–1.

Table 8–1. Examples of Errors in Complex Phoneme Sequences

Target Word	Phonetic Transcription
suspicious	/ˈspɪ.səs/—WSD, PS
joystick	/ˈdʒɔɪ.kɪk/—CR, A
Saturday	/ˈsæ.ɚ.deɪ/—PO
prediction	/pə.ˈdɪ.ʃən/—CR, PO
appreciated	/ˈpi.ʃeɪ.əd/—WSD (2), PO

Note. A, assimilation; CR, cluster reduction; PO, phoneme omission; PS, phoneme substitution; WSD, weak syllable deletion.

Young (1987) recommends using backward chaining (described in more detail in Chapter 3) to suppress cluster reduction and weak syllable deletion. In Young's research, visual supports in the form of *rebus pictures* were used to train accurate production of clusters. Rebus pictures are incorporated into articulation therapy by using simple drawings and/or letters that are combined to represent a specific word, thus reducing the complexity of the target word. To represent the word *slip*, for example, the clinician could use pictures of a snake or a leaky tire for /s/ and a picture of lips for "lip," then producing the word from back to front (e.g., Say "lip." Now say "s-lip"), eventually reducing the gap or segmentation between /s/ and "lip." Figure 8–2 illustrates how rebus pictures can be used along with backward chaining to facilitate accurate production of both initial and final clusters.

Forward chaining and backward chaining (described in Chapter 3), as well as rebus pictures, described earlier, can be beneficial to improving production of complex multisyllabic words by reducing phoneme and syllable omissions and phoneme substitutions. The word *evacuation* could be represented with rebus pictures as shown in Figure 8–3 using a backward chaining technique.

When looking for sources of materials for the target stimuli, be sure to choose targets for which the child can be sufficiently challenged. You can collaborate with the child's classroom teacher and explore the child's textbooks because appropriate treatment targets may be abundant in the child's curriculum materials (e.g., conduct, flexible, multiply, slumber, continent, contrast, experience, persuade). A list of multisyllabic words (useful for addressing syllable stress) that would be appropriate to work on production of complex phoneme sequences can be found in the online materials.

As children acquire new phonemes, they often demonstrate confusion during production of words or sentences that contain both a phoneme which historically had been difficult and their former phoneme substitution for that error phoneme. Provide additional practice with words and sentences containing both the error and substitution phonemes when the child is ready for this increased challenge.

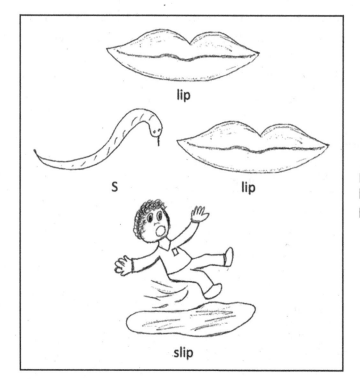

Figure 8–2. Using rebus pictures and backward chaining to facilitate accurate production of clusters.

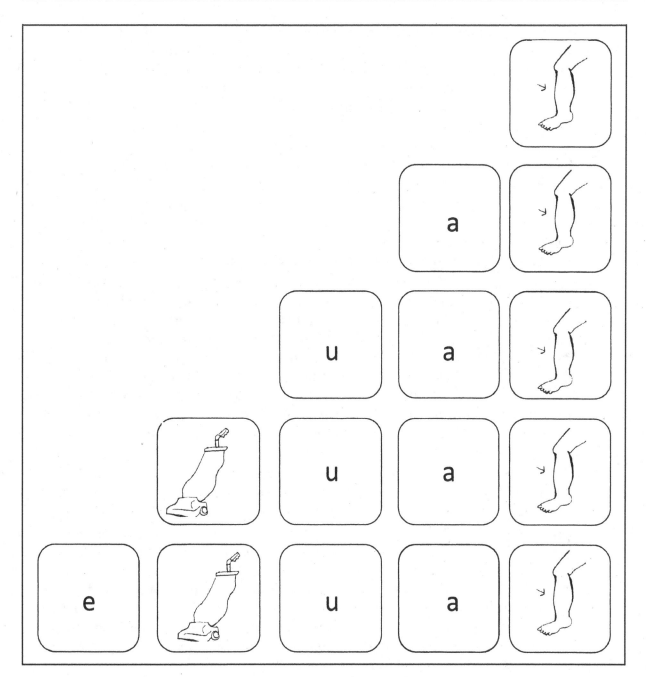

Figure 8–3. Using rebus pictures and backward chaining to facilitate accurate production of multisyllabic words.

Voicing Errors

Voicing errors, particularly substitution of voiced stops /b, d, g/ for their voiceless cognates /p, t, k/ in the initial position of syllables, are a residual challenge for some school-age children with CAS (e.g., /dim/ for *team*; /baɪgɪŋ lat/ for *parking lot*). To support the accurate production of voiceless plosives in the syllable initial position, a combination of speech discrimination and speech production activities as shown in the following sequence is beneficial.

1. **Discrimination using minimal pairs.** The use of minimal pair pictures to teach voicing contrasts (e.g., Paul/ball, time/dime, coat/goat) can be incorporated into

treatment both for auditory discrimination and production activities. Begin by showing the child both pictures of the contrast pair and then asking the child to point to the picture of the word that is named. This activity can be extended to phrase- and sentence-level discrimination practice by having the child point to the picture corresponding to spoken sentences (e.g., "Point to the picture that shows, 'I see a coat.' Point to 'I see a goat.'")

2. **Discrimination of correct versus incorrect productions.** Beginning at the single-word level, ask the child to determine if the clinician's production of the target word was correct or incorrect (e.g., "This is a picture of a coat. Clap your hands each time you hear me say the word incorrectly. See if you can catch me each time. Let's begin. Coat, coat, coat, goat." Child claps. "Excellent! You caught me when I mixed up my words. Let's try another one.")

3. **Production practice with aspiration in single words.** When the child is able to discriminate between the two words of each of the contrast pairs with a high level of accuracy, begin a variety of production activities. An early step in production practice for reducing voicing of initial stop consonants would be to increase the length and amount of aspiration following production of the voiceless phoneme. According to Ladefoged (2001), voiceless stop phonemes are aspirated in syllable initial position, as in "pan" [pʰæn], "top" [tʰap], and "coat" [kʰot]. By extending the length of the aspiration, the child is more likely to produce the voiceless phoneme correctly because the aspiration separates the voiceless phoneme from the voiced vowel that follows. Over time, the child would be asked to shorten the length of aspiration until the child's production more closely approximates the adult production of the target word.

4. **Single-word production practice using minimal pairs.** The child produces contrast pairs using the stop cognates: /p, b/, /t, d/, and /k, g/ (e.g., pay-bay, pack-back, toe-dough, time-dime, come-gum, coat-goat).

5. **Sentence-level production practice.** Several minimal pair pictures are turned face down, and the child is asked to choose one of the pictures and name that picture or use the word in a sentence, such as "I am holding a picture of a *coat*." The clinician, who has an identical set of pictures, shows the child the picture of the word the child produced. If the child makes the voicing distinction correctly, the clinician's picture will match the picture the child is holding. If the child's production is inaccurate, it would be apparent the child did not make the voicing adjustment to achieve the semantic distinction between the contrast pairs.

6. **Sentence-level production practice using both words of contrast pairs.** The child can practice producing sentences containing both words of the contrast pairs. For *coat* and *goat*, the child may say, "The silly *goat* wore a *coat*."

Vowel Errors

Children with CAS may continue to demonstrate vowel distortions, even as they get older. If vowel disorders persist in older children, it is essential to incorporate vowel identification and discrimination activities into treatment, as accurate vowel production is particularly important for literacy skill development. Be sure to embed spelling instruction into the vowel production activities. A more thorough discussion of intervention for vowels can be found in Chapter 5.

Challenges With the Suprasegmental Features of Speech

School-age children with CAS may continue to demonstrate prosody differences and intonation patterns that give their speech a robotic or unusual sounding quality. Some of these differences may include the following:

- use of excessive equal stress or incorrect application of lexical stress, particularly in complex, multisyllabic, or less familiar words
- limited application of phrasal and contrastive stress in sentences
- gaps between sounds and syllables
- ineffective use of rising and falling intonation in sentences
- poor use of variations in tone of voice that reflect mood or feeling or denote sarcasm or irony

The Rapid Syllable Transition Treatment (ReST) program (described in greater detail in Chapter 4) is designed to address ongoing segmental and sequencing errors, as well as establish smoother coarticulatory transitions from syllable to syllable and correct syllable stress assignment (Murray et al., 2015). Chapter 5 offers detailed recommendations for treatment of these suprasegmental features of speech.

Reduced Comprehensibility

Older children with CAS may have attained a fair level of speech intelligibility, but their speech intelligibility may deteriorate when they are sharing a lot of information, speaking out of context, or using a rapid rate of speech. This can cause a communication breakdown. Children can be taught to be more aware of when a communication breakdown has occurred by encouraging the child to watch the communicative partner's face and judge by the facial expression if the message was understood or listen to the partner's responses and decide if the listener is understanding them.

When a communicative breakdown has occurred, the child can be taught to utilize some simple cueing strategies such as those listed in Box 8–2 to increase the comprehensibility of their communication.

Case Study

Kai is a 14-year-old boy with a complex communication profile, including CAS. Kai is working on increasing his comprehensibility in conversational interactions and organizing his language to formulate verbal narratives. The SLP requests that Kai's mom **share information** regarding highlights about Kai's week that Kai may want to talk about via text prior to sessions. When Kai struggles to organize his language or make himself understood during conversation, the SLP can then **ask leading questions** or **choice questions** based on the information shared by Kai's mom (e.g., *Was the party at someone's house or at a restaurant? Whose house was the party at?*). When a word comes up that the SLP is not able to understand, Kai is encouraged to **use gestures** to "act out" what he is trying to say, to **spell** it, or to use his cell phone to **locate a picture on the internet** referencing what he is struggling to explain. After creating a graphic

■ Box 8–2. Strategies for Increasing Comprehensibility

- Work on reducing the rate of speech.

- Use gestures and pantomiming to act out the ideas being shared.

- Repeat the part of the message that was misunderstood with greater emphasis and clarity (e.g., Child—"I'm going to be a **bot** for Halloween." Clinician—"Oh, like a robot?" Child—"No, a **BAT**.")

- If the child can type or write, encourage the child to write it down or type out the word(s) that are not being understood.

- Ask the child to pull up an image on the internet of what they are referring to.

- Use synonyms for words that are not being understood.

- Prepare for your session by asking the caregiver to share some information and details about a topic the child may want to talk about, as having a sense of the topic and a few details can support the comprehensibility of the speech of children whose conversational speech clarity is poor.

- Be sure the child is aware of what the goals and expectations are for each activity during the session.

- Teach the child to provide an initial statement about the topic of the conversation, such as establishing the people, setting, situation, time frame, or other key pieces of information prior to launching into a story. For example, the child can prepare the listener by saying, "Something really **funny** happened at **lunch today**." When the listener acknowledges that they understand the child will be telling a **funny** episode, the episode will relate to an experience the child had during **lunch**, probably in the school cafeteria, and the episode happened **today**, the child then can begin to tell the story. Figure 8–4 illustrates a sample topic board used by a child in a lunch group to help establish the topic of a conversation prior to beginning the conversation.

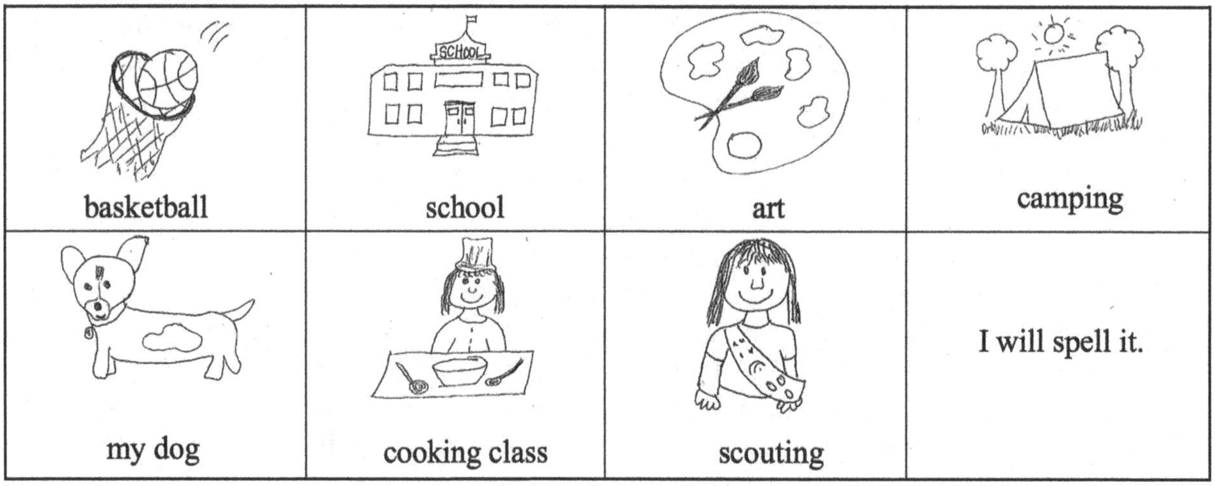

basketball	school	art	camping
my dog	cooking class	scouting	I will spell it.

Figure 8–4. Topic board for conversational initiation.

organizer about the topic, the SLP **reminds Kai of his speech goals** and **highlights those letters or words representing challenging phonemes and phoneme combinations**; those targets are then practiced in isolation and short phrases. Finally, Kai is able to formulate the verbal narrative in response to a conversation question, "What did you do over the weekend?" and focus on both the language formulation and the clarity of his speech simultaneously. Kai would not have been successful in this final step if the groundwork had not been laid earlier in the session.

During a recent session, Kai wanted to share information about a dance he had attended recently with some friends. Because **his mother had sent a brief text message** about the event and who attended, it was possible to get the gist of many of the details about the event, even those his mother had not shared. When discussing some of the songs the DJ played at the event, the SLP had trouble understanding the name of a singer. Kai checked his cell phone and was able to **pull up a picture** of the artist along with the artist's name, allowing the flow of the conversation to continue. When talking about the food, Kai talked about pizza, and the SLP thought Kai said he had eaten pizza at the event. The SLP asked Kai what type of pizza he had eaten and Kai quickly shook his head and **used emphatic stress** to say he did NOT eat any of the pizza. While Kai was listing some of the friends he saw at the dance, the SLP was having trouble understanding some of the names. The SLP said, "Wow, you said that so fast, I couldn't keep up. What can you do to help me understand the names of your friends?" Kai replied, "Slow down," and then started listing the names again, but at a much **slower pace**, waiting between each name for the SLP to repeat the name and write it on the graphic organizer. The conversation was much more robust and comprehensible because Kai employed several strategies for increasing comprehensibility.

Supporting Generalization

Shifting to activities that support generalization is an important step in the treatment process. As mentioned earlier, it is not unusual for a child to demonstrate a high level of accuracy during more structured activities or simply when in the presence of the clinician. When a child is able to produce a target utterance with a very high level of accuracy in structured, connected speech activities, it is advisable not to discontinue treatment prematurely, but to continue to find ways to challenge the child so the child can maintain their learning and generalize their skills. Following are several recommendations to help achieve generalization and maintenance of speech skills in older children. Chapter 3 also provides further information about working at the child's optimal challenge point.

Incorporating a Distraction

One way to increase the level of challenge in treatment is to introduce some type of distraction within the treatment activity. The distraction could involve incorporating a motor activity into the speech task (e.g., practicing the target utterances while building a block tower or playing a game like Jenga). Another way to incorporate distraction into the treatment activity is to set up activities that require the child to give a considerable amount of attention to the *content* of the message. When the child needs to concentrate hard on *what* the child is saying, the child has less available attention to apply to *how* the child is articulating the message. Activities that challenge the child's memory or provide substantial cognitive-linguistic challenges offer a distraction for the child.

Reducing the Level of Structure

The clinician can challenge the child further by reducing the amount of structure within the treatment framework, such as engaging in conversational speech activities or asking the child to summarize a story or movie. Structured language activities provide a more predictable framework for the communicative interaction, whereas conversational speech activities are less predictable and offer a more uncertain structure. Activities with reduced linguistic structure may include asking the child to summarize a story the child has read, explain a movie the child has seen, describe a setting in great detail, or explain the sequence and rules for playing a game that is unfamiliar to the adult. It requires that the child think back and recall visual details or other details of a past event. It also requires the child to use decontextualized language to express these ideas in a logical sequence and with sufficient detail so the listener can make sense of the child's message. The attention to detail required of the child in these less structured activities is substantial, resulting in less available attention to concentrate on *how* the message is being articulated. When linguistic and speech demands are both high, opportunities for generalization are greater.

Varying the Treatment Context

The clinician can vary the context of the treatment by changing the setting (working in the hallway, on the playground, or in the cafeteria) or interacting with peers or less familiar persons in the setting. A less familiar person will not provide the same types of cues as the clinician, and this decreased reliance on cueing is an important part of the generalization process.

Table 8–2 provides several examples of activities to help promote generalization. Many of these activities also may serve as appropriate homework activities for families during later stages of treatment. During generalization activities, it is important to have an adult monitor the child's speech production practice rather than have the child practice alone. The monitor may be the clinician, but it also may be a teacher, teacher assistant, or a parent. If someone other than the clinician is acting as the adult monitor, it is important that the individual is well aware of the expectations for the child. For example, a child may be working on reducing the deletion of syllables from multisyllabic words during paragraph reading. If the child has not mastered the /θ/ phoneme yet, the adult monitor may be marking words with incorrectly produced /θ/ phonemes as incorrect, even though the child's goal was to reduce syllable deletion. This could be discouraging for the child. Be sure the adult monitors are keeping data and providing feedback on the appropriate treatment goal(s) for the activity.

Language Difficulties

Children who exhibit both speech and language challenges are at greater risk for exhibiting "significant reading and spelling difficulties through adulthood" (Lewis & Freebairn, 1992). Thus, it is crucial that both speech and language goals be addressed from early on in treatment. Ideas for supporting early language development were addressed in Chapter 6.

Table 8–2. Sample Generalization Activities for Speech

Read aloud. The child reads aloud for 5–10 min (stopping at 1-min intervals) from an age-appropriate textbook or novel. The child is encouraged to read at a regular pace, not too fast or too slow. At each 1-min interval, an adult monitor will write down any words that were pronounced incorrectly and review these words with the child. During the early stages of read-aloud activities, it may be beneficial to look through the reading materials ahead of time with the child to identify and highlight the words with which the child may demonstrate difficulty, and the highlighted words would vary depending on the goals and needs of the child. Eventually, the use of a highlighter would be faded to promote greater generalization. A bookmark can also be inserted into a book to read for homework practice, and the child or parent can chart the child's production accuracy of those target words.
Favorite songs. The clinician can print out lyrics to the child's favorite songs and highlight the target words to focus on during singing. The child can keep the lyric pages in the car or in their room to refer to when singing aloud.
Summarize. The child reads aloud for 3–5 min, stopping at 1-min intervals. At each 1-min interval, the child is asked to summarize that section of the book in the child's own words. The adult keeps track of the words produced incorrectly and reviews these words with the child. It may be beneficial to preview potential challenging words prior to reading; however, as mentioned earlier, the preview will be faded eventually as the child's generalization improves.
Magazine picture story. The child looks through pictures in a magazine that has photos that are interesting to the child, which may be a gaming magazine, sports magazine, or other type of magazine about a subject of interest to the child. The child is encouraged to make up a story about an interesting picture of 1–3 min in length. The adult monitor keeps track of the child's performance and reviews this with the child at the end of the story.
Tag team story. The child creates a story with a partner, either a peer or an adult monitor. The individuals take turns telling parts of a story. Each time the storyteller comes to a logical story transition point, the storyteller tags the partner who continues the story to the next logical transition point. The length of the story can be predetermined either by a specified number of minutes or a specified number of turns. The adult monitor keeps track of challenging words throughout the story and shares these with the child at the completion of the story. Icons, such as those from Story Grammar Marker or Story Champs, can be incorporated into these story activities to help reinforce concepts of what makes a narrative. For example, one child could be given the icon of setting, characters, problem, solution, etc.
I'm going on a picnic, on a trip, to a party, etc. Play the memory game, "I'm going on a picnic" (or any version of this game). Each person is asked to name something they would bring to the given event, and the other participants add to the list (e.g., Player 1: "I'm going on a picnic, and I'm bringing a brown picnic basket." Player 2: "I'm going on a picnic and I'm bringing a brown picnic basket and a tennis racquet." Player 1: "I'm going on a picnic and I'm bringing a brown picnic basket, a tennis racquet, and a pitcher of lemonade.") To encourage practice on the targeted goals, the clinician could ask the child to only add items to the list that contain the target phoneme or syllable structure, such as *items that begin with /r/ or items that are at least three syllables in length.*
Conversation time. The family is asked to set aside two to three times during each day to have conversation time and focus on accuracy of speech production during the conversation. The conversational topic can be randomly selected or can be chosen from a topic jar. A topic jar is simply a container with a list of numerous conversational topics that would be of interest to the child. The conversation can be 3–5 min in length. During the conversation, the adult monitor keeps track of challenging words and reviews these with the child.

continues

Table 8–2. *continued*

Conversation time with a distraction. Incorporate a distraction during the "conversation time" activity, such as throwing a beanbag or ball back and forth, building a block tower, or playing tic-tac-toe.
How do I get there or how do I do it? The child describes to an adult monitor the directions you would follow to get to a location you visit often, explains the rules of how to play a game, or describes a sequence for completing an activity. The adult monitor keeps track of challenging words and reviews these with the child. These types of activities reinforce development of expository skills, which is academically appropriate for school-age children.
Tongue twisters. Search online for tongue twisters for the target phoneme on which the child is working. Practice some of these tongue twisters, until they can be said fairly easily. Several English as a Second Language (ESL) websites provide samples of tongue twisters, many of which target specific speech sounds. Children may attempt to memorize some short tongue twisters as a way to practice without the written letter cues.
Rote counting and other counting variations. The child practices counting various sets of numbers or skip counting in specific ways depending on the target goals. Some counting sets that target specific articulatory goals include the following: • /f/—count by fives from 5 to 100 or count each number from 40 to 60 • /s/—count from 60 to 80 • /v/—count by 10s starting with 7 (7, 17, 27, 37...) or by fives from 5 to 100 • /ɚ/—count from 30 to 50 • /tw/ clusters—count from 20 to 30 • "th"—count by 10s starting with 3 (3, 13, 23, 33...) count from 30 to 39
Mad Libs. You can use premade Mad Libs books or find them online and use them with a word bank that focuses on the target stimuli you would like the child to work on. For example, if the child is working on multisyllabic words, you would provide the child with a list of multisyllabic nouns, verbs, adjectives, etc., from which to choose words to fill in the Mad Lib stories. Some children may prefer to make up their own. The child could think of words ahead of time so more time could be devoted to practice. One online resource for generating Mad Libs is Mad Takes and can be found at https://www.madtakes.com/libs/187.html
Summer reinforcement. School speech-language pathologists (SLPs) or private SLPs whose clients do not receive services in the summer can provide calendars with practice words or activities to complete throughout the summer.

This section addresses ongoing challenges in the areas of morphology, syntax, and vocabulary and ways to treat these areas in the context of speech treatment.

Delays in Grammatical Skill Development

As children with CAS get older, they may continue to demonstrate syntactic and morphological errors that should have been resolved. Omission or incorrect use of morphological markers, such as those denoting verb tense (walk*s*, push*es*, help*ed*, talk*ing*), plurality (hat*s*, dress*es*), and possession (Mommy*'s*, Liz*'s*, Frank*'s*), are observed in some children in early elementary grades and beyond. Gender pronoun errors may be noted when a child either uses the incorrect form of the gender pronoun (e.g., "**Her** went to the party.") or switches the gender type (e.g., "I saw Suzie, but **he** didn't see me."). Omission of function words, such as articles "a" and "the," auxiliary verbs "is" and "can," and prepositions "in" and "to," may persist for children with a history of CAS and language impairment.

Difficulties also may be noted in children's ability to formulate more complex syntactic constructions and to use and comprehend many *literate text features*. Literate text features (described later in this chapter) support a child's ability to comprehend written text and to write in a more literary and less conversational style. Helping children learn to use more advanced language, or "literate language," is important because it is the bridge between conversational-type language and the language that is used in books and school instruction. According to Westby (1991) referencing Pellegrini (1985), the four features of literate language that differentiate it from conversational language include wider use of the following linguistic structures:

- conjunctions other than "and," "then," "and then"
  - coordinating conjunctions (e.g., but, so, yet)
  - subordinating conjunctions (e.g., because, before, after, while, until, if, although)
- mental and linguistic verbs
  - mental verbs (e.g., decided, knew, thought, forgot)
  - linguistic verbs (e.g., said, announced, reported, yelled, grumbled, asked)
- adverbs and adverbial clauses, including these different types of adverbs
  - time (e.g., before work, at 6:00, when he was angry)
  - manner (e.g., quickly, emphatically, wickedly)
  - place (e.g., in the ocean, by the door, to the office)
  - frequency (e.g., every morning, once in a while, often, each evening)
  - degree (e.g., extremely, almost)
  - purpose (e.g., to explain what happened, to keep the sun out of his eyes, to help his mom)
- elaborated noun phrases
  - modifiers (e.g., *big, red* house)
  - qualifiers (e.g., the house *next to the park)*

By using literate language features, the speaker (or writer) can use greater clarity and specificity that is consistent with decontextualized language. Conducting a language sample in which the communicative interaction is related to things that are not present or to events in the past or future would be a useful way of assessing a child's ability to use and comprehend more complex morphology and syntax. Story retelling also may be a useful diagnostic tool for evaluating a child's use of decontextualized language and literate language features. If deficits are observed in the child's understanding and/or use of literate language structures, these structures can be incorporated into the context of treatment using books, pretend play, and structured language activities. Examples of teaching the use of literate language elements in various treatment contexts are described in Table 8–3.

Table 8–3. Examples of Teaching the Use of Literate Language Elements in Various Treatment Contexts

Teaching subordinating conjunctions in the context of a children's storybook.
The book, *"The Mountain that Loved a Bird"* by Alice McLerran, is a story about a mountain that makes the acquaintance of a bird who happens to land on it. A number of subordinating conjunctions are incorporated into the text of the book. Syntactic structures from the book could be used to elicit similar structures from the client(s). The clinician could lead a discussion about how the mountain pleaded with the bird to visit for as many years as she could. The mountain told the bird she would feel upset if the bird eventually stopped coming, but she would feel even more upset if the bird never came again. A sentence frame such as, "I would feel _____ if _____, **but** I would feel even _____ **if** _____" could be used to facilitate production of the conjunctions "if" and "but."
Teaching a child to use mental verbs in the context of a board game.
While playing a board game the child and adult can take turns guessing what number will be rolled on the die (e.g., Teacher: "I *predict* I will roll a six." The teacher rolls a four. "I *thought* I would roll a six, but I rolled a four. I *guessed* the wrong number. Bobby, it's your turn to roll. Tell me what you *predict*.") After providing the above model, the adult would encourage the child to produce the same series of mental verbs—in this case, *predict, thought, guessed*—on each subsequent turn. The repetitive practice of the target linguistic structures within a semi-structured intervention activity will support the child's use of these structures in more spontaneous language.
Teaching a child to use adverbial clauses in the context of play.
When equipping superheroes for an adventure the adult may model, "My superhero needs a cape **to help him fly**. He can fly **above the mountains**. Tell me what your superhero needs." If the child replies, "x-ray glasses," the adult could respond, "to do what?" thus encouraging the child to use an adverbial clause such as, "to help him see through walls."
Teaching a child to use elaborated noun phrases in the context of structured language activities.
The clinician and child can create a dinosaur town on a large sheet of paper. Using Google® Images or other search engine, the clinician can print out pictures of many different dinosaurs with a number of shared characteristics (e.g., color, size, horns, wings, sharp teeth). The child is asked to describe which dinosaur should be placed on the picture next, and needs to describe the desired dinosaur with sufficient detail. If the child responds by providing a description that does not provide enough detail to distinguish the desired dinosaur from other dinosaurs, the adult could elicit a more elaborate noun phrase. For example, the child says, "I want to put a purple dinosaur on the top of the tree" the adult could respond, "Hmm. I see three purple dinosaurs. I'm not sure which one you want." The child could elaborate by saying, "The big, purple dinosaur with little, red spots on his tail." The adult would then have sufficient information to give the child the desired dinosaur to add to the picture scene.

Difficulty Attaining Higher-Level Vocabulary

Children with receptive and expressive language challenges may demonstrate deficits in vocabulary that impact their ability to comprehend both literary and expository text well. Although they may have an understanding of more common words used in conversational speech, such as *walked, pretty,* or *quickly,* they may have less familiarity with words that are more precise and have greater nuance of meaning: verbs like *sped, lumbered, prowled, crept*; adjectives like *exquisite, fashionable, radiant, sublime*; and adverbs like *speedily, rapidly, briskly, hastily*. Beck and McKeown (1985) introduced the concept of tiers of vocabulary. The words *walked, pretty,* and *quickly* would be considered Tier I vocabulary, whereas words carrying greater nuance, such as *prowled, radiant,* and *hastily,* would be considered Tier II words. In the Beck and McKeown vocabulary hierarchy, topic or subject-specific academic vocabulary words (e.g., isotope, parabola, uvula) are considered Tier III vocabulary. High-quality children's literature, even literature for young children, is an abundant resource for facilitating learning of more nuanced Tier II vocabulary. For example, the picture book, *Zinnia and Dot* (Ernst, 1992), written for children ages 5 to 7 years, contains numerous Tier II vocabulary words and figures of speech, including *rare, irritable, smooth, shimmer, insisting, quarreling, brilliant, shrieked, strutted, without a doubt, admit*. Although children need to learn vocabulary in all tiers, SLPs, teachers, and parents can use high-quality children's literature to introduce and establish deeper understanding of Tier II vocabulary. Tier II vocabulary also can be integrated into conversational interactions. Rather than only using the more common and simple vocabulary in conversations with our students with language impairments, less common and more nuanced vocabulary can be introduced by linking an unknown word to a familiar word. Multiple exposures of words also are beneficial. The following conversation demonstrates how a parent could introduce the word *irritable* to a child by linking it with a more familiar word, *grumpy*:

Parent: "I'm sorry I yelled at you. I'm feeling a bit grumpy and *irritable* today."

Child: "That's okay, Mommy."

Parent: "I guess I'm in a bad mood. I should not yell at you just because I'm feeling *irritable* and grumpy. I'll try not to be so *irritable* anymore."

Child: "Thank you, Mommy."

A variety of robust vocabulary instruction activities described by Beck et al. (2002, 2013) can help children develop a greater depth of understanding of Tier II vocabulary, thus supporting reading comprehension and academic achievement. A few examples of some of the robust vocabulary instruction activities described in Beck et al. include the following:

- **Child-friendly definitions.** Provide a child-friendly definition of the instructional word. Link the word to familiar vocabulary and concepts, and offer multiple exposures of the word. For example, a teacher may say, "If you *admire* something, it means you like it very much or you think it is wonderful. You can *admire* a thing, such as a beautiful garden. You also can *admire* a person, such as an athlete or a military hero. For instance, I *admire* the pictures in the book we are reading. I think they are very beautiful. I also *admire* the author of the book. I *admire* her because she writes interesting stories and draws beautiful pictures for her books. She is one of my favorite authors."

- **Relate to the child's experiences.** Relate a new word to the child's experience. "I *admire* Suzie Goodartist, the illustrator of this book. Tell me something or someone you *admire*. You can begin by saying, "I *admire* _____."

- **Thinking questions.** Ask thinking questions. "Would you *admire* someone who is mean to you? Do people often *admire* others who do heroic things?" Children can be encouraged to use the new vocabulary in sentences. "I *admire* people who do heroic things, but I don't *admire* people who are mean."

- **Choice questions.** Ask choice questions. "Which would you *admire* more, a paper someone scribbled on or a painting in a museum?"

Refer to Beck et al. (2002, 2013) for a more thorough discussion of robust vocabulary building activities.

Reduced Motivation

As children with CAS get older, they may begin to tire of ongoing speech therapy or may feel embarrassed about having to leave class and go to speech therapy. Rather than blaming the child, the SLP can pose some reflective questions such as those in Table 8–4 and consider changes to the program that may facilitate motivation.

Social Communicative Challenges

It is not unusual for children with severe speech sound disorders to exhibit accompanying difficulties with social and conversational interactions. They may struggle with conversational reciprocity, narrative production, managing communicative breakdowns appropriately, and using appropriate eye contact. Children with global apraxia may also have difficulty using appropriate body language, posture, and facial expressions.

Some factors that can influence the social communication challenges of children with highly unintelligible speech include the following:

- **fewer early social language experiences than peers** that cause children to lag behind their peers in social interaction.

- **concomitant challenges** in social communication due to underlying neurodevelopmental differences

- **history of limited social success** that can impact the self-esteem of children with speech impairment (Rice et al., 1991), leading to self-consciousness or a lack of confidence in social interactions

- **accompanying expressive language disorder** that makes it difficult to participate in conversation with the same degree of nuance and fluidity as peers

- **limited expressive vocabulary** that limits the child's ability to express a wide range of communicative functions

Basic Elements of Conversational Reciprocity

When children demonstrate limited spontaneous conversational interactions, adults frequently attempt to facilitate interaction by using persistent questioning (e.g., "How was school today?" "Did you have gym?" "What did you eat for lunch?" "Whom did you play with at recess?").

Table 8–4. Questions to Consider Regarding Reduced Client Motivation

Questions	Reflections on What Can be Changed
Are the intervention activities, or at least the reinforcers, motivating for the child?	If not, speak with the child or the child's family about the kinds of things the child may prefer to do or a reward system the child may find more motivating.
Are the target utterances chosen for treatment functional and motivating for the child?	If not, speak with the child, teacher, and/or parent about what treatment targets would be more functional for the child, so the child can see the benefits of the work the child is doing in therapy.
Is the treatment schedule keeping the child from participating in a favored activity?	If so, consider shifting the child's treatment schedule to one that enables the child to participate in a favored activity.
Does the child know their goals and is the child aware of the progress they are making?	If so, be sure it is clear the child knows and understands their goals and is aware of the progress they are making. Use charts, graphs, or other visual systems to show the child their progress over time.
Are the target utterances too difficult?	If so, simplify the stimuli to work within the child's zone of proximal development (see Chapter 3).
Is the child attending sessions regularly?	If not, work with the family to determine ways to increase consistent attendance or consider having some of the sessions be remote sessions.
Is the child practicing regularly at home?	If the child is not practicing regularly at home, speak with the family to determine what may be limiting carving out time for home practice. See Chapter 13 for more ideas for home practice.
Is it difficult to get the child's attention or to encourage the child to put forth maximum effort during the session?	If so, speak with the child or the family about things that are highly motivating for the child, such as earning a certificate for an extra book at story time, a special snack, or a 2-min break during the session.
Are the number of practice trials in the session sufficiently high?	If not, reflect on ways to use your time more efficiently in the sessions.
Does the child have any input into the target utterances chosen for intervention?	If not, encourage the child and/or caregivers to provide input about important and functional utterances that can be used as stimuli. The child may share specific words that have been difficult for them. Perhaps it is something they tried to order in a restaurant, but the server did not understand the order, the name of a teacher or classmate, or some words from a unit of Social Studies. These words could be added to the list of target utterances for intervention.

During reciprocal conversations, the participants do not require constant questions to keep up their end of the conversation, as they use these conversational elements:

- produce *supportive responses* and *comments* (e.g., *Oh, nice!; Too bad; Sorry to hear that; Cool!*)
- *ask relevant questions* to get more information (e.g., *You're going on a trip? Where are you going?*)
- *add related information* related to the conversational topic (e.g., *Oh, my cousin lives in Florida!*)

Strategies to Support Conversational Reciprocity

Helping children use these three elements of conversation will dramatically improve their ability to participate in conversational interactions. Strategies such as *modeling, coaching,* and *suggesting* can be incorporated into treatment to facilitate the development of these conversational tactics. Examples of each strategy are described in Table 8–5. When children become more adept at conversational reciprocity, it helps their communicative partner recognize they are . . .

LISTENING

and

INTERESTED

in what their partner has to say.

Discrete Practice Activities to Facilitate Conversational Reciprocity

In addition to the strategies described earlier that can be incorporated into real-time conversations, discrete practice activities can be used to facilitate extra practice opportunities in conversational reciprocity. Several discrete practice activities are described next.

Using Cue Cards to Facilitate Comments, Questions

Activities can be set up to provide the child with multiple opportunities to practice commenting, asking related questions, and sharing information. Cue cards can be beneficial when children struggle to think of what to say during conversations.

To increase commenting and asking relevant questions, structured practice activities can be set up involving the child choosing an appropriate comment or question from a set of possible choices (such as comments listed in Box 8–3 or questions listed in Box 8–4) in response to various statements such as those listed as follows that are read by the clinician or a peer:

- "Then the bee landed right on my arm!"
- "My soccer team won both games this weekend."
- "My mom won't let me go to the mall without an adult."
- "I'm having a birthday party and I was hoping you could come."
- "Some of the kids from our soccer team will be there."

Table 8–5. Strategies for Facilitating Conversational Reciprocity

Strategies	Descriptions	Examples
Modeling	*Model the conversational tools you want the child to use.*	**Commenting** Child: "I got a trophy for soccer." Speech-Language Pathologist (SLP): "WOW! That is so cool!"
		Related questions Child: "I got a trophy for soccer." SLP: "Nice! How big is it?"
		Sharing related information Child: "I got a trophy for soccer." SLP: "Nice! When I was young, I got a trophy for baseball once."
Coaching	*Instruct/coach the child to use a specific conversational tool.*	**Commenting** Child A: "I'm going to soccer after speech." SLP: "Tell your friend, 'That's cool.'" Child B: "That's cool."
		Related questions Child A: "I'm going to soccer after speech." SLP: "You can ask your friend if he has a good team." Child B: "Do you have a good team?"
		Sharing related information Child A: "I'm going to soccer after speech." SLP: "You can tell your friend what you're doing after speech, too." Child B: "Oh, I have soccer after speech, too."
Suggesting	*Give the child a reminder of a conversational tool that could be used.*	**Commenting** Child A: "I hurt my foot at soccer." SLP: "What could you say to your friend?" Child B: "Oh, sorry to hear that."
		Related questions Child A: "I hurt my foot at soccer." SLP: "What could you ask your friend?" Child B: "How did you get hurt?"
		Sharing related information Child A: "I got hurt at soccer." SLP: "Can you tell your friend about how you got hurt last week." Child B: "Oh, I hurt my knee at soccer last week."

■ **Box 8–3.** Multiple Choice Comment Cue Card

Great!
Wow!
Cool!
Awesome!
Sorry
That's too bad.
Oh, scary!

■ **Box 8–4.** Multiple Choice Question Cue Card

Who?
What?
Where?
When?
Why?
How?

- "I'm not going to be at school tomorrow."
- "I'm going on vacation."

Learning to share related information requires the child to make contingent responses. To make a contingent response, the child needs to (a) listen carefully to their communicative partners; (b) use reciprocal, topic-related responses; and (c) be flexible as conversations tend to flow to tangentially related or different topics. When first teaching children to share related information in conversation, discrete activities can be used. Some discrete activity strategies are listed next.

Word Association Strings

Word associations require only single-word responses, thereby limiting the amount of expressive language required. Each of the skills required for use of contingent responses (careful listening, reciprocity, flexibility) are needed during word association games. Consider the following word association string. When multiple meaning words are used, the child is forced to use flexible thinking and move in a new direction. The child's responses are italicized.

zoo → *monkey* → elephant → *trunk* → car → *HUH?* → car → *drive* → truck →

big → little → *ant* → uncle → *HUH?* → uncle → *man* → Superman → *hero*

Building and Describing

During building activities, discussion can occur around what is happening in the here and now and what the conversational partners are thinking, doing, and observing related to the ongoing activity. Because conversations regarding remote events are more challenging, it may be more manageable to introduce contingent responses in the context of creative activities, such as building a block tower or a potato head. Using building and describing activities is an easy way to help the child learn to be more contingent. Notice the use of emphatic stress on the words in bold. The use of stress helps bring the child's awareness to specific information in the sentences and then make related responses about that information. Examples include the following:

building potato heads (SLP: *My potato wants **blue** shoes.* Child: ***Green** shoes*)

building simple block towers (SLP: *I'll put on a **blue** block.* Child: *I'll do a **red** block.*)

building with Legos, Magna Tiles, or other building sets (SLP: *I think I'll build a **robot**.* Child: *I'm going to make a **skyscraper**.*)

drawing pictures (SLP: *I can't decide if I want to draw a **cat** or a **dog**.* Child: *Let's draw a **cat**.* SLP: *Okay. My cat's name is **Charlie**.* Child: *My cat is **Snowball**.*)

Reducing Direct Questioning

During each of these conversations, there was an emphasis on reducing the amount of direct adult questioning in favor of facilitating responses that were elicited in the context of the conversation. Children with expressive communication challenges may become dependent on direct questioning and not recognize opportunities to share their comments, questions, and related information or ideas spontaneously within the context of a conversation. Question comprehension, while an important skill, is only one piece in the flow of a robust conversation. We want to be sure our clients are learning to be *conversant* and not just *respondent*. As clinicians, we can help children learn to be more contingent in their responses by

- **COMMENTING** more and **QUESTIONING** less to promote a natural sharing of ideas and opinions, for example,

  Clinician: "Batman is the coolest because he doesn't have any magical powers. He's more realistic."

  Child: "No, Superman is cooler. He can fly."

- **PAUSING** to gain the child's interest and attention and possibly open an opportunity for the child to share ideas, for example,

  Clinician: "I think Elmo wants to sit next to, hmmm . . ."

  Child: "Big Bird."

- Using appropriate **VOCAL INFLECTION** on key words as a way to "suggest" an appropriate response, for example,

  Clinician: "*I think the spinner is going to land on red.*"

  Child: "*I think it's gonna be blue.*"

- **MUSING** and **WONDERING** about things as a way to invite the child to share ideas in an indirect way, for example,

  Clinician: "Hmm . . . I can't decide which color eyes to put on my pumpkin."

  Child: "Yellow eyes."

  Clinician: "I need to pick a name for this pumpkin."

  Child: "Call him 'Boo.' He's scary looking."

We can also coach caregivers and school staff to reduce the tendency to use direct questioning by teaching them to use comments, pauses, vocal inflection, and musing/wondering during conversational interactions and play. Discrete practice activities, such as those described next, that utilize visual supports can facilitate reciprocal conversational interaction.

Tracking the Use of Conversation Extenders

When children have become more adept at making supportive comments, asking related follow-up questions, and sharing their own related ideas, you can incorporate visual tools to help children track their use of these conversation extenders. For instance, during a conversation, each participant can use different colored chips (or other marker) and place a chip on the corresponding type of conversation extender that they used (as shown in Box 8–5). This allows the clinician and child to observe conversational trends (e.g., monopolizing the conversation or adding little to the conversation; asking a lot of questions, but sharing very little relevant information or the reverse). When the participant makes an off-topic remark, a chip can be placed outside of the boxes, and that trend can be noted as well.

The Conversation Train

In the Conversation Train activity, each participant is provided with a set of "trains" (blocks, paper strips) of a specific color. The use of this simple visual tool supports longer conversational interaction for many children who struggle with maintaining conversations for more than a couple of turns. The steps for playing the Conversation Train are as follows:

- The conversational participants set "trains" side by side for each conversational turn.
- When someone interrupts the person who is speaking, a "talk over" (T.O.) card is set vertically on top of the speaker's paper strip or block.
- When an individual makes an off-topic comment, their "train" falls off the track (placed off to the side) or a lightning bolt image is set atop the "train".
- Children should not be the only ones who talk over their conversational partners or make off-topic responses. Children enjoy "catching" adults when they forget the rules, too.

After the Conversation Train activity is completed, the participants can observe trends within the conversation. Was one participant interrupting a lot? Was there give-and-take in the conversation or did one participant do most of the talking? Figure 8–5 illustrates a short Conversation Train.

■ Box 8–5. Conversation Cue Cards

Making Comments	Asking Related Questions	Sharing Related Ideas

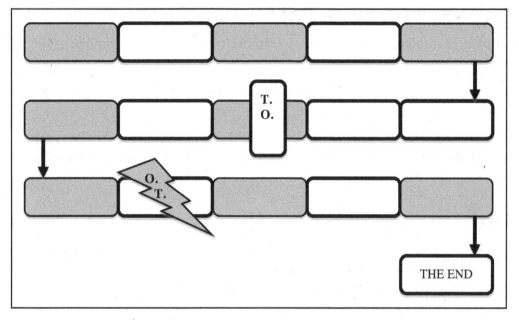

Figure 8–5. The conversation train.

Facilitating Development of Narrative and Expository Skills

Narrative skill development is important as it allows us to accomplish a variety of interactions:

- report about past events
- tell a sequential story
- summarize a book, movie, television show, or favorite game/app
- tell interesting stories about ourselves or others

Families of children with severe communication impairments may have difficulty eliciting information about what is happening when their children are away at school or visiting a friend. Children may have stories they would like to share but not have the robust language skills to share them. When children demonstrate limitations in their ability to report about past events, clinicians can help to build children's narrative development by scaffolding, beginning with simple narratives in which the child converses about immediate past events and working toward reporting about more remote events, as follows:

- Report about *immediate* past events.
- Report about *recent* past events.
- Retell stories with and without visual cues.
- Create novel stories with a partner.
- Create novel stories independently.
- Report to family or classmates about more *remote* events.

Reporting About an *Immediate* Past Event

A number of activities can be used to help children practice reporting about an immediate past event.

Telephone

After the child completes an activity, have the child pretend to call a family member on a toy telephone and tell the person what they did (e.g., "Hi, Daddy. I made a block tower for the dinosaurs.")

Simon Says

The child is asked to follow a one- or two-part instruction, such as "Simon says, hop on one foot and shut your eyes." After the child completes the action(s), ask the child to tell the parent or peers what they did (e.g., "I hopped on one foot and shut my eyes.")

Hide 'n Seek

Hide the child's target picture cards or objects. When the child finds a picture or object, ask the child to bring it back and tell what the child did (e.g., "I found a cupcake under the table.")

Reporting About Recent Past Events

Reporting about a recent past event is similar to reporting on immediate past events. The only difference is that the time lapse between the event and the reporting is extended.

Speech Therapy Summary

At the end of the treatment session, ask the child to report to their teacher or parent about the activities completed during the session (e.g., "I made a potato head. I played the hiding game with a flashlight. Then I made a zoo for the animals.") This summary report can be completed with or without the benefit of a visual schedule.

Activity Summary

After completing a multiple-step activity, the child is asked to report about what was done. For example, the child is given a worksheet with target utterance pictures. The child is asked to color, circle, underline, and/or cross out various pictures one-by-one (e.g., "Find the picture of something you use to unlock a door and circle it. Find a picture of an insect that makes honey and color it orange."). After the child completes the entire worksheet, the child can tell what they did (e.g., "I circled the key. I colored the bee orange."). Another example is having the child feed some farm animals. After all the animals have been fed, the child can report on what each animal ate (e.g., "The cow ate corn. The pig ate grapes. The sheep ate cookies.").

Teach Me How to Do It

After setting up a game or completing a simple project, ask the child to explain each step to the clinician, the parent, or a peer. After setting up the game Kerplunk, for example, the child can say, "First, I put the sticks in the holes. Then I put all the marbles in the hole on top. Last, I pulled the sticks out and the balls fell down."

Retelling Stories

The benefit of working on story retelling is that the child is learning to connect ideas together in a logical sequence using multiple sentences.

Sequential Picture Stories

Sequential story picture cards come in various levels of difficulty, from as simple as two-picture sequences to lengthier eight-picture sequences. The child puts the pictures together in the correct order and then tells the story as a whole, using the pictures as a cue. After telling the story with the pictures, the pictures can be removed, and the child can retell the story again without the benefit of the visual picture cues.

Repetitive Line Stories

Toys or magnetic pictures can be used to tell stories with repetitive lines. The syntactic structure of repetitive line stories stays the same throughout most of the story, thereby reducing the linguistic load for the child. Familiar children's stories frequently contain repetitive lines (e.g., "Someone's been eating/sitting on/sleeping on . . . " from *Goldilocks and the Three Bears*). The following is an example of a repetitive line story using toy props:

> All the animals wanted to ride in the boat. The zebra got in the boat. The giraffe got in the boat. The gorilla got in the boat. The hippo got in the boat. The elephant got in the boat. Uh, oh, too many animals. YIKES! The boat tipped over. All the animals got wet.

> The linguistic structure of these stories can be made simpler or more complex, depending on a child's language capacities.

Sequenced Event Stories

Props and pictures can be used as needed to work on retelling familiar children's stories (e.g., *Red Riding Hood*) or telling new stories. The difference is that greater linguistic variety is evident in the sequential story than the repetitive line story, making it more challenging for children with expressive language impairments. The following story is based on an activity from *Language Exercises for Auditory Processing—Preschool Edition (LEAP-P,* Mattes & Schuchardt, 1997). Facilitating the use of connecting structures, such as conjunctions, is important in narrative skill development and should be modeled and taught when appropriate.

> Pitney Pig was very hungry, *so* he decided to eat some dinner. He ate spaghetti and salad for dinner. He was still hungry, *so* he ate some oranges and pears for dessert. *But* Pitney

was a very sloppy pig. He spilled spaghetti and salad all over the kitchen floor, *so* he swept the floor with a broom *and* washed the floor with a mop. *When* his mother came home she was so happy *because* the kitchen was all cleaned up.

Creating Novel Stories With a Partner

Partnering to tell a story allows the child to develop the ability to formulate novel ideas in the context of a story format without the child having to construct an entire story independently. Partner stories require each participant to demonstrate careful listening and flexibility because they need to expand on what the other participants have just said. The clinician can incorporate linguistic components (e.g., "first" "next" "after that," "finally," "suddenly something very scary happened," "It would have been perfect, but") that cue the child about the sequential nature, conflicts, and resolutions of the story. Begin with stories that mimic either familiar stories or familiar events for the child. The following is an example of a partner story based on an event familiar to the child: going to a movie theatre. After completing a portion of the story, the teller can pass a token to or tag the next storyteller to indicate that it is their turn.

"Two brothers went to see a movie. The movie was called . . .

Star Trek . . .

First they had to . . .

Buy some tickets . . .

Then they wanted some food, so . . .

They got popcorn and M&Ms and soda . . .

Next they went into the theater and . . .

Sat down in the back row . . .

The older brother liked the movie, but . . .

The younger brother didn't like it . . .

Because it was too scary. After the movie . . .

They went out for pizza. THE END"

Another option in partner storytelling could be to incorporate speech target stimulus words into the story. To do this, choose several of the child's target stimulus pictures and lay them on the table. The story moves back and forth between the clinician and the child or between two peers. Each time the child has a turn to tell a new part of the story, a new stimulus word is chosen and needs to be incorporated into the story. The stories may be silly, but that is okay. An additional way to structure an activity like this would be to go back to the beginning each time a new part of the story is added. This provides children multiple opportunities to use the same sentence structures and target words repeatedly.

Describing a Personal Experience or Series of Events

It is not unusual for children to be vague when asked, "What did you do at school today?" Choosing not to be forthcoming, however, is far different from being unable to formulate ideas to describe prior events. The systematic practice of reporting back on immediate and recent past events and learning how to connect ideas to tell a sequential story, which were described previously, will support the final goal of reporting about a personal experience or sequence of events. Visual cues may provide meaningful support for children who demonstrate challenges with recall.

Home-School Notebook

A home-school notebook is a beneficial support system for children, parents, and staff to relay information to the various individuals involved with the child on a day-to-day basis. To support the use of narratives by children, a teacher or parent can share information about the events of the weekend, school day, or any special activities or significant events that occurred during the course of the day. Children can refer to the notebook to trigger the recall of the day's events to respond to the parent's questions about the school day. For parents or teachers, the notebook can provide ideas for questions to help scaffold children's information sharing. For instance, if the parent indicated in the home-school notebook that the family went to a circus over the weekend, the teacher may begin by asking the child what the child did over the weekend. If the child does not provide a response, the teacher can probe further, "Did you go anywhere special with your family this weekend?" If further probing is required, the teacher may say, "Your parents wrote in your book that you saw a special show with people and animals doing tricks. Can you tell me about it?" Photographs or other remnants also can be added to the home-school notebook that may spark conversation about special events and activities.

Video Sharing

Short video segments of special activities can be shared between the child's family, school, and therapy. Digital video is easy to download onto the computer then send via email to and from parents, teachers, and clinicians, sparking conversation about the special events.

Independent Reporting

After children have developed the capacity to share information about events or daily activities with support, they may be ready to report about prior events independent of visual cues and supports. Repeated practice and provision of supports can be used as needed to make it easier for children with speech and language impairments to formulate increasingly complex personal narratives. The same holds true for conversations. It is difficult for children with language impairments to develop more advanced conversational skills without systematic practice.

Put "conversation time" or "sharing time" on the child's daily speech schedule so it becomes an anticipated activity. For children who are reluctant to share personal information, keep the conversation or sharing activity relatively short, even just a couple of minutes, and have them build up to conversations of increased length and complexity. The clinician should remind children when they leave therapy sessions or upon seeing them in the school building, that the clinician or teacher will be interested in hearing all about an upcoming activity, such as a school dance, a soccer game at recess, or a visit to Grandma's. Provide an environment in which (a) children recognize that individuals are interested in what they have to say and (b) supports and scaffolds are provided as needed; these will help to set the stage for greater willingness to engage in conversation and storytelling. With repeated practice, children's conversational and narrative skills will become increasingly complex and robust, building a sense of confidence and competence.

Games and Activities to Promote Social Interaction

SLPs, teachers, and parents can structure activities that promote enjoyable social interactions between children with communicative challenges—even children with rather limited expressive language—and their peers. As children acquire more language, they may be highly unintelligible in contexts that require a more open-ended style of interaction. Finding activities that are more structured, in which the language is somewhat more predictable, should allow for greater social engagement with reduced frustration. Although the ultimate goal in social interaction is flexible, novel communicative interactions, children with limited language may benefit from structure and predictability. Some of the activities listed here require limited or no language, making them beneficial for children with severe expressive language deficits. Other activities would be more appropriate for children with more expressive language.

Facilitating Social Interaction in Children With Limited Expressive Language

A child can participate in a variety of games and activities that address social communication, even if the child has limited expressive language.

Simple Board Games

Playing simple board games can promote reciprocal interaction in children with limited expressive communication. Board games typically evoke the following beneficial responses:

- elicit verbal interactions that are predictable and repetitive
- incorporate a set vocabulary
- utilize language that can be anticipated and practiced ahead of time

Children can be taught several key words and phrases that would be used within the context of games in general ("My turn." "Your turn." "I won!") or that could be applied to specific games ("I got red." "I got a match." "I'm ahead of you."). Picture boards with key words and phrases can be provided for children who are not able to express their ideas verbally.

Dyad or Small-Group Activities

The following games and activities can be played with a partner or in a small group with limited or no language required:

- Yes-no game. This game is played using only gestures, no words. A ball or beanbag is rolled or tossed among the players. The "passer" must make eye contact with the "receiver" to ask (using a gesture such as a shoulder shrug or pointing toward another player) if the receiver wants the ball. The receiver can choose to nod or shake their head. If the receiver shakes their head, the passer must gesture to another participant.

- Rock/paper/scissors
- Gestures game. Several easy to act out action or animal picture cards are placed face down in the center of the table. The player chooses a card and, without revealing it to anyone, acts out the card's action (e.g., brushing teeth, washing hair, sleeping, blowing out candles on a birthday cake) or pretends to be the animal shown on the card. The other participants try to guess the card.
- Tic-tac-toe
- Cooperative block tower. Two or more children build a block tower together. Each participant takes a turn placing a block of their choice on the tower. Children can ask one another for the required blocks (e.g., "blue square," "Give me a yellow rectangle.") either verbally or by pointing to picture symbols, so the children practice asking questions and listening to one another.
- Cooperative Potato Head or other character. This is similar to the cooperative block tower. Children can either build one character together or build individual characters. The interactions involve asking one another for the parts they need to build their characters.
- Mirror-mirror. This is a nonverbal game in which children take turns being the leader. The leader performs movements, and the follower acts out (mirrors) what the leader is doing. Children love to perform silly actions while learning to observe one another carefully.

Small- or Large-Group Activities

These activities also require limited or no language but can be played in the context of a small or large group:

- Balloon in the air. The group works cooperatively to keep a balloon in the air and not let it touch the ground.
- Act it out pairs. Each child is given a picture card of an animal or action to act out. Someone else in the game also has the same card. All the players begin acting out the picture shown on the card and try to find the person in the room with the matching card.
- Change the action or change the leader game. This game is similar to "Mirror-mirror" described earlier. The group stands in a circle, and the participants mirror the actions of the leader. When the leader tosses a beanbag or ball to another participant, that participant becomes the new leader.

Facilitating Social Interaction in Children With Greater Language Proficiency

After children have developed the ability to use spontaneous connected speech, other types of games and activities can be used to address social communication needs.

Activities That Show Off a Child's Knowledge or Passion

With the right support, children often are eager to demonstrate what they know. They may have a great deal of knowledge about a specific topic or have a strong interest in a particular area. Set up opportunities for children to show off their knowledge using activities such as the following:

- Collection sharing. The child may bring in a collection to school and tell their peers about what they collect and how they became interested in this collection.

- Show-and-tell. Show-and-tell activities can be incorporated into treatment groups or classrooms. The child can describe the hidden object, and the other students can try to guess the object. An alternative would be for the observers to ask yes-no questions in a 20-questions format to try to guess the object.

- Jeopardy! Create a Jeopardy! game, similar to the television game. Devote specific columns to topics about which the individual children have specific knowledge or interest, thus allowing the child to shine.

Barrier Games

The following barrier games/activities require the child to increase specificity in language and to increase sensitivity to the needs of the listener with regard to speech clarity:

- Describe how to draw it, build it, make it. Children are provided with the necessary tools to draw, build, or create something. With a screen between the paired children, one child tells how the item is created one step at a time, while the partner creates the item exactly as indicated by the child. After the screen is removed, the two creations can be compared. The complexity of language required for these activities can be simplified or increased by limiting or increasing the variety of objects available to the children. For example, if a child is giving instructions for decorating a tree, the sentence could be, "Put three yellow stars on the tree" or "Put two orange cats under the tree." The child can ask for clarifications of instructions as needed. If the child gave instructions to a peer, and the instructions are not clear enough, the peer may request clarification (e.g., Child A: "Put the hat on the doll." Child B: "Which hat?" Child A: "The one with the green feather.") Activities may include the following:
    - creating holiday and seasonal decorations (tree, pumpkin, snowman, outdoor seasonal scene)
    - making pretend meals (pizza, hot dogs, hamburgers, sandwich, salad, soup, ice cream sundae) with the requested toppings or ingredients
    - decorating or dressing a paper doll or pet
    - building a block tower
    - sketching a picture drawing
- Barrier-type board games for purchase. Each of these games provides a structured way for two participants to communicate by asking questions or giving instructions to one another:
    - MagneTalk (Super Duper, Inc., http://www.superduperinc.com/)

- Guess Who? (Hasbro, http://www.hasbro.com)
- Battleship (Hasbro, http://www.hasbro.com)

Role-Play Activities

Role-play activities can provide opportunities to expand expressive communication by using scenarios familiar to the children. Vocabulary and typical questions and responses appropriate to a given scenario may be practiced ahead of time for children who need some preteaching. Because the topic is defined, the impact of the child's limited speech intelligibility may be reduced. Giving the child roles in familiar play scenarios (e.g., grocery store clerk, waiter, ice cream parlor scooper, mechanic, car dealer, doctor, schoolteacher, pet store owner, firefighter) that are manageable offers opportunities for the child to participate more fully in the interaction. Costumes, hats, props, and puppets—even simple stick puppets—can provide additional cues to help children maintain interaction and facilitate language use.

This chapter stressed the importance of looking at the whole child as they get older to address their ongoing communication challenges. By addressing articulation, language, and social communication, the child will continue to develop greater communicative competence to achieve their full potential both educationally and socially.

References

Baker, E. (2021). Minimal pairs intervention. In A. L. Williams, S. McLeod, & R. J. McCauley (Eds.), *Interventions for speech sound disorders in children* (2nd ed., Chapter 3). Brookes Publishing.

Baker, E., Williams, A. L., McLeod, S., & McCauley, R. (2018). Elements of phonological interventions for children with speech sound disorders: The development of a taxonomy. *American Journal of Speech-Language Pathology, 27*, 906–935. https://doi.org/10.1044/2018_AJSLP-17-0127

Beck, I. L., & McKeown, M. G. (1985). Teaching vocabulary: Making the instruction fit the goal. *Educational Perspectives, 23*, 11–15.

Beck, I. L., McKeown, M. G., & Kugan, L. (2002). *Bringing words to life: Robust vocabulary instruction.* Guilford Press.

Beck, I. L., McKeown, M. G., & Kugan, L. (2013). *Bringing words to life: Robust vocabulary instruction* (2nd ed.). Guilford Press.

Bleile, K. (2018). *The late eight* (3rd ed.). Plural Publishing.

Ernst, L. C. (1992). *Zinnia and Dot.* Viking Press.

Ladefoged, P. (2001). *A course in phonetics* (4th ed.). Harcourt.

Lewis, B. A., & Freebairn, L. (1992). Residual effects of preschool phonology disorders in grade school, adolescence, and adulthood. *Journal of Speech and Hearing Research, 15*, 819–831. https://doi.org/10.1044/jshr.3504.819

Lundeborg, I., & McAllister, A. (2007). Treatment with a combination of intra-oral sensory stimulation and electropalatography in a child with severe developmental dyspraxia. *Logopedics Phoniatrics Vocology, 32*, 71–79. https://doi.org/10.1080/14015430600852035

Mattes, L. J., & Schuchardt, P. R. (1997). *Language exercises for auditory processing: Preschool edition.* Academic Communication Associates.

McNeill, B. C., & Gillon, G. T. (2021). Integrated phonological awareness intervention. In A. L. Williams, S. McLeod, & R. J. McCauley (Eds.), *Intervention for speech sound disorders in children* (2nd ed., pp. 111–139). Brookes Publishing.

Murray, E., McCabe, P., & Ballard, K. J. (2015). A randomized controlled trial for children with childhood apraxia of speech comparing Rapid Syllable Transition Treatment and the Nuffield Dyspraxia Programme (3rd ed.). *Journal of Speech, Language, and Hearing Research, 58*(3), 669–686. https://doi.org/10.1044/2015_JSLHR-S-13-0179

Pellegrini, A. D. (1985). Relations between preschool children's symbolic play and literate behavior. In L. Galda & A. D. Pellegrini (Eds.), *Play, language and stories: The development of children's literate behavior.* Ablex.

Perzas, R. F., Magnus, L. C., & Hodson, B. W. (2021). The cycles approach. In A. L. Williams, S. McLeod, & R. J. McCauley (Eds.), *Intervention for speech sound disorders in children* (2nd ed., pp. 251–278). Brookes Publishing.

Preston, J. L., Brick, N., & Landi, N. (2013). Ultrasound biofeedback treatment for persisting childhood apraxia of speech. *American Journal of Speech-Language Pathology, 22*, 627–643. https://doi.org/10.1044/1058-0360(2013/12-0139)

Rice, M., Sell, M., & Hadley, P. (1991). Social interactions of speech and language-impaired children. *Journal of Speech and Hearing Research, 34*, 1299–1307. https://doi.org/10.1044/jshr.3406.1299

Secord, W. A., Boyce, S. E., Donohue, J. S., Fox, R. A., & Shine, R. E. (2007). *Eliciting sounds: Techniques and strategies for clinicians* (2nd ed.). Thomson Delmar Learning.

Westby, C. (1991). Assessing and remediating text comprehension problems. In A. Kamhi & H. Catts (Eds.), *Reading disabilities: A developmental language perspective* (pp. 199–260). Allyn & Bacon.

Williams, A. L., & Sugden, E. (2021). Multiple oppositions intervention. In A. L. Williams, S. McLeod, & R. J. McCauley (Eds.), *Intervention for speech sound disorders in children* (2nd ed., pp. 61–89). Brookes Publishing.

Young, E. C. (1987). The effects of treatment on consonant cluster and weak syllable reduction processes in misarticulating children. *Language Speech, and Hearing Services in Schools, 18*, 23–33. https://doi.org/10.1044/0161-1461.1801.23

Treating Children With Co-Occurring Disorders

As mentioned in earlier chapters, childhood apraxia of speech (CAS) often co-occurs with other disorders that may be impacted by or unrelated to CAS. Children with CAS are at greater risk for difficulties with *phonological and phonemic awareness and literacy*, especially if the child with CAS also has an accompanying language disorder (Miller et al., 2019; Zaretsky et al., 2010). CAS often co-occurs with *expressive language disorder* that may or may not be impacted by the child's sensorimotor planning and programming difficulties (Ekelman & Aram, 1983; Lewis et al., 2004). Chapter 7 provides a more thorough discussion of the types of phonological awareness and early literacy challenges facing children with CAS, as well as suggestions for working with these challenges in the context of speech sensorimotor planning treatment. Facilitation of expressive language in younger children is addressed in Chapter 6 and in older children in Chapter 8.

This chapter addresses some of the other co-occurring challenges that children with CAS may experience including dysarthria, attention deficit hyperactivity disorder (ADHD), social-emotional differences, autism spectrum disorder (ASD), and developmental coordination disorder (DCD). While there are other challenges that may co-occur with CAS (e.g., seizure disorders, hearing loss, cleft lip/palate, genetic disorders), this chapter's discussion is limited to co-occurring dysarthria, ADHD, social-emotional differences, ASD, and DCD.

It behooves us as speech-language pathologists (SLPs) to complete a thorough speech and language evaluation, to observe the child carefully, and to ask the caregivers and teachers questions that may help uncover the broader challenges the child is experiencing at home, in school, and in the community. It also is important to recognize the secondary impacts on the child's social and emotional functioning that may occur in children who struggle to speak intelligibly or whose speech and language is significantly delayed. A holistic approach to evaluation was described in Chapter 2. By looking at the whole child and practicing diagnostic therapy by regularly observing the ongoing and changing needs of the child, the SLP can make appropriate referrals and recommendations, determine the relative contribution of each of the child's areas of challenge, prioritize treatment goals, and support the family in understanding the complex needs of their child.

Addressing the Needs of Children With
Co-Occurring Developmental Dysarthria and CAS

As described in Chapters 1 and 2, children may have co-occurring developmental dysarthria and CAS. Whereas CAS implies challenges at the level of sensorimotor planning and programming, developmental dysarthria implies damage to the central or peripheral nervous systems impacting the *execution* of speech movement. Dysarthria impacts any one of or combination of the speech subsystems (respiration, phonation, resonance, articulation, and prosody; Pennington & Hodge, 2021) to varying degrees. Although all dysarthrias are characterized by imprecise articulation, the specific features for different subtypes depend on which neural substrates (e.g., cranial nerves, *basal ganglia* control circuit, cerebellum) are affected and the resulting degree of impairment (Skinder-Meredith & MacLeod, 2013). For example, if the cerebellum is impacted, we would expect to see an *ataxic dysarthria*, which is characterized by disordered prosody, poor respiratory-phonatory coordination, and scanning speech. If cranial nerves are damaged, we may observe weakness and decreased range of motion, coordination, speed, and/or stability in the structures they innervate. When dysarthria is suspected, a thorough examination of each of the speech subsystems is essential (see Chapter 2 for more detail). Table 2–24 in Chapter 2 provides a comparison of CAS, dysarthria, and severe phonological disorder. Note that errors of consonant and vowel distortion are a common feature in the speech of children with dysarthria, along with voicing errors and phoneme substitutions and omissions. Children with dysarthria exhibit reduced strength and coordination of the speech musculature; often have difficulty controlling rate, rhythm, and prosody; and often have hypernasality and voice quality differences (e.g., strained, breathy, harsh). Although dysarthria may impact any or all of the speech subsystems, Lee et al. (2014) and Allison and Hustad (2018) reported that the articulatory subsystem had the most significant impact on the speech intelligibility of children with dysarthria and cerebral palsy (CP).

Research regarding treatment to improve speech intelligibility and communication in children with dysarthria is limited. However, there has been some recent research to help guide SLPs in treatment for children with dysarthria. Three approaches to treatment of developmental dysarthria, the *Speech Systems Approach, Lee Silverman Voice Treatment (LSVT LOUD),* and *Speech Intelligibility Treatment,* are described here.

Pennington and Hodge (2021) describe a Speech Systems Approach to treatment of developmental dysarthria and provide evidence of its positive outcomes for children with CP and dysarthria (Pennington et al., 2010, 2013). This approach supports outcomes as presented in the International Classification of Functioning, Disability and Health, Children and Youth version in *Body Function* by increasing the child's control of speech systems, *Activities* by increasing overall speech intelligibility, and *Participation* by increasing the child's frequency of communication in a wider variety of contexts. The program achieves these outcomes by supporting a child's ability to (a) maintain a sufficiently loud voice so they can be heard; (b) use a rate of speech that facilitates articulatory accuracy in production of words and phrases; and (c) chunk utterances into shorter, more manageable phrases. The child's perception is also targeted in treatment to help the child recognize when their speech is clear versus imprecise and weak.

Rather than being a speech sound intervention, the focus of the Speech Systems Approach is on increasing overall intelligibility by teaching the child strategies to increase the clarity of speech and develop an automaticity in remembering to use the strategies that are practiced during treatment in other settings. Simple cues are provided in treatment to help focus the child's attention on loudness (e.g., loud, strong voice), rate (e.g., slow, steady), and chunking (e.g., short). Many of the suggestions provided in Chapter 5 on establishing vowels and natural prosody will be helpful for children with dysarthria as well.

Another approach for children with dysarthria that has gained some attention is the Lee Silverman Voice Treatment (LSVT LOUD). By increasing loudness, researchers have found that there is a spreading effect to the articulatory system in some children with CP and Down syndrome (Fox & Boliek, 2012; Langlois et al., 2020). Information regarding training and certification in LSVT LOUD can be found at the LSVT Global website (https://www.lsvtglobal .com/Therapists_Professionals#trainingCertificationSection).

Levy et al., (2021) provided Speech Intelligibility Treatment (SIT) to children with CP and dysarthria in an intensive summer camp program (i.e., 6.5 hours/day, 5 days/week, for 3 weeks). The children were provided with instruction to "speak with your big mouth and strong voice," (p. 2302) beginning with word-level productions and moving up to their higher linguistic level in playful and social activities. The "big mouth" instruction was used to facilitate increased articulatory excursion for more precise articulation. The children were cued to use a "strong voice" to increase vocal intensity and raise "amplitude across the speech production system" (p. 2302). The overriding goals of the SIT program were to improve the children's speech intelligibility and encourage increased participation in communicative interactions through intensive and repetitive practice. Although there was considerable variability among the participants, the children enrolled in the program demonstrated gains in intelligibility and communicative participation.

Hodge and Wellman (1999) and Skinder-Meredith and MacLeod (2013) provide recommendations for treatment of each of the speech subsystems for children with dysarthria. They recommend providing treatment that helps support increased muscle strength (so the child can use greater physiological effort during speech), normalization of tone, and improvement of the coordination of the speech musculature. Increasing loudness is also recommended, along with improving vocal quality and prosody, and increasing the child's phonological and phonetic repertoire.

Table 9–1 provides a summary of suggestions for treatment of each of the speech subsystems when working with children with dysarthria.

For children who have CAS as well as dysarthria, it is important to address the child's sensorimotor planning as well as speech execution to achieve speech that is as intelligible as possible. A special emphasis on increased respiratory effort (say it louder, say it with intent), reduced rate of speech, and chunking of phrases to speak within the limits of respiratory control will be required. As with any child with CAS, careful selection of target utterances that match the child's sensorimotor speech capacities will be important, as will the use of multisensory cueing to facilitate increased accuracy of productions.

Keep in mind that at different points in the child's development, the focus of treatment may shift from addressing sensorimotor planning and programming (CAS) to addressing motor execution (dysarthria) depending on the relative contribution of various factors to the child's current speech status at a specific time. Also know that children don't "grow out of" dysarthria, and the focus of treatment for some children with CAS and dysarthria may be on achieving the highest level of intelligibility possible rather than expecting absolute accuracy. For some children, the use of augmentative and alternative communication (AAC) as a primary means of communication or to augment speech when communication breakdowns occur will need to be implemented as part of the treatment program.

Table 9–1. Treatment to Address the Speech Subsystems for Children With Dysarthria

Speech Subsystem	Suggestions for Treatment
Respiration	Provide seating that supports the child's posture. Consult with a physical therapist (PT) or occupational therapist (OT) to ensure the child's positioning is ideal for speech practice.
	Have the child practice using quick, deep inhalations followed by longer, controlled exhalations. Consult with a PT or OT for recommended activities to facilitate better respiratory capacity and breath control.
	Incorporate tactile feedback to help the child better associate the internal sensation of controlled exhalation during sustained frication of /s/ while they have one hand on their abdomen and one hand on their chest. Encourage slow, sustained production while they feel the contraction of their muscles.
	Control the length of the phrase chunks to match the child's respiratory capacity. Practice taking breath breaks at natural pauses in longer utterances.
Phonation	Establish greater physiological effort to increase the intensity of the voice and to sustain the loudness for longer breath groups.
	Incorporate visual feedback for maximum sustained phonation. This can become a game or a contest to see who can sustain the longest and with the loudest voice. The Bla Bla Bla app provides a visual representation of amplitude and is ideal for young children. The Voice Analyst app provides information on pitch, amplitude, and duration and is more appropriate for school-age children. Audacity software could also be used to show duration and amplitude.
	Work on producing a habitual pitch that is more acceptable (not too high or too low) and variations in pitch range.
	Address voice quality if voice is breathy, hoarse, harsh, or strained. Use relaxation techniques if the voice is strained or pushing (adduction) techniques if the voice is breathy.
	Work on voice onset time (VOT) to establish more accurate voiced/voiceless contrasts of phonemes.
Resonance	Increase jaw opening to increase oral resonance if the child is hypernasal.
	Decrease rate of speech to allow velopharyngeal mechanism more time to get to the correct aperture for appropriate resonance.
	Refer to an ENT for visualization of the velopharyngeal movement to see if a palatal lift or surgery to reduce hypernasality and nasal emission is warranted.

Table 9–1. *continued*

Speech Subsystem	Suggestions for Treatment
Articulation	Control the rate of speech to support increased speech intelligibility.
	Control the phrase length and the numbers of syllables per breath so the child does not run out of breath and speak on residual air, which can cause speech to be rushed and reduce intelligibility.
	Teach the child to use exaggerated speech movements to increase articulatory distinctions between phonemes.
	Facilitate articulatory precision using phonetic contrasts of consonants related to place (e.g., /t/ vs. /k/), manner (e.g., /m/ vs. /b/) and voicing (e.g., /t/ vs. /d/).
	Work on vowel contrasts for diphthongs vs. monophthongs (e.g., /aɪ/ vs. /ɑ/), tense vs. lax (e.g., /u/ vs. /ʊ/), central vs. the corner vowels (i.e., /i/, /u/, /æ/, and /ɑ/) (e.g., /ʌ/ vs. /æ/).
	Address accuracy of vowel production as needed (see Chapter 5).
	Work on prosody to facilitate more natural sounding speech (see Chapter 5)

In addition to direct speech practice, overall comprehensibility can be improved by teaching the child to incorporate strategies including introducing the topic before speaking about the topic (or using a topic board to inform the listener of the topic); checking on the listener to see if the listener seems to be following along; and using gestures, pointing, and facial expressions to help the listener understand the intent of the message. The communicative partners also can support the child by reducing distractions and background noise, looking at the child while they are talking, letting the child know when you do not understand them, asking the child yes-no or choice questions to check in and see if you are understanding the child's message, and repeating the part of the message you understood, so the child can fill in the portion that was not intelligible.

Attention Deficit Hyperactivity Disorder

A subgroup of children with CAS exhibit challenges with attention. Some of these children may be diagnosed with ADHD, exhibiting inattention, hyperactivity, or both. Lewis et al. (2012) examined the prevalence of ADHD in children with speech sound disorders (SSDs) of varying levels of severity. Their findings were interesting. ADHD was found to be more prevalent in children with more severe SSDs; however, this higher prevalence was limited to children with co-occurring language impairment (LI) and SSD. That is, children with SSD and co-occurring LI were at higher risk for ADHD. In addition, they found that children were more likely to have ADHD with inattention when both parents had histories of SSD. They suggest that children should be monitored for attention problems when there are risk factors such as two parents with a history of SSD or when children have both SSD and LI. When ADHD is suspected, it is appropriate to recommend that the child be seen by the family physician, developmental pediatrician, or pediatric neurologist who can make a definitive diagnosis.

For children to be full participants in the treatment process, attention to the task and to the clinician's face is vital. When children struggle with attention during the session, this can be challenging for the clinician and, perhaps, frustrating for the child. To support attention, provide activities that are intrinsically motivating. The activities should be predictable in that the child has a clear understanding of the expectations and their role in the activity. Keeping the activities short is also recommended for keeping children on task. Visual cueing systems to show the order of activities in the session can be beneficial, as the child can anticipate what is coming up, including when they may expect a short break (as illustrated in Figure 9–1). The activities themselves should have a clear beginning and a clear ending, so the child is not left hanging, not knowing when the activity will be over.

Some games and toys provide clear visual cues about how long the activity will go or how many turns the child will need to take before the activity is over. For example, a cupcake tin with a target utterance in each tin (that can be traded for playdough to make "cupcakes") provides the child with a clear, visual representation of how many more utterances will need to be practiced before moving on to the next activity. A game such as Jumping Jack by Goliath requires the child to place 12 carrots into the grass prior to pulling the carrots out one-by-one until the bunny pops out of the grass. This provides a naturalistic way for the child to keep track of how many targets will be practiced for that activity. A simple 10 × 10 matrix can be used with each of the 100 boxes crossed off as the child produces the targets—a 5 × 5 or a 2

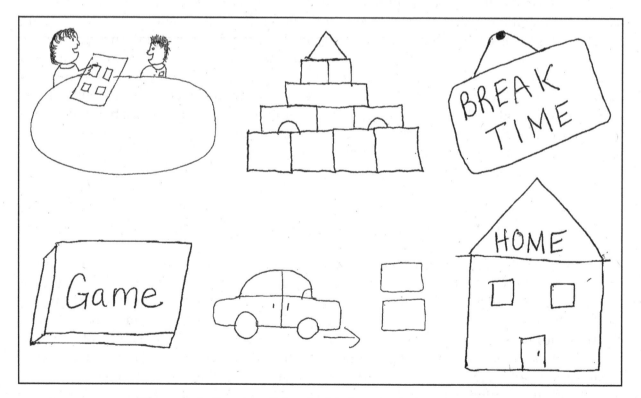

Figure 9–1. Sample activity schedule for speech therapy session.

× 5 matrix may be more appropriate for children who would find 100 boxes overwhelming. External reinforcers that are motivating for the child may prove to be beneficial in facilitating task completion. For example, a 2 × 5 token reinforcement chart can be created with tokens such as chips or blocks placed in each box. As the child completes a set of target utterances, the tokens are moved over to a companion chart showing what the child is working toward. After the child has placed all tokens on the companion chart, the child earns the reinforcer, as shown in Figure 9–2. Ask the child or consult with the parents about what is motivating for the child and find ways to incorporate motivating activities or themes into the treatment sessions.

Social-Emotional Wellness in Children With CAS

Children with CAS may experience difficulty with peer social engagement and/or emotional stress as a result of limited early vocal behaviors, limited experiences and opportunities to practice interacting verbally with peers during preschool years, and teasing or rejection of communication attempts by peers (Lewis et al., 2021; Rice et al., 1991; Tarshis et al., 2020). Parents of children with CAS express concern about their child's communication challenges and ability to produce intelligible speech, as well as their child's peer interactions (Rusiewicz et al., 2018).

Tarshis et al. (2020) describe the social interaction that begins during infancy, when children coo, cry, and babble, as the beginning of a social interaction feedback loop. Family members share emotional affect through words, smiles, or looks of concern to match the baby's emotional state. When babies and toddlers babble, parents imitate the babble and comment on what the child is looking at and doing. As a child learns to speak, caregivers react to their words, and the child responds (verbally or gesturally) to the caregiver's reaction, creating reciprocal circles of communication (Greenspan et al., 1998), thus strengthening the feedback loop. For children who do not babble as babies and do not speak intelligible words

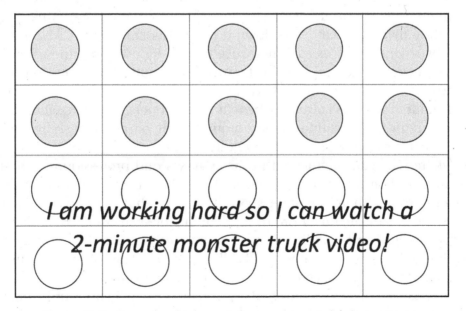

Figure 9–2. Example of token reinforcement materials in treatment.

during their toddler and preschool years, the feedback loop is weak. Parents tend to speak less to the child and share fewer reciprocal interactions. This lack of exposure can impact the child's social competence, self-esteem, and social problem solving. During the preschool years, Rice et al. (1991) observed that children with speech and language disorders tended to direct their verbal interactions to the adults in the preschool environment (rather than their peers), further limiting opportunities for peer social interaction, reciprocity, and social problem solving. As children get older and reach adolescence, the ramifications of poor verbal communication put these youngsters at risk for challenges in areas of psychosocial development. Adolescents with a history of CAS and those with a history of SSD and LI were more likely than their peers without communication disorders to have ADHD, social problems, and thought problems (Lewis et al., 2021).

Tarshis et al. (2020) recommend that when babies are at risk for severe communication stressors, including motor-speech impairment, parents should be provided with guidance about facilitating reciprocity and social engagement with their children. Parents can learn social and communicative routines, such as those described in Chapter 6 that are the foundation of Babble Boot Camp. As children begin to develop intentional communication, incorporating functional utterances (or manual signs) into treatment is essential to provide young children with skills to communicate and interact with their family and their peers. Consider power words/phrases like *"hi," "I do," "me too," "my turn," "not yet,"* and *"oh no,"* and provide realistic opportunities to practice using these targets in naturalistic activities. By delivering some of the treatment minutes in the context of the classroom or in dyads or small groups, the child has opportunities to navigate peer social interactions in a supportive environment and practice using their target utterances and gestures to take turns, share materials, and join their peers in cooperative play. Some of the other excellent recommendations put forth by Tarshis et al. to support the social development of toddlers and preschoolers with CAS include encouraging and facilitating children's attention to other communicative partners; creating opportunities for nonverbal interactive/cooperative play routines where a child and a caregiver/therapist or a child and their peers can play as social partners; layering in language to these play routines and adding small variations to the play routines in subsequent sessions; and creating opportunities for children to take on nonverbal or low verbal roles in play routines. For example, if the play routine involves racing cars down a ramp, the child with CAS may take on the role of Starter by saying, "go," as each new race begins. By using routines, the child has an opportunity to practice functional target utterances over multiple sessions to build repetitive practice opportunities, but in socially interactive ways.

Parents of children with CAS also may benefit from support. Rusiewicz et al. (2018) recommend guiding parents to or creating support groups where parents can share concerns about having a child with severe communication challenges. Apraxia-Kids offers Facebook groups for families where they can interact with other parents and professionals. These Facebook groups offer information and resources relevant to CAS. In addition to the "Apraxia Kids Official Support Group," there are other specialty groups that provide support for families with more specific needs, such as a group for "Parents of Teens and Tweens with Apraxia" and one for "Severe/Profound Childhood Apraxia of Speech (ages 5–12)." Rusiewicz et al. also recommend that SLPs assess not only the child's speech skill development, but use tools to measure functional outcomes, such as the Focus on the Outcomes of Communication Under Six (FOCUS) that assesses how well the child is improving in their communication and participation in real-world settings.

When working with school-age children and adolescents, particularly those with ongoing speech and language challenges, it is important for the SLP to be aware of the impact that long-term communication challenges can have on the child's social and emotional development (Lewis et al., 2021). The child may be comfortable with the SLP and the family who provide a safe and nurturing communicative environment; however, the child may be struggling socially and emotionally in other environments (classroom, community). Open a dialogue with the child and/or the family to discover if there are situations and settings where the child is less attentive, less comfortable and confident, and perhaps, more anxious. Make appropriate referrals to mental health professionals, such as a social worker, counselor, or psychologist, who can provide support for the child who is struggling with social and emotional differences. When possible, connect with the child's mental health professional to learn strategies that can be incorporated into treatment to support the child emotionally when they are struggling to communicate to help reduce the child's frustration and build resilience. Within the context of treatment, the SLP can incorporate target utterances that give the child a way to express their feelings of stress and frustration (e.g., *"This is hard." "I don't want to do it." "I'm worried about ___." "I need help with ___." "I feel stuck."*) and the internal sensations they may be feeling (e.g., *"I have a headache." "My stomach hurts."*). Providing functional phrases that promote resilience may also be useful (e.g., *"I can do it." "It was hard, but I did it." "I'll take a deep breath and try again."*). These types of strategies do not take the place of a mental health professional but may provide a way for children to express their emotions when they are experiencing frustration with the challenges with communication.

For children who have anxiety centered on communication, Kotrba (2015) has many tools to guide parents, teachers, and therapists to help the child work through the "worry monster." Although her resources are written for children with selective mutism, they still apply broadly to children who struggle with anxiety in general. One helpful technique is to name the emotion. There is an adage that says, "name it to tame it." If we name it the "worry monster," it can be thought of as something that you and the child can talk about and confront together. For example, if the child is looking anxious, you could state, "Hmmm, it looks like the worry monster is peeking out again. What should we tell him?" Power phrases like *"Go away!"* and *"You're not the boss of me!"* could be empowering. When it comes to anxiety, it is helpful to remember that it is a physiological response. We cannot make it entirely go away, but we can help lessen it to the point of it being tolerable.

Building resilience is beneficial for children who experience anxiety. It can be useful to think of resilience as an emotional muscle, and anxiety can be reduced by building the "resilience muscle." It is similar to working out, but instead of lifting weights, we are coaching the child through anxiety triggers in a gradual manner to help desensitize the child to what is perceived as worrisome. In the anxiety cycle illustrated in Figure 9–3, one can see how the avoidance of an anxiety-producing situation only fuels more anxiety, which leads to increased avoidance.

Parents, teachers, and therapists can work together with the child to figure out what the child's triggers are and make a plan to systematically work through them. Consider a child who is finding it difficult to engage with their peers due to anxiety. Step 1 could be to have them wave to a peer without looking at them; Step 2 could be to look at a peer and wave at them; Step 3 could be to wave and whisper "hi"; Step 4 would be to wave and say "hi" audibly; Step 5 could be to say "hi" and make a comment; and so on. By confronting the anxiety in a safe and supportive environment through purposeful and sequential practice opportunities,

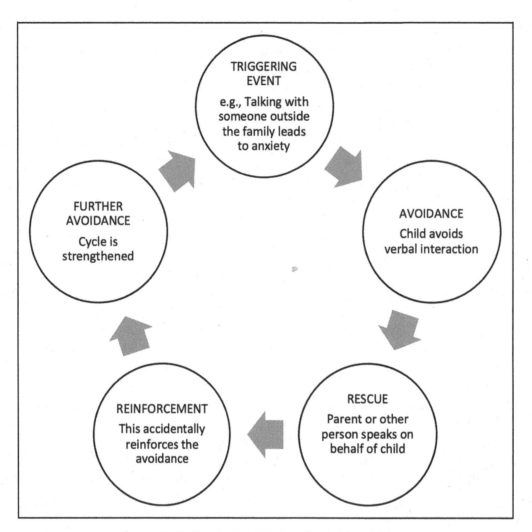

Figure 9–3. The Anxiety Cycle, adapted for children.

the anxiety cycle is disrupted, and the child can experience success in being able to do hard things. Each step will take multiple trials before the anxious feeling subsides, but when the child gets to experience that they were able to get through it, it can serve as encouragement that they can in fact do hard things. Kotrba (2015) and others who address the communication anxiety with children with speech and language disorders explain that the role of the adult is to be the child's cheerleader for any step made along the way. For example, in the previous situation, think of the child getting up the courage to wave to a peer but then looking away as soon as they did it. Rather than expressing disappointment, the adult can provide affirmation. "I'm proud of you. I know that was hard for you to do and you did it. What do you think we could try next time?" It is recommended that the SLP consult with a mental health professional (school counselor, social worker, psychotherapist) who can provide additional ways to support the child who is experiencing emotional, social, and functional impacts as a result of their communication challenges.

It takes a child with CAS a lot of work to improve speech, and there are many understandable moments when the child may want to quit or not try due to fear of failure. Luckily, many wonderful children's books have been published to help children understand they are

■ Box 9–1. Books for Young Children That Address Emotional Well-Being

The most magnificent thing by Ashley Spires

You are awesome by Susann Hoffmann

Resilience by Jayneen Sanders and Sofia Cardosa

A perfectly messed up story by Patrick McDonnell

A little SPOT of flexible thinking: A story about adapting to change by Diane Alber (Diane Alber has a series of books to help children have a growth mindset.)

I can do hard things: Mindful affirmations for kids by Gabi Barcia

Worry says what? by Allison Edwards and Ayesha Rubio

The Awfulizor (truth Tellers) by Kristin Maher

Wilma Jean the worry machine by Julia Cook

I have ants in my pants by Julia Cook

I can handle it and *I can handle it 2* by Laurie Wright and Ana Santos

not alone and that there are ways to get through making mistakes, taking on new challenges, and handling their fear and anxiety. Box 9–1 offers a list of books that can be beneficial in addressing the child's emotional well-being.

Addressing Speech Sensorimotor Planning in Children With ASD

Individuals with a diagnosis of ASD exhibit deficits in social interaction and communication, along with restricted interests and repetitive behaviors (American Psychiatric Association, 2013). Communication differences in children with autism may be quite severe. Approximately one-third to one-half of individuals with autism never develop functional speech (Wetherby et al., 2000). Those who do develop speech often exhibit challenges in the use of speech for more socially communicative purposes.

Rogers and Bennetto (2000) theorize that imitation of motor movements and oral/motor praxis challenges are core features for many individuals with ASD. Although it is recognized that underlying praxis problems contribute to the lack of speech development in some children with ASD, Wetherby et al. (2000) point out that "the transitions to intentional and symbolic communication provide the biggest obstacles to achieving communicative competence" (p. 128). Therefore, when evaluating children with autism who have sensorimotor speech planning deficits, it is important to recognize that a child's sensorimotor planning capability constitutes only one domain that may impact communication. Cognitive, social, emotional, and linguistic factors also impact communicative competence (Wetherby et al., 2000).

A thorough, multidisciplinary evaluation is needed to assess the extent to which each deficit area (e.g., sensorimotor planning and imitation; use of intentional communication for a broad range of functions; understanding of the symbolic nature of language; the capacity to share enjoyment and interests with others; cognition, receptive and expressive language; language processing and processing speed; working memory) impacts overall communication. Determining the extent to which deficits in any of these areas contribute to the child's communicative challenges will help prioritize goal setting for treatment planning.

Establishing Priorities in Treatment

In treatment of a child with ASD who has underlying speech praxis problems, it is critical that the treatment be socially relevant with an emphasis on helping the child with ASD learn to use speech for a wide range of communicative functions. Treatment of the speech praxis challenges outside a socially relevant context does little to help the child with social communicative challenges learn to use language purposefully. Individuals with combined CAS and autism benefit from a balanced program that provides opportunities for repetitive practice (to address the motor-speech challenges) in the context of a dynamic socially relevant environment (to address the social communication challenges).

When careful consideration is given to the "whole child," and each of the child's needs are determined following the evaluation process, it may become apparent that the child is not ready to work on speech imitation. For example, a motor-speech evaluation may reveal significant challenges with speech praxis. The language evaluation also may reveal significant difficulties learning the shared meaning for symbols (words, gestures, pictures). That is, the child may not associate a spoken word, picture, or manual sign (e.g., "milk") with what it represents (e.g., sippy cup). In this case, the initial treatment priority would be to help the child establish the cognitive-linguistic capacity for symbol use. Similarly, an evaluation of a child may reveal that the child makes limited attempts at social interaction. The treatment focus for this child would be on establishing joint attention and engagement, rather than trying to focus too early on imitation of sounds and words.

Specific Treatment Considerations for Children With ASD

After a child has begun to demonstrate greater social connectedness and recognize that sounds, words, gestures, or pictures can be used intentionally to express ideas, speech praxis goals can begin to be addressed. The following is a list of several specific considerations when developing and implementing treatment programs for children with ASD who also have CAS. Although each of these concepts is relevant to children with more typical social profiles, they take on greater significance when applied to children with ASD. They include the following:

- careful selection of target utterances
- careful selection of reinforcers
- balance of drill–based treatment strategies with social-pragmatic approaches
- carryover of skills learned to other settings
- use of augmentative communication

Each of these considerations is detailed in the following sections.

Select Target Utterances Carefully

When selecting target utterances for treatment, it is important to choose targets that are

- within the child's motoric capacities (including the child's phonemic and phonotactic repertoire)
- motivating for the child to increase the child's willingness to put forth the effort required to achieve success (e.g., favorite toys and food, familiar routines and enjoyable interactive games and activities)
- supportive of the child's use of language for a wide range of communicative functions (e.g., requesting favorite toys and activities, protesting, social communication such as greeting, commenting, getting attention, sharing information)

In addition to choosing appropriate target utterances for the treatment sessions, the activities used as teaching opportunities need to match the child's social, linguistic, cognitive, and motor abilities. The child needs to have a reason to communicate and something to communicate about. Imposing activities that "most" young children find desirable may backfire if the activities are not of interest to the child. Rather than attempting to resist the child's repetitive interests, try to use these strong interests to stimulate intentional communication. The child who repeatedly rolls toy cars off the edge of a table may be willing to produce target utterances such as, "uh oh," "go," "ready, set, go," "more," "more car," "blue car," or "give me a car" if the clinician is the purveyor of the desired cars. Playfully blocking the cars from rolling off the table may facilitate "move," "move your hand," or "move please." Consideration of the child's most immediate needs and strongest interests is essential when selecting target utterances for children with ASD.

Provide Meaningful and Motivating Reinforcers

Consider activities that are naturally reinforcing for the child (e.g., building a train track; rolling marbles down a marble run; completing a puzzle) and incorporate relevant treatment targets into these play activities. If the child can participate in some drill-type treatment prior to incorporating the target stimuli into play activities, provide quick reinforcers that are motivating to the child.

Balance Drill–Based Treatment Strategies With Social-Pragmatic Approaches

Beiting and Maas (2021) completed a preliminary investigation of treatment for three children with ASD and CAS. Their Autism-Centered Therapy for Childhood Apraxia of Speech (ACT4CAS) incorporated seven components that addressed the unique difficulties of children with severe social communication differences and CAS. These seven components included the following:

- **providing drill-based practice** to increase production attempts and establishment of the child's new sensorimotor plans
- **incorporating target stimuli into play-based practice** to encourage the child to maintain attention to the tasks, reduce the child's frustration, and facilitate generalization of newly acquired speech skills

- **focusing on production of functional target utterances** to promote increased opportunities to generalize the targets in home practice and to motivate and engage the child with more naturalistic speech/language opportunities

- **using prerecorded video models** to reduce reliance on real-time eye contact for children whose eye contact may be fleeting and to provide multiple exemplars of the speech targets by providing models produced by a range of speakers

- **incorporating visual supports** to increase the predictability of the session sequence through use of a visual schedule and to improve language comprehension through pairing of target utterances with video models and pictures

- **utilizing a hierarchy of prompts and cues** to support a higher degree of accuracy of productions, stabilize the child's sensorimotor plans, and increase opportunities to provide positive reinforcement

- **completing an initial assessment of preferences** to provide reinforcers that are maximally rewarding for the child and decrease the child's likelihood to become frustrated during challenging tasks

Many of the treatment elements overlap with DTTC (Strand, 2020). For example, the child is provided a similar hierarchy of cueing, ranging from simultaneous production with tactile support to prompted production without a model. In addition, parents are encouraged to participate and learn a variety of treatment and cueing strategies to increase the quality of the home practice program. The results of this preliminary treatment study were mixed. One child demonstrated improvement on some of the treatment targets, but the other two children did not. This may have been due to the limited number of treatment sessions, the severity of the children's communication skills, and these participants not being able to complete the study. The theoretical underpinnings of the program are strong. For example, ACT4CAS incorporates principles of motor learning and the key elements of DTTC, which have been shown to be effective in treatment of CAS. It also uses additional visual supports, such as a graphic schedule and video modeling, which have proven to be beneficial for children with ASD. Adapting the live modeling of the target utterance to video modeling is worthy of further investigation, as it is well supported in the literature for teaching children with ASD interactive play, social, and daily living skills from preschool through adult ages (Cox & AFIRM Team, 2018; Miltenberger & Charlop, 2015; NPDC, 2010). The adaptation of using video modeling may be beneficial to other children as well, especially for children who have better focused attention to a video-recorded presentation of the target utterance than a live model. Having parents as the recorded model may also help the child be more attentive and engaged. The one disadvantage, however, is the ability to change the rate of the video model when making sure the child's articulatory positions are in the correct place before moving on to the next sound. If nothing else, video modeling can be beneficial during the pre-practice phase of showing the child what the movement sequence will look like ahead of time.

Provide Opportunities for Carryover

One area of significant challenge in working with children with ASD is facilitating generalization and more spontaneous use of language learned during treatment into other settings. To promote carryover, it is important to

- Maintain open communication by sharing videos of sessions with caregivers and providing written communication to keep families and school teams aware of the goals and expectations.

- Demonstrate cueing techniques to parents and encourage parents to practice these strategies with the child.

- Incorporate the target stimuli into a variety of activities and, when possible, other settings so the child can make broader associations between the target utterances, what they represent, and their functional use.

- Systematically fade the multimodal cues and feedback to minimize cue dependency and feedback dependency (see Chapter 3).

- Choose activities that are meaningful and highly motivating to the child and structure the environment, so the child has a *need* to communicate (e.g., store favorite toys out of reach, have an essential piece of a toy/game omitted from the storage container to facilitate requesting).

- Provide sufficient practice opportunities to build muscle memory by keeping the activities quick and simple and providing opportunities for drill-based practiced as a warm-up.

Incorporate Augmentative Communication Into Treatment as Needed

Honoring communicative intent is critical in establishing meaningful communication in children with ASD. Therefore, providing children who have limited, inconsistent, or no verbal language with other means to express ideas is important for promoting communicative competence. AAC may take a variety of forms, including utilizing meaningful gestures and sign language, nonelectronic picture communication such as picture boards or the Picture Exchange Communication System (Frost & Bondy, 2002), and voice output communication devices. In Chapter 6, the positive impact on speech development for children using AAC was discussed. There may be transitional periods in which the child is using the verbal mode of communication in some situations and AAC in other situations. Situations of heightened stress, communication with unfamiliar listeners, repairs of communicative breakdowns, and attempts to express more complex ideas than the child's current speech motor system allows may require ongoing use of AAC.

DCD in Children With CAS

Some children with CAS may present with general clumsiness (e.g., tripping, bumping into furniture) and slow and inaccurate performance of gross and fine motor skills (e.g., kicking, throwing, catching a ball; using tools for cutting, drawing, and writing; riding a bike). If you ask a child to run down the hallway and watch the child's gate pattern or observe the child drawing a picture, you may see some of these features. When these deficits are significant enough that they interfere with the child's self-care (e.g., brushing teeth, using eating utensils), performance in school, or participation in play and leisure, but the challenges are not linked to a neuromuscular condition or an intellectual disability, the child could be diagnosed with

DCD. If you observe or the parent reports these types of clumsiness and coordination issues, you will want to refer the family to a pediatrician, developmental pediatrician, and/or a pediatric occupational therapist (OT) or physical therapist (PT) for an evaluation.

A study by Iuzzini-Seigel (2019) found that children with CAS + LI performed more poorly on coordination and balance tasks compared to children with SSD alone or typically developing children. In fact, all of the CAS + LI children in the study scored within the disordered range on the Movement Assessment Battery for Children, Second Edition (Henderson, Sugden, & Barnett, 2007). Duchow et al. (2019) compared the responses of parents of children with suspected CAS (sCAS) to parents of typically developing children on a DCD parent questionnaire. Their findings confirmed those of Iuzzini-Seigel, with 49% of children with sCAS and 9% of typically developing children being at risk for DCD.

Missiuna and Campbell (2014) summarized some of the broader implications for children with DCD. These include more limited physical activity and reduced physical fitness, as well as an increased likelihood of becoming overweight. Because children with DCD often face bullying and struggle to keep up with other children at school or in recreational activities, they are at increased risk for anxiety and depression. Given the potential social and emotional outcomes of children with DCD and CAS, it is imperative that we work with families, school personnel, OTs, and PTs to establish ways to mediate challenges faced by children who struggle with coordination and communication. OTs and PTs can provide recommendations regarding the child's seating arrangements when the child is seated at a desk, table, or on the floor. Schools can be encouraged to provide a laptop for taking notes, utilize a note-taker, or allow the child to record lectures to reduce the stress of writing. Adaptations can be made to gym class, so the child feels more secure and less anxious during ball activities. CanChild, a research center housed within the School of Rehabilitative Science at McMaster University, recommends encouraging children to participate in lifestyle activities "that do not require constant monitoring and feedback" (CanChild, 2022), such as running, swimming, and cycling. We have personally observed this in some of our older children with CAS and DCD who have taken up running, cycling, and skiing for recreation and fitness, activities that have brought significant joy and self-esteem to their lives.

In summary, a sensorimotor speech disorder may influence other areas of development, such as literacy, language, and social-emotional well-being. In addition, children with CAS can have co-occurring disorders in areas that impact attention, motor coordination, strength and coordination of speech movements, social interaction, and psychosocial development. It is imperative that SLPs be aware of the concomitant challenges that may be affecting children with CAS and make referrals when appropriate. Children with more complex medical and developmental differences will require a team approach to intervention that can identify the current challenges in all areas of development, determine the relative contribution of each of the areas affecting the child's current status, and recognize potential future issues that may impact the child's overall well-being.

References

Allison, K. M., & Hustad, K. C. (2018). Data-driven classification of dysarthria profiles in children with cerebral palsy. *Journal of Speech, Language, Hearing Research, 61,* 2837–2853. https://doi.org/10.1044/2018_JSLHR-S-17-0356

American Psychiatric Association. (2013). *Diagnostic and statistical manual of mental disorders* (5th ed.). https://doi.org/10.1176/appi.books.9780890425596

Beiting, M., & Maas, E. (2021). Autism-centered therapy for childhood apraxia of speech (ACT4CAS): A single-case experimental design study. *American Journal of Speech-Language Pathology, 30,* 1525–1541. https://doi.org/10.1044/2020_AJSLP-20-00131

CanChild. (2022). *Developmental coordination disorder: Management.* https://canchild.ca/en/diagnoses/developmental-coordination-disorder/management

Cox, A., & AFIRM Team. (2018). *Video modeling.* National Professional Development Center on Autism Spectrum Disorder, FPG Child Development Center, University of North Carolina. http://afirm.fpg.unc.edu/video-modeling

Duchow, H., Lindsay, A., Roth, K., Schell, S., Allen, D., & Boliek, C. (2019). The co-occurrence of possible developmental coordination disorder and suspected childhood apraxia of speech. *Canadian Journal of Speech-Language Pathology and Audiology, 43,* 81–93. https://cjslpa.ca/files/2019_CJSLPA_Vol_43/No_2/CJSLPA_Vol_43_No_2_2019_MS_1159.pdf

Ekelman, B. L., & Aram, D. M. (1983). Syntactic findings in developmental verbal apraxia. *Journal of Communication Disorders, 16,* 237–250. https://doi.org/10.1016/0021-9924(83)90008-4

Fox, C. M., & Boliek, C. A. (2012). Intensive voice treatment (LSVT LOUD) for children with spastic cerebral palsy and dysarthria. *Journal of Speech, Language, and Hearing Research, 55,* 930–945. https://doi.org/10.1044/1092-4388(2011/10-0235)

Frost, L., & Bondy, A. (2002). *The picture exchange communication system training manual.* Pyramid Educational Products.

Greenspan, S. I., Wieder, S., & Simons, R. (1998). *The child with special needs: Encouraging intellectual and emotional growth.* Addison-Wesley.

Henderson, S. E., Sugden, D. A., & Barnett, A. L. (2007). *Movement Assessment Battery for Children-2, Second edition (Movement ABC-2).* The Psychological Corporation.

Hodge, M. M., & Wellman, L. (1999). Management of children with dysarthria. In A. J. Caruso & E. A. Strand (Eds.), *Clinical management of motor-speech disorders in children* (pp. 209–280). Thieme Medical.

Iuzzini-Seigel, J. (2019). Motor performance in children with childhood apraxia of speech and speech sound disorders. *Journal of Speech, Language, and Hearing Research, 62,* 3220–3233. https://doi.org/10.1044/2019_JSLHR-S-18-0380

Kotrba, A. (2015). *Selective mutism: An assessment and intervention guide for therapists, educators & parents.* PESI Publishing & Media.

Langlois, C., Tucker, B. V., Sawatzky, A. N., Reed, A., & Boliek, C. A. (2020). Effects of an intensive voice treatment on articulatory function and speech intelligibility in children with motor speech disorders: A phase one study. *Journal of Communication Disorders, 86.* https://doi.org/10.1016/j.jcomdis.2020.106003

Lee, J., Hustad, K. C., & Weismer, G. (2014). Predicting speech intelligibility with a multiple speech subsystem approach in children with cerebral palsy. *Journal of Speech, Language, and Hearing Research, 57,* 1666–1678. https://doi.org/10.1044/2014_JSLHR-S-13-0292

Levy, E. S., Chang, Y. M., Hwang, K., & McAuliffe, M. J. (2021). Perceptual and acoustic effects of dual-focus speech treatment in children with dysarthria. *Journal of Speech, Language, and Hearing Research, 64,* 2301–2316. https://doi.org/10.1044/2020_JSLHR-20-00301

Lewis, B. A., Benchek, P., Tag, J., Miller, G., Freebairn, L., Taylor, G., Iyengar, S. K., & Stein, C. M. (2021). Psychosocial comorbidities in adolescents with histories of childhood apraxia of speech. *American Journal of Speech-Language Pathology, 30,* 2572–2588. https://doi.org/10.1044/2021_AJSLP-21-00035

Lewis, B. A., Freebairn, L. A., Hansen, A. J., Iyengar, S. K., & Taylor, H. G. (2004). School-age follow-up of children with childhood apraxia of speech. *Language, Speech, and Hearing Services in Schools, 35,* 122–140. https://doi.org/10.1044/0161-1461(2004/014)

Lewis, B. A., Short, E. J., Iyengar, S. K., Taylor, H. G., Freebairn, L., Tag, J., . . . Stein, C. M. (2012). Speech-sound disorders and attention-deficit/hyperactivity disorder symptoms. *Topics in Language Disorders, 32,* 247–263. https://doi.org/10.1097/tld.0b013e318261f086

Miller, G. J., Lewis, B., Benchek, P., Freebairn, L., Tag, J., Budge, K., Iyengar, S. K., Voss-Hoynes, H., Taylor, H. G., & Stein, C. (2019). Reading outcomes for individuals with histories of suspected childhood apraxia of speech. *American Journal of Speech-Language Pathology, 28,* 1432–1447. https://doi.org/10.1044/2019_AJSLP-18-0132

Miltenberger, C., & Charlop, M. (2015). The comparative effectiveness of portable video modeling vs. traditional video modeling interventions with children with autism spectrum disorders. *Journal of Developmental and Physical Disabilities, 27*, 341–358. https://doi.org/10.1007/s10882-014-9416-y

Missiuna, C., & Campbell, W. N. (2014). Psychological aspects of developmental coordination disorder: Can we establish causality? *Current Developmental Disorders Reports, 1*, 125–131. http://dx.doi.org/10.1007/s40474-014-0012-8

National Professional Development Center on Autism Spectrum Disorders (NPDC). (2010). *Evidence-based practice brief: Video modeling.* https://autismpdc.fpg.unc.edu/sites/autismpdc.fpg.unc.edu/files/imce/documents/VideoModeling_Complete.pdf

Nikopoulos, C. K., & Keenan, M. (2004). Effects of video modeling on social initiations by children with autism. *Journal of Applied Behavior Analysis, 37*, 93–96. https://doi.org/10.1901/jaba.2004.37-93

Pennington, L., & Hodge, M. M. (2021). Intervention strategies for developmental dysarthria. In A. L. Williams, S. McLeod, & R. J. McCauley (Eds.), *Interventions for speech sound disorders in children* (2nd ed., pp. 601–625). Paul H. Brookes.

Pennington, L., Miller, N., Robson, S., & Steen, N. (2010). Intensive speech and language therapy for older children with cerebral palsy: A systems approach. *Developmental Medicine and Child Neurology, 52*, 337–344. https://doi.org/10.1111/j.1469-8749.2009.03366.x

Pennington, L., Roelant, E., Thompson, V., Robson, S., Steen, N., & Miller, N. (2013). Intensive dysarthria therapy for younger children with cerebral palsy. *Developmental Medicine and Child Neurology, 55*, 464–471. https://doi.org/10.1111/dmcn.12098

Rice, M., Sell, M., & Hadley, P. (1991). Social interactions of speech- and language-impaired children. *Journal of Speech, Language, and Hearing Research, 34*, 1299–1307. https://doi.org/10.1044/jshr.3406.1299

Rogers, S. J., & Bennetto, L. (2000). Intersubjectivity in autism: The roles of imitation and executive function. In A. Wetherby & B. Prizant (Eds.), *Autism spectrum disorders: A transactional developmental perspective* (pp. 79–107). Paul H. Brookes.

Rusiewicz, H. L., Maize, K., & Ptakowski, T. (2018). Parental experiences and perceptions related to childhood apraxia of speech: Focus on functional implications. *International Journal of Speech-Language Pathology, 20*, 569–580. https://doi.org/10.1080/17549507.2017.1359333

Skinder-Meredith, A., & MacLeod, A. (2013). Motor speech disorders in children. In B. Peter & A. MacLeod (Eds.), *Comprehensive perspectives on child speech development and disorders: Pathways from linguistic theory to clinical practice* (pp. 411–442). Nova Science.

Strand, E. A. (2020). Dynamic temporal and tactile cueing: A treatment strategy for childhood apraxia of speech. *American Journal of Speech-Language Pathology, 29*, 30–48. https://doi.org/10.1044/2019_AJSLP-19-0005

Tarshis, N., Garcia Winner, M., & Crooke, P. (2020). What does it mean to be social? Defining the social landscape for children with childhood apraxia of speech. *Perspectives of the ASHA Special Interest Groups, SIG 2, 5*, 843–852. https://doi.org/10.1044/2020_PERSP-19-00116

Wetherby, A. M., Prizant, B. M., & Schuler, A. L. (2000). Understanding the nature of communication and language impairments. In A. M. Wetherby & B. M. Prizant (Eds.), *Autism spectrum disorders: A transactional developmental perspective* (pp. 109–141). Paul H. Brookes.

Zaretsky, E., Velleman, S. L., & Curro, K. (2010). Through the magnifying glass: Underlying literacy deficits and remediation potential in childhood apraxia of speech. *International Journal of Speech-Language Pathology, 12*(1), 58–68. https://doi.org/10.3109/17549500903216720

10

Considerations in Treatment of Childhood Apraxia of Speech Via Telepractice

I n the 1990s, the American Speech-Language-Hearing Association (ASHA) began investigating the viability of treatment via telepractice in the fields of speech-language pathology and audiology. ASHA (n.d.) defines *telepractice* as "the application of telecommunications technology to deliver professional services at a distance by linking clinician to client, or clinician to clinician for assessment, intervention, and/or consultation." ASHA now provides a Practice Portal defining the roles and responsibilities and ethical considerations of telepractice practitioners.

Recent studies are just beginning to show the benefits of telepractice treatment in children with childhood apraxia of speech (CAS). In a study of five children receiving Rapid Syllable Transition Treatment (ReST) four sessions per week for 3 weeks via telepractice, all the participants demonstrated gains in their imitation of pseudowords during treatment, as well as their production of untreated pseudowords and real words. Some of the children maintained their skills 4 months posttreatment, but the group did not show ongoing improvement posttreatment (Thomas et al., 2016). Grogan-Johnson et al. (2013) compared the progress of children with articulation disorders receiving in-person speech therapy services to those receiving telepractice therapy services. They found that children in both groups made improvement, and no difference in the progress between the groups was noted, thus supporting the use of telepractice for children with articulation disorders.

Proponents of telepractice services have pointed to the need to offer quality speech-language pathology services to individuals living in rural communities or others who have limited access to these services. In 2020, however, the need for telepractice services grew exponentially because of the COVID-19 pandemic. Clinicians were suddenly thrust into a situation of quickly getting up to speed in telepractice service delivery to keep their clients from losing valuable treatment services. Legislatures in many states required insurance companies to cover claims for services provided via telepractice just as they would for in-person services. As school districts began instituting remote learning options, school-based clinicians began providing telepractice services for their students. Training institutions also had to quickly adapt by learning and then teaching their student clinicians how to implement telepractice with telesupervision. In addition, the Commission for Academic Accreditation changed their guidelines so that students could more easily obtain clinical hours using this service delivery model.

 This chapter provides recommendations for telepractice service provision in general, as well as specific considerations for treating children with CAS. In writing this chapter, we acknowledge that regulations and technology including computers, peripheral equipment, software, and videoconferencing technology are constantly changing. Therefore, it is important for readers of this chapter considering implementing telepractice to recognize that some of the information provided here may no longer be applicable or accurate.

General Considerations for Telepractice

When implementing telepractice, consideration should be given to the hardware and software required, as well as setting up the teaching and learning spaces.

Hardware and Software Considerations

- Set up the device (computer or tablet) close to the WiFi router if possible.
- If the internet connection is unstable, try connecting the device to the router using an ethernet cable.
- When possible, choose a device with a larger screen, such as a computer or a tablet with a large screen. Cell phone screens may work, but it will be difficult for the child to watch the clinician's face on the small screen.
- Tablet computers, such as iPads, may work, but some applications may not work as smoothly as they would on a computer. In addition, some applications such as screen sharing or giving the child control of the screen may not work as well on a tablet.
- Be sure the device is fully powered or plugged into a power source.
- The child and the SLP should be using a good quality headset with a microphone for optimal sound quality and audibility. If an e-helper needs to help with the session, a headphone splitter can be used so two sets of headsets can be plugged in.

Setting Up the Teaching and Learning Spaces

- Find a quiet place to work with limited distractions (radio, television, people coming and going).
- Sit in a well-lit area with light in front of the computer to light up your face. If lighting is not ideal, you may be able to adjust for low light with the application you are using. For example, Zoom's video settings have a feature that will adjust for low light.

- Encourage the client to use a table/desk and chair, rather than sitting on the floor or on a bed.
- If your background is distracting, consider using a virtual background if the platform you are using allows for it.
- For younger children, an e-helper can assist the child in getting set up on the video communication platform. Some children will either require or benefit from the e-helper being on hand to facilitate the child's participation in the learning, while others may be able to participate without an e-helper once they are set up.
- Prior to starting each session, check your computer connection and log in a few minutes early to be sure your video screen and microphone are working. Open each of the games and activities you are planning to use during the session and have a few extra activities readily available in case one or more of your activities are not working or if the child is reluctant to engage with the activities you chose.

Telepractice Provision for Children With CAS

Not all children will be ideal candidates for telepractice. There are several internal (child-based) factors that will determine if a child with CAS would benefit from telepractice services including the child's age, their vision and hearing status, and their ability to attend to the screen and participate in a remote learning session. Other factors include access to a reliable internet connection, the availability of a learning environment with limited distractions, and an e-helper who can be available to support the child who may struggle to participate without support. Telepractice for children with CAS offers several benefits, as well as a few challenges.

Benefits of Telepractice for Children With CAS

There are many benefits of telepractice services for children with CAS and their families, including the following:

- Telepractice offers the benefit of reduced travel time. Because there is no travel time, there may be more opportunities for families to schedule shorter, more frequent sessions. By cutting out travel time, there also may be more flexibility in the days/ times the sessions are scheduled. Some clients we worked with during 2020 using a telepractice model were able to participate in three 30-min sessions, rather than the two 45-min sessions they were receiving prior to shifting to telepractice.
- Telepractice services may support better adherence to the therapy schedule by reducing interference with getting the child to therapy (e.g., transportation, illness of other members of the family, weather).
- Telepractice provides increased opportunities for the child's caregivers to participate in and observe the child's sessions. Because the therapy sessions occur in the child's natural environment, there are greater opportunities for carryover and generalization of skills.
- During telepractice sessions, the clinician has opportunities to coach caregivers in the use of treatment strategies (auditory, visual, and tactile cues). The clinician can coach

the caregivers in using cueing strategies in real time, rather than having the caregivers just watch the clinician provide the cues. For example, if the child would benefit from simultaneous production or a tactile cue to facilitate lip rounding, the clinician can cue the caregiver in how to provide the cues to the child (e.g., "Benny, look at mom's face. You and mom can say, "*go home*," together. Mom will help you with your circle lips if you need it.")

- Some children may find telepractice to be quite motivating, especially children who have an inherent interest in screens.

- The clinician can bring greater attention to their face by getting close to the camera, where getting this close-up view in person would feel awkward, not to mention not recommended by the Centers for Disease Control and Prevention (CDC) guidelines.

- The availability of a wide range of motivating and age-appropriate activities may enhance the child's motivation. During telepractice, the clinician can use novel teaching strategies and materials, by using the screen-sharing function to share PowerPoint or Google Slides, YouTube videos, enjoyable online games, and activities, as well as creative green-screen activities. If you are looking for innovative ideas for telepractice, consider participating in one of the many Facebook telepractice groups for speech-language pathologists (SLPs) that gained popularity during the COVID-19 pandemic.

Challenges in Provision of Telepractice

There also are some inherent challenges in providing CAS treatment through telepractice, including the following:

- Some families may have limited access to a computer or may not have a stable internet connection.

- Families may have difficulty finding a place to set up that offers limited distractions.

- It may be difficult to manage the behavior of some children or work with children who are easily distracted in their home environment.

- During treatment for children with CAS, the clinician often uses tactile cues. In telepractice, the clinician is no longer able to provide these tactile cues. Nevertheless, many parents are open to and do well with learning to provide some tactile cues through coaching.

- There also are limitations in the use of simultaneous production as a cueing strategy, because only one user's computer microphone is active at a time. This does, however, open up opportunities to coach parents to use simultaneous productions and to vary their rate and prosody when modeling target utterances. Our experience has been that parents improve and develop greater confidence in the provision of these cueing strategies with practice.

- A comprehensive motor-speech evaluation via telepractice would be difficult, as the child's ability to benefit from certain cueing strategies, specifically simultaneous productions and tactile cues, would be impossible in a remote assessment situation.

Engaging Children With CAS in Treatment Via Telepractice

Following are ideas to keep the child engaged and make the sessions as productive as possible:

- Evaluate the appropriateness of your online materials to be sure they match the child's age, cognitive, and linguistic levels. Also consider if the materials you choose are culturally appropriate for the individual client.

- Reach out to the child and the family to learn more about the child's interests. Use these interests in designing engaging activities to motivate the child to work through challenging tasks. For example, a child may have a goal to produce their name accurately. If the child loves superheroes or princesses, the clinician can use the screen-share function to show pictures of different superheroes. As each superhero comes on the screen, the child can "introduce" themselves to the superhero.

- Have a few more activities ready for the child to do during the session than would be required, so if one activity is a flop, you can easily move to another activity that may be more engaging for the child.

- Have all your screen-share activities open on your screen and ready to go, so you do not take up valuable session time hunting for the activity you want.

- Communicate with the caregivers in advance of the session if there is anything you want them to have available during the session (e.g., worksheet, picture cards, game, toy, paper, markers).

- Keep things positive by working at the child's optimum challenge point and by providing reinforcers that are meaningful for the child. Some children are happy to work hard for verbal feedback and reinforcement. Others may need tangible reinforcers such as earning stickers, earning points toward a small prize or a privilege at home, or being given an opportunity to watch a short video at the end of the lesson.

- Consider allowing the child to have a fidget or comfort item available to hold during the session as long as the item does not present a distraction.

- Provide the child with opportunities to make choices during the session.

- Take short movement breaks during the session to break up the monotony of sitting for extended periods of time. Movement breaks may involve a quick game of Simon Says, running in place, or doing a few yoga stretches.

- Keep the treatment activities relatively short to reduce boredom and keep the child interested and engaged.

Building Your Telepractice Toolbox

There are many ways to engage children with CAS in telepractice. Using a platform with screen-sharing capabilities allows you to create and then share personalized materials using Microsoft Word and PowerPoint, Google Docs, and other applications. Personalized materials can be as simple as a Word document (as in the example in Table 10–1) or more visually enticing with fun graphics and color. Table 10–1 is an example of a simple Word document

Table 10–1. Sample Shared Document for Online Treatment With Older Child

GOALS:
• Increasing accuracy of syllable stress assignment
• Reducing distortion of /i/ vowel
• Improving vowel-to-vowel juncture
• Controlling phrase length and taking breaths as needed
• Smooth coarticulatory transitions

CHALLENGE WORDS AND PHRASES			PRACTICE SENTENCES
how was *howuzz*	weekend *weekend*		How was your **wee**kend?
meet you *me chew*			I'll meet you at Starbucks.
we are *we yarr*	Florida ***floor** ruh duh*	vacation *vay **kay** shin*	We are going to **Flo**rida // for va**cat**ion soon.
I am *eye yam*	going *go wing*		I am going // to grandma's new house.
Tallahassee *tal luh **hass** see*			My grandma lives // in Talla**hass**ee.
spend time *spenn time*	Ethan ***ee** thin*		I like to spend time // with **E**than.
doing *do wing*	speech *sp**ee**ch*		What are you doing // after sp**ee**ch today?
you enjoy *you win **joy***	reading *ree ding*	poetry ***poe** wit tree*	Do you enjoy // **ree**ding poet**ry**?

shared during a telepractice session with a teen with CAS and mild dysarthria working on segmental and suprasegmental goals in functional sentences. Alternate spelling, highlights, breath pause markers (//), and bold print are used in this document to cue the youngster about his speech goals and facilitate accurate, smooth, and efficient productions of the target stimuli.

To achieve repetitive practice of functional phrases, you can incorporate the client's target phrases into social stories presented via PowerPoint or Google docs. Stories can be illustrated with clipart and photographs of the child's favorite people, pets, activities, and places. Write the story in a manner that encourages variable practice. For example, in a story where the child is asking friends to play, the main character asks, "Wanna play?" in a shy voice and then in a brave confident voice. To encourage multiple repetitions, stage loud events in the background of the narrative (e.g., a plane flying overhead or a jackhammer), to create situations where the child has to produce their phrase multiple times to be heard and needs to place more stress on the word heard incorrectly. For example a character could mis-hear one of the words and respond, "Do I wanna BAY?" The main character then responds, "No, wanna PLAY?"

For a quick visual feedback tool, create a simple sorter to provide general feedback on the child's target utterances. The sorter can be made on a PowerPoint slide. Place a picture on one side to represent "needs work' (e.g., Olaf in pieces) and one on the other side to represent ''you got it!" (e.g., Olaf all put together and smiling). Have ten virtual tokens prepared (e.g., colored circles to look like chips or other small shapes) and place a token on the side of the screen that shows the child's performance after each repetition. After the 10 tokens are placed, the child can then continue to work to acquire all the tokens on the "you got it" picture.

It can take time to locate picture stimuli for individualized activities. To increase work efficiency, it can be helpful to create online files with pictures representing target stimuli sorted by phoneme, syllable shape, functional phrases, and so on. The same picture can be placed in multiple files (e.g., a picture of a child walking toward a house can be used to represent "go home" and be placed in files for CVCVC, /o/, /g/, /h/, and /m/). Whether you upload your own pictures/photos or find clipart from online sources, the sorting process allows you to easily access the pictures to incorporate into your games and activities to create personalized materials for your clients. For repetitive practice, the same set of picture resources could be incorporated into a variety of activities within a Google document or a PowerPoint document. Quick and simple activities may include hiding pictures behind a shape and giving clues to guess the picture; completing fill-in-the-blank sentences by choosing a target picture; showing two or three pictures on one slide and then hiding one of the pictures on the next slide and having the child guess which picture is missing; and tic-tac-toe.

Online Resources

Digital visual biofeedback applications (e.g., *Waveform, Spectrogram, and Pitch Display* (WASP2), *Audacity*, *Voice Analyst*, *Bla Bla Bla*) can be used for individuals who benefit from analysis of acoustic signals to help judge their speech production accuracy. For *WASP*, you can provide the link to the web version (https://www.speechandhearing.net/laboratory/wasp/) in the chat box so the child can open it on their computer and share their screen with you. This will allow for better sound capturing since it will be done directly from their microphone. *Audacity* would need to be downloaded onto the client's computer or the recording would come through your computer. This still works. It just will not be as clean of a signal. Apps like *Voice Analyst* and *Bla Bla Bla* can be shared when using Zoom by going to the share iPhone or iPad option. If the client's family has these apps, you can show them how to share it from their end. If not, you can share and record the child's voice from your computer.

Following is a small sampling of the enormous number of online resources for telepractice. Many of these websites offer free or low-cost online resources that are suitable for therapy or for reinforcement. Some resources, such as Wheel of Names, Match the Memory, and Jeopardy Labs, can be customized to meet the needs of specific children.

- *Wheel of Names* provides a platform to create spinners with pictures, words, phrases, or sentences (https://wheelofnames.com/).

- *Jeopardy Labs* allows you to create Jeopardy games or use the library of Jeopardy games on the website, to practice specific target utterances at single-word, phrase, and sentence level (https://jeopardylabs.com/).

- *Match the Memory* allows you to create online matching games for target utterance practice (https://matchthememory.com/).

- *Ultimate SLP* offers a large selection of games to address speech and language, many of which can be customized for practice of specific target utterances (https://www.ultimateslp.com/).

- *Simply Speaking SLT* offers a wide variety of games to address speech and language, many of which can be customized. Many of games are quite similar to popular children's board games, so will be familiar to the children (https://simplyspeaking slt.com/).

- *Boom Learning* offers a huge selection of ready-made activities to support development of specific skills, including an ever-growing library of activities for children with CAS (https://wow.boomlearning.com/). When looking through the online store, use the search feature to locate materials for children with CAS. You can preview the activities before purchasing.

- *Teachers Pay Teachers* is a huge clearinghouse of learning tools, many of which are online tools, for teaching. You can use key words to search for activities specific for children with CAS, phonological, or articulation problems (https://www.teachers payteachers.com/).

- *Open Library* is a free platform for open access to a huge selection of e-books that can be borrowed for up to 14 days (https://openlibrary.org/).

- *Kids Poki* provides a large selection of fun games for young children to stimulate language and conversation (https://kids.poki.com/).

- *ABCYa* offers a wide selection of learning games and reinforcement activities (https://www.abcya.com/).

- *LessonPix Custom Learning Materials* provides low-cost membership to access a large range of templates and materials to create customized speech, language, and learning activities (https://lessonpix.com/).

- *Flyleaf Publishing* provides access to print and online decodable books for children in early elementary school and emergent readers (https://flyleafpublishing.com/).

- *Really Great Reading* provides movable letter tiles, which can be used to promote phonemic and phonological awareness. (https://www.reallygreatreading.com/lettertiles/)

Whether you are providing telepractice by choice or by necessity, it can be a powerful and effective way to treat children with CAS. As technology continues to improve, there will no doubt be increasingly effective online tools available for treatment, as well as assessment.

References

American Speech-Language-Hearing Association. (n.d.). *Telepractice* [Practice portal]. https://www.asha.org/Practice-Portal/Professional-Issues/Telepractice/

Grogan-Johnson, S., Schmidt, A. M., Schenker, J., Alvares, R., Rowan, L. E., & Taylor, J. (2013). A comparison of speech sound intervention delivered by telepractice and side-by-side service delivery mod-els. *Communication Disorders Quarterly, 34*, 210–220. https://doi.org/10.1177/1525740113484965

Thomas, D. C., McCabe, P., Ballard, K. J., & Lincoln, M. (2016). Telehealth delivery of Rapid Syllable Transitions (ReST) treatment for childhood apraxia of speech. *International Journal of Language and Communication Disorders, 51*, 654–671. https://doi.org/10.1111/1460-6984.12238

The Changing Needs of Children Over Time

Children grow and change over time. As they do, their needs and priorities will change as well. It is not unusual for children diagnosed with childhood apraxia of speech (CAS) to participate in direct speech and language treatment for extended periods of time, typically measured in years rather than months. Over the course of treatment, the goals and structure of the treatment program, as well as the methods used to address the child's goals, will change substantially. The 3-year-old child with a diagnosis of CAS may receive four individual, 30-min treatment sessions per week with an emphasis on facilitating speech praxis. As the child gets older, he may have developed fairly good control over sensorimotor speech planning but may be exhibiting notable deficits in syntax and morphology and residual articulation and/or phonological errors. Social and academic challenges may emerge along the way. The structure of treatment may shift to dyad or small-group sessions to address the child's articulation, language, academic, and social challenges. After significant progress has been made, it will be reasonable to reduce the number of weekly treatment minutes. The types of programs or treatment methods appropriate for a child exhibiting severe speech praxis challenges will be quite different from a child with some residual articulation errors.

 Although the diagnosis is important, it is the child's speech and language behaviors, not the diagnostic label, that will drive the treatment plan and determine the appropriate treatment methods.

Treatment Planning Considerations for Children With CAS

There are many things to consider when planning treatment programs for children with CAS. Several considerations are listed here, followed by a case study of a child with CAS. The case study is used to illustrate a child's changing needs and priorities over the course of several years. Considerations in treatment planning include the following:

- Be sure to look at the whole child. Consider the child's needs in the areas of oral praxis, speech praxis, prosody, resonance, voice, fluency, receptive and expressive language, social language, academics, and pre-academics when planning treatment. Determine what the primary issues are that are impacting the child's development (both speech/language and other areas of development) and set priorities for addressing these needs.

- In terms of speech, there is a balance between working on developing increasingly complex phoneme sequencing abilities and facilitating an expanded repertoire of phonemes.

- When choosing which phonemes to address, consider what we know about normal phoneme development, as well as the specific abilities of the child. Consider the child's stimulability when selecting phonemes for treatment and incorporate phonemes with varied place, manner, and voicing features to expand flexibility in coarticulation.

- After the child has developed the ability to produce targets with simple phonotactic complexity, continue increasing the complexity of phoneme sequences by facilitating the production of multisyllabic words, clusters, and more complex phoneme transitions, such as shifting between coronal and dorsal phonemes (e.g., /t/ to /k/ as in "talk").

- Begin to address language, particularly phrase production, early in the treatment process. Use simple and functional phrases and carrier phrases such as, "I want _____," "Help me," "Go home," "No _____," "I do it," and "Hi _____." Target a variety of parts of speech (nouns, verbs, prepositions, descriptive terms, etc.) to facilitate an easier transition into phrases.

- As a child's expressive language develops, keep an eye on any emerging challenges in syntax, morphology, and grammar, and address deficits in these areas as needed.

- Incorporate phonological awareness and early literacy activities into the context of speech praxis treatment beginning in preschool.

- Watch for possible literacy problems, and work in collaboration with the child's educational team to address any needs that arise.

- Goals related to prosody should be embedded in treatment throughout the course of therapy.

Case Study

A case study is used in Tables 11–1 through 11–9 to illustrate the changing nature of treatment over time (from 9 months through 14 years of age) for a girl whose brother has a diagnosis of severe CAS. The family and the brother's private speech-language pathologist (SLP) had been proactively keeping an eye on the child's development and decided to intervene at 9 months when the child exhibited no consonants in babbling and use of only vowel-like vocants during vocalizations. At each stage of development, the child's present level of performance will be described, along with recommendations for treatment that are priorities for the child at that moment in time. Basic treatment goals and possible methods for treatment are listed. The treatment goals listed in this case study are basic goal areas that will be addressed for this child. Goals that are developed for Individualized Education Programs and treatment plans, however, need to be written with greater clarity and specificity. Goal writing will be addressed in greater detail in Chapter 12.

Table 11–1. Mishka, Age: 9 Months

Present Level of Performance	
Vocalizations	Vocalizations consist of vocants (vowel-like productions); no canonical babbling
Verbal behavior	No true words
Imitation	Very limited gross motor imitation; no oral/facial or vocal imitation
Muscle tone/ strength	Within normal limits
Feeding	Within normal limits
Receptive language	Appears age-appropriate
Gestural communication	Uses a small number of gestures intentionally (e.g., pointing, shaking head no)
Social interactive skills	Excellent
Frustration	Generally happy demeanor

Diagnosis
Delayed early vocal development (b/c of limited babbling)

History
Older brother diagnosed with severe CAS—Family proactively following Mishka's development

Recommendation
Participate in modified parent-child dyad training with SLP trained in Babble Boot Camp (see Chapter 6), The Hanen Program (http://www.hanen.org/Programs/For-Parents/It-Takes-Two-to-Talk.aspx) or other program to facilitate early communication development.

Treatment Goals

Increase imitation

- Gross motor movements
- More subtle movements
- Oral/facial movements

Increase intentional communication

- Gestures
- Manual signs

Increase volubility and variety of vocalizations and babbling

continues

Table 11–1. *continued*

Treatment Methods

Facilitate imitation by

- Imitating the child's movements and sounds
- Praising the child's efforts at imitation
- Securing the child's attention prior to modeling movements or sounds
- Describing what the child is doing motorically (to support later cognitive controls)
- Interspersing movements the child can imitate consistently (e.g., clapping, banging on the table, raising arms above head) with more challenging movements (e.g., wiggling fingers, protruding tongue, saying "ah")
- Modeling and shaping social interactions (e.g., waving, blowing kisses, peek-a-boo)

Increase intentional communication by

- Modeling signs, gestures, and words in a slower, more dramatic manner
- Using hand-over-hand procedure to guide the production of simple gestures and manual signs (more, eat, mine, all done)
- Associating manual signs with spoken words

Facilitate vocalizations by

- Using amplification tools or toys that are activated in response to voice to stimulate vocalizations
- Reinforcing the child's vocalizations
- Imitating the child's vocalizations
- Modeling simple vocalizations the child has already produced
- Associating a vocalization with a specific event (e.g., "uh oh" each time the car crashes; lip pops each time a bubble is popped)
- Pausing and looking at the child expectantly after several models of the preceding vocalizations to give the child time to motor plan the vocalizations

Table 11–2. Mishka, Age: 2 Years, 0 Months

Present Level of Performance	
Vocalizations	Increased vocalizations and canonical babbling with a wider range of phonemes
Verbal behavior	Five or fewer true words; difficulty coordinating the timing of respiration, phonation, and articulation, resulting in *silent posturing* (positioning articulators as if to speak, but without vocalizing)
Imitation	Body imitation and oral/facial imitation improving; difficulty imitating true words, but beginning to imitate some vocalizations/sound effects (e.g., siren, baby crying)
Gestural communication	Uses several manual signs and gestures intentionally with a model and spontaneously
Frustration	Occasional tantrums when unable to be understood

Diagnosis

Expressive language delay; Suspected CAS (sCAS)

Recommendation

Begin direct one-to-one speech-language therapy 3×/week

Treatment Goals

Establish volitional verbal imitation

Increase phoneme repertoire

- Vowels
- Consonants

Increase repertoire of simple syllable shapes

Develop a core spoken vocabulary of functional words and phrases that incorporate simple word shapes and phonemes

Increase overall linguistic skills using multimodel communication that includes

- Spoken words
- Natural gestures
- Sign language
- Picture boards

continues

Table 11–2. *continued*

Treatment Methods

Address verbal imitation by

- Reinforcing verbal attempts
- Modeling a core vocabulary of simple syllables and words during play activities
  - Securing the child's visual attention when modeling core vocabulary
  - Keeping the core vocabulary set small
  - Using a reduced rate and greater vocal inflection for core vocabulary words
- Describing what the child is doing motorically (to support later cognitive controls)
- Interspersing sounds the child can imitate consistently with new sounds

Establish an increased phoneme repertoire and syllable-shape repertoire to facilitate the production of a functional vocabulary by

- Utilizing a multisensory treatment program that incorporates the principles of motor learning that would be appropriate for younger children (see Chapter 4)
- Introducing core vocabulary books to label and point to familiar people, objects, and places

Support multimodal communication by

- Modeling the use of sign language, gestures, and picture selection within the context of playful and functional activities
- Quickly and consistently reinforcing the use of words, signs, gestures, and picture selection

Reinforce speech-language development by

- Coaching parents in the use of early speech-language stimulation strategies during play and familiar routines and provide a manageable home practice program

Table 11–3. Mishka, Age: 2 Years, 9 Months

Present Level of Performance	
Vocalizations	Good volitional control over vocalizations
Verbal behavior	Produces many true words using the phonemes (/b, d, m, n, h, w/ and /i, u, o, a, ʌ/ and syllable shapes (C, CV, CVCV—mostly reduplicated); a great deal of homonymy exists due to limited phonetic inventory.
Imitation	Verbal imitation is progressing
Gestural communication	Beginning to use several signs spontaneously

Recommendations
School speech-language treatment: two times per week individual; one dyad session
Private speech-language treatment: two times per week individual

Treatment Goals
Increase phonetic inventory   • Vowels   • Consonants   • Syllable shapes
Reduce homonymy
Expand expressive vocabulary
Develop functional phrases and simple carrier phrases
Increase variety of novel phrases using a wider range of semantic relations

Treatment Methods
Support continued expansion of phonetic inventory and reduced homonymy by   • Focusing on phoneme sequencing/coarticulation, repetitive practice, and multisensory cueing (Chapter 3)   • Using a multisensory, evidence-based treatment program (see Chapter 4)

continues

Table 11–3. *continued*

Treatment Methods *continued*

Expand expressive vocabulary by giving thoughtful considerations to selection of target utterances (Chapter 3), including

- Syllable shape and phoneme repertoire
- Linguistic needs (vocabulary to support semantic relations)
- Environmental factors (family, neighborhood)
- Motivation (interests)
- Social needs (vocabulary to support a wide range of social language functions)

Develop phrase use by

- Expanding syllable shapes (see Chapter 6)
- Teaching vocabulary that supports semantic relations
- Using multimodal communication (see Chapter 6)
  - Manual signs
  - Gestures
  - Picture selection
  - Verbal communication

Table 11–4. Mishka, Age: 3 Years, 9 Months

Present Level of Performance	
Verbal behavior	Uses speech almost exclusively to communicate; connected speech is highly unintelligible; speech sound repertoire is expanding to include /p, b, t, d, m, n, w, h/, as well as /f, s/ in final position of a few words, and many vowels, with the exception of lax front and back vowels, rhotics, and some diphthongs; syllable shapes are expanding but exclude clusters; persistent vowel distortions in connected speech
Expressive language	Speaks in phrases of two to four words using telegraphic language patterns
Receptive language	Difficulty with comprehension of spatial concepts (e.g., under, next to, behind, in, out, by)
Social interaction	Prefers interacting with adults; shy and hesitant to interact with peers

Recommendations
Enroll in blended preschool classroom composed of seven children with special needs and seven typically developing children five mornings per week
School speech-language treatment 150 min per week: 90 min per week individual to address speech praxis and language   30 min small group or dyad to facilitate social interaction   30 min per week classroom-based instruction to address receptive and expressive language
Private speech-language treatment: two times per week one-to-one

Treatment Goals
Increase comprehension and use of spatial concepts
Increase speech intelligibility by   • Increasing consistency of syllable shape productions in phrases and sentences   • Increasing consistent use of phonemes within her repertoire in phrase- and sentence-level productions   • Expanding contexts of /f/, and /s/, and expanding phoneme repertoire to include other fricatives   • Controlling rate of speech to reduce phoneme and syllable omissions and vowel distortions   • Reducing reliance on multisensory cueing for accurate speech production

continues

Table 11–4. *continued*

Treatment Goals *continued*

Expand expressive syntax and morphology

- Articles (a, the)
- Copular and auxiliary verbs (is, are)
- Negatives (not, don't, no)
- Verb tense markers (ing, s)
- Plural "s" marker
- Possessive "s" marker
- Prepositions
- Early conjunctions (and, then)

Increase responses to peers' language and initiation of language toward peers

---

Treatment Methods

Expand basic concepts vocabulary, syntax, and morphology by

- Using play-based language therapy
- Expanding syllable shapes to include clusters (e.g., CVCC) to support morphological markers (e.g., cups, runs, Mom's)

Facilitate increased consistency and expansion of phonetic inventory at the phrase and sentence level by

- Using multisensory, evidence-based treatment programs
- Focusing on phoneme sequencing, repetitive practice, and multisensory cueing (Chapter 3)
- Providing visual cues to reduce rate of speech

Expand phoneme repertoire by

- Using traditional phonetic placement strategies
- Choosing *facilitating contexts* (phonemes before or after the target phoneme that help facilitate the accurate production of the target phoneme)

Facilitate social language development with peers by participation in a social language group and increasing opportunities to participate in dyads in the classroom

Table 11–5. Mishka, Age: 5 Years, 0 Months

Present Level of Performance	
Verbal behavior	Significant improvement in speech praxis; continued difficulty with complex, multisyllabic words and clusters; needs reminders to reduce speaking rate in order to increase intelligibility; expanded use of /s/ and /f/ to initial position of words and more final position contexts; beginning to produce /k/, /g/, and /ʃ/ in some contexts; not stimulable for /θ, ð, tʃ, dʒ, l, r/
Expressive language	Some residual morphological and syntactic errors
Receptive language	Goal met
Social interaction	Improved interaction with peers, but needs continued attention
Academic	Poor phonological awareness and phonemic awareness

Recommendations

Continue blended preschool program

School speech-language treatment 160 min per week:

    30 min per week dyad to address articulation/praxis, expressive language

    40 min per week individual to address articulation/praxis and phonological awareness

    30 min per week small group or dyad to facilitate social interaction

    60 min per week classroom-based instruction to address expressive language and phonological awareness

Private speech-language treatment: two times per week one-to-one

Treatment Goals

Increase speech intelligibility

- Increase phoneme repertoire
- Reduce phoneme/syllable omissions in connected speech
- Increase production of clusters in initial and final position of words
- Increase accurate production of multisyllabic words
- Increase consistency of /s/, /f/, /k/, /g/, and /ʃ/

Improve morphology and syntax skills

Improve phonological awareness skills in combination with articulation/ praxis skills

Improve social interaction skills with peers

continues

Table 11–5. *continued*

Treatment Methods

Address speech intelligibility through

- Phonetic placement techniques
- Use of facilitating contexts
- Visual, tactile, and cognitive cueing strategies to support production of multisyllabic words

Address rate control through

- Modeling
- Visual cueing
- Reinforcement of reduced rate in utterances of increased length

Address morphology and syntax through

- Language therapy
- Facilitation of the more complex syllable shapes required for production of various morphological markers

Address phonological awareness using Integrated Phonological Awareness or other similar programs

Facilitate social language development with peers through participation in a social language group (see Chapter 8 for treatment suggestions)

Table 11–6. Mishka, Age: 6 Years, 0 Months

Present Level of Performance	
Speech	Stimulable for /θ, ð, tʃ, dʒ/, but inconsistent
	Not yet stimulable for /r, ɚ/
	Difficulty with multisyllabic words
	Prosody differences (related to syllable stress of multisyllabic words; rhythm; syllable segregation)
Expressive language	Significant improvement in morphology and syntax; difficulty with organization and complexity of narrative language
Social interaction	Greatly improved
Academic	Improved phonological and phonemic awareness, but not grade/age appropriate

Recommendations
School speech-language treatment 90 min per week in small group or dyad to address articulation and narrative skill development
Learning resource assistance 120 min per week to address phonological awareness and early literacy
Private speech-language treatment discontinued

Speech-language Treatment Goals

Increase speech intelligibility

- Increase consistency and accuracy of production of /θ, ð, tʃ, dʒ /
- Attempt to elicit /r, ɚ/

Improve prosody

Improve narrative language development

Treatment Methods

Address speech intelligibility through

- Phonetic placement techniques
- Use of facilitating contexts and chaining methods (see Chapter 8)
- Contrastive techniques (e.g., minimal pairs)
- Practice of target phonemes in utterances of increased length with decreased structure and cueing

Address prosody using ReST (see Chapter 4)

Facilitate improved narrative language skills (see Chapter 8) by

- Retelling stories
- Using pictorial graphic organizers to organize basic components/features of narrative language (e.g., characters, setting, problem, solution, ending)
- Reporting back about prior events (see Chapter 8)
- Incorporating conjunctions into language to establish greater cohesion of ideas (so, then, but, because, when, first, next, later, etc.)

Table 11–7. Mishka, Age: 7 Years, 0 Months

Present Level of Performance	
Speech	Stimulable for /r/, but not consistent
	Improved segmental accuracy of multisyllabic words, but continued difficulty with prosody, especially syllable segmentation of complex words
Narrative language	Narrative skills improving but continue to require treatment
Academic	Literacy skills remain below grade level
Recommendations	
School speech-language treatment 60 min per week to address articulation and narrative skill development	
Learning resource assistance 120 min per week to address literacy	
Speech-Language Treatment Goal	
Improve narrative language development	
Treatment Methods	
Improve consistency and accuracy of /r/ production by	
• Using shaping, chaining, facilitative contexts	
• Increasing complexity of target utterances; reducing feedback and cueing	
Improve prosody using ReST	
Facilitate improved narrative language skills by	
• Retelling stories with greater complexity	
• Reporting back about prior events using greater complexity	
• Incorporating coordinating and subordinating conjunctions into language to establish greater cohesion of ideas	

Table 11–8. Mishka, Age: 8 Years, 6 Months

Present Level of Performance	
Articulation	Articulation goals were met
Narrative language	Narrative skills goals were met
Academic	Literacy skills remain below grade level
Recommendations	
School-based speech-language treatment discontinued	
Learning resource assistance 120 min per week to address literacy	

Table 11–9. Mishka, Age 14 Years, 6 Months

Present Level of Performance	
Speech	Mishka's high-school theater class teacher recommended that she speak with the SLP to work on enunciation; screening results showed a reduction in speech intelligibility when attempting to speak quickly and when pronouncing complex multisyllable words; speech prosody differences also were noted; reduced rate supported better speech intelligibility

Recommendation
Mishka did not qualify for school-based speech and language treatment services.
Private treatment was initiated for one, 60-min session per week to address enunciation and prosody

Speech-Language Treatment Goals
Improve speech intelligibility in connected speech
Improve speech prosody

Treatment methods
Facilitate improved speech intelligibility by using a variety of methods, including • Practicing tongue twisters • Practicing producing multisyllabic words in phrases and sentences of increased complexity; incorporating stimuli selected from Mishka's textbooks and conversational topics related to school, family, and current events • Reducing habitual speaking rate • Using strategies to repair communicative breakdowns **Address speech prosody (stress and intonation)** using strategies described in Chapter 5

The case study illustrates the importance of how the treatment of CAS evolves as the child's needs change. The SLP working with children with CAS should become acquainted with a variety of treatment programs (see Chapter 4) to meet the needs of younger and more severely impaired children, as well as programs and strategies that meet the needs of older children who exhibit challenges with prosody, acquisition of later developing phonemes, phonological development, and/or phonological awareness.

12

Developing Meaningful Goals and Collecting Data

Speech-language pathologists (SLPs) working in a wide range of settings develop treatment plans or Individualized Education Programs (IEPs) for individuals on their caseloads. Writing appropriate goals and objectives helps establish a roadmap for treatment and keeps the individuals on the client's team (client, parents, teachers, other therapists) informed of the direction of treatment. The long-term goals for treatment describe what skills the child will achieve by the end of a designated time frame (e.g., the length of a school year). Short-term objectives or benchmarks clarify the steps the child will take toward achieving the long-term goals and should align closely with the long-term goals.

Determining how the child's progress toward the goals will be measured is important. When goals are written with clarity and specificity, the method(s) used to measure progress will need to align with what that goal is measuring. For instance, if the goal for a child who is minimally verbal is to increase the number of vocalizations/verbalizations within a session, the progress charting could simply be a tally sheet with a tally mark used each time the child vocalizes or verbalizes during the session. If the goal is to increase intelligibility of functional phrases during game play with peers, a simple tally sheet would not suffice. You could create a progress monitoring form listing the functional phrases used during the lesson and mark if the peer was able to understand the child's productions of these phrases. This type of data-keeping would help determine which functional phrases are stable and which need more work.

Another consideration in development of goals and objectives is the impact those goals will have not only on the child's sensorimotor speech skills (as measured in percent consonants and vowels correct), but also on the effectiveness of the child's communication skills, how that impacts the child's engagement with family, peers, and others in the community, the child's self-esteem, and the child's social development. This holistic, person-centered approach to goal development and data collection aligns with the World Health Organization International Classification of Functioning, Disability, and Health.

This chapter describes the features of well-written goals and provides suggestions for improving clarity when writing goals. Considerations in progress monitoring are discussed later in the chapter.

Writing Smart Goals

The term SMART goal is an acronym originally developed for creating goals for businesses (Doran, 1981); however, this term has been expanded for a wide range of purposes, including developing educational and therapeutic goals. The acronym, SMART goal, varies somewhat depending on the setting in which it is used. Figure 12–1 shows a description of SMART goal features (Oklahoma State Department of Education, 2014) that can be applied to developing speech and language goals in a wide range of treatment settings.

Specific

SMART goals should be *specific*. The goals should specify what the child will do, under what conditions, in what context, and with which individuals. If specific cues will be provided, this also should be stated in the goal.

When goals are specific, they are written clearly and unambiguously. The goals should not be open to interpretation. It may be difficult for the person writing the goal to recognize that a goal is unclear or ambiguous. Farquharson et al. (2014) reviewed articulation goals written by SLPs and reported that the majority of goals tended to lack clarity; that is, the speech behaviors targeted in the goals would be difficult for teachers, caregivers, and perhaps other SLPs to understand and address. Sometimes lack of clarity is a result of using speech-related terminology that is not parent/teacher friendly. Lack of clarity also can be a result of ambiguity. Consider the goals in Box 12–1 for a child with childhood apraxia of speech (CAS) who is working on phonological awareness. The first goal lacks specificity, and the second goal is far more specific because it expresses a clear idea about how the child will demonstrate the skills being taught and the conditions in which the child will demonstrate the skill. If the clinician is clear about what the child is expected to do, it is easier to establish goals that are clear, specific, and less ambiguous.

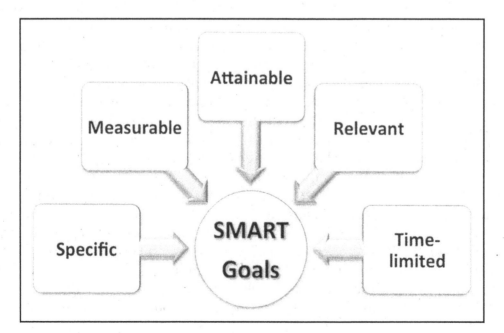

Figure 12–1. Five features of SMART goals.

■ Box 12–1. Sample Goals Contrasting Specificity

The child will identify the letters corresponding to the final phonemes of CVC words with 80% accuracy.	**After listening to the clinician** produce a CVC word from the target utterance list, the child will **identify the letter corresponding to the final consonant sound of the word (from these sounds—p, b, m, t, d, n, f, s) when presented with a choice of three different consonant letters** with at least 80% accuracy in 20 trials over three consecutive sessions.

Measurable

SMART goals need to be *measurable* and should contain actions words that can be measured. Goals that incorporate vague or abstract terms such as "learn," "understand," or "know" describe actions that are difficult to define and measure. In the sample goals in Box 12–2, the child is working on improving speech prosody. The way the first goal is written is too abstract and would make it impossible to measure progress. The second goal includes an action word that is measurable and allows the clinician to create a charting system for progress to be measured.

■ Box 12–2. Sample Goals Contrasting Measurability

The child will demonstrate an understanding of the use of syllable stress in words with trochaic versus iambic stress patterns.	Following a clinician model, the child will produce correct trochaic and iambic syllable stress in two-syllable words in short phrase-level productions (e.g., Sit at the **table**. I made a mi**stake**.) in at least 9/10 trochaic and 9/10 iambic stress words over two consecutive sessions.

Attainable

SMART goals should be *attainable* and *realistic*. Attainable goals are those that can be accomplished by the child in the specified period of time. Although it may be the hope of the clinician and the family that the child will attain a complete phoneme repertoire and produce words with complex syllable shapes accurately in conversational speech, it is unlikely that these goals will be attainable within one school year. The first goal in Box 12–3 illustrates a goal that is not a realistically attainable annual goal for a minimally verbal 3-year-old child with CAS. The second goal is more realistic, and it is far more likely that the child will attain the goal.

■ Box 12–3. Sample Goals Contrasting Attainability

The child will establish accurate production of all consonant and vowel phonemes in English in conversational speech with 90% accuracy.	The child will accurately **produce at least 20 functional words containing phonemes within the child's repertoire in CV, VC, CVC, and/or reduplicated CVCV shapes** (e.g., mom, dada, no, whee, me, boo boo, hi, bye, up) **following a model with 80% accuracy** over two consecutive sessions.

Relevant With a Clear Rationale

It is important that SMART goals be *relevant* for the child's academic, social, and functional growth and development. In other words, your *rationale* for including specific goals on the IEP should be clear. To test whether a goal is relevant and has a clear rationale, you should be able to ask *why* the child is working on the specific goal and come up with a meaningful reason.

It also is important not to confuse **goals** with the **methods/strategies** used to achieve the goals. Consider a child who demonstrates weak syllable deletion during multisyllabic word production. One method a clinician may employ to facilitate accurate production of multisyllabic words would be to tap out or count the syllables in the word. Although syllable counting may be an appropriate **strategy** for the child, the ability to count syllables is not a *relevant* goal. The relevant goal would be to reduce omission of weak syllables in multisyllabic words. The goals in Box 12–4 illustrate a contrast between a goal without clear rationale and a goal that is meaningful and has a strong rationale. When writing a goal, you should be able to tag on the phrase, "and this is an important skill for the child to develop because . . . "

■ Box 12–4. Sample Goals Contrasting Functional Relevance

The child will count the number of syllables of words containing three to four syllables with 80% accuracy.	During a 2- to 3-min speech sample (i.e., retelling a story, describing a recent event), the child will **produce three- and four-syllable words without omission of weak syllables** while independently using a syllable counting cueing system as needed in at least 8/10 trials over two consecutive sessions.

Time-Limited

A clear time frame should be established when writing SMART goals, and the time frame should be *time-limited*. Time frames often are determined by the specific setting in which the clinician is working. School SLPs generally follow a 1-year time frame. The time frame for developing and updating treatment plans in clinics or hospital settings may be dictated by the client's insurance plan requirements. Insurance plans may require treatment plans to be reviewed and revised annually, semi-annually, quarterly, or even monthly.

Short-term objectives or benchmarks can help to specify the smaller steps that will be used to measure ongoing progress toward a long-term goal; these benchmarks also have specified dates for expected achievement. Children with CAS do not develop skills all at once, so benchmark goals or short-term objectives will reflect the smaller steps of progress along the way. There are several ways that benchmarks can be used when writing goals. Often benchmarks are developed that reflect increasingly higher levels of accuracy (e.g., 40% accuracy by March, 60% accuracy by June, and 80% accuracy by September). Although this is a popular way for clinicians to set intermediate steps (benchmarks) toward achievement of a long-term goal, there are other ways to measure progress toward a goal that encourage higher accuracy levels throughout the treatment process, including the following:

- fading cueing (e.g., with simultaneous production and tactile cueing; following a direct model; without a model)

- increasing the complexity of skill development (e.g., in CV words; in CVCV words; in CVC and CVCVC words)
- establishing the skill in more challenging linguistic contexts (e.g., in single words; in two- to three-word phrases; in sentences)
- establishing the skill in more challenging environmental contexts (e.g., in varied settings, with less familiar communicative partners)
- adding a distraction (e.g., while throwing a ball back and forth, while building a block tower)

Tables 12–1 to 12–4 show examples of four different long-term goals along with benchmarks for fading cueing, increasing the complexity of skill development, establishing the skill in more challenging linguistic contexts, and establishing the skill in more challenging environmental contexts. The level of accuracy for each of these goals remains high all along the way, but the complexity levels or contexts may be increasingly challenging, or the amount of cueing provided may be reduced over time.

Table 12–1. Setting Benchmarks by Establishing the Skill in More Challenging Linguistic Contexts

Establishing the Skill in More Challenging Linguistic Contexts	
Present Level of Performance: Michael is able to produce final consonant clusters in single words with a direct or delayed model with 90% accuracy and without a model with 40% accuracy.	
Long-Term Goal	By June, 2024, during story retelling activities, Michael will produce final consonant clusters in sentences containing one or more of the following: third person singular verb tense, regular past tense, and plurality in four- to six-word sentences (e.g., "The bunny **hops** in the garden. Then he **digs** up **carrots**. Then he eats the **carrots**." "The dog **chased** the cat. Then the cat **climbed** a tree. Then the dog **walked** away.") independently in at least 8 of 10 trials over three consecutive sessions.
Benchmarks	By October, 2023, when responding to questions about pictures, Michael will produce final consonant clusters in single words containing third person singular verb tense, regular past tense, and plurality (e.g., hops, hopped, cats) (e.g., Q: *What does the bunny do every day?* R:"**hops**" Q: *What did the bunny do this morning?* R:"**hopped**" Q: *What hid in the box?* R: "**kittens**") independently in at least 8 of 10 trials over three consecutive sessions.
	By January, 2024, during picture description activities, Michael will produce final consonant clusters in two- to three-word sentences containing third person singular verb tense, regular past tense, and plurality (e.g., "The bunny **hops**." "Bunny **hopped** home." "**Cats** sleep.") independently in at least 8 of 10 trials over three consecutive sessions.
	By April, 2024, during picture description activities, Michael will produce final consonant clusters in words containing third person singular verb tense, regular past tense, and plurality in four- to six-word sentences (e.g., "The bunny **hops** in the grass." "Bunny **hopped** all the way home." "My **cats** sleep on my bed.") independently in at least 8 of 10 trials over three consecutive sessions.

Table 12–2. Setting Benchmarks by Fading Cues

Fading Cues	
Present Level of Performance: John is able to produce variegated CV.CV word shapes consisting of phonemes within his current phoneme repertoire with visual (V), auditory (A), and tactile (T) cueing and reduced rate with 60% accuracy.	
Long-Term Goal	By June, 2023, during structured speech drills, John will produce variegated CV.CV word shapes in single words containing phonemes within his repertoire /p, b, t, d, m, n, w, j ("y sound"), i, eɪ, ɑ, oʊ, u, aɪ/ independently (without cueing) at a normal rate of speech with at least 80% accuracy over two consecutive sessions.
Benchmarks	By March, 2023 during structured speech drills, John will produce variegated CV.CV word shapes in single words containing phonemes within his repertoire (see above) with V, A, and T cueing (direct model and tactile cue) as needed at a reduced rate with at least 80% accuracy over two consecutive sessions.
	By April, 2023, during structured speech drills, John will produce variegated CV.CV word shapes in single words containing phonemes within his repertoire (see above) with V and A cueing (direct or delayed model) as needed at a reduced rate of speech with at least 80% accuracy over two consecutive sessions.
	By May, 2023, during structured speech drills, John will produce variegated CV.CV word shapes in single words containing phonemes within his repertoire (see above) with V and A cueing (direct or delayed model) as needed at a normal rate of speech with at least 80% accuracy over two consecutive sessions.

Table 12–3. Setting Benchmarks by Increasing the Complexity of Skill Development

Increasing the Complexity of Skill Development	
Present Level of Performance: Malcolm is able to produce CV words with consonants /p, b, t, d, m, n, h, w/ and vowels /i, ei, ɑ, o, u ai/ independently with 55% accuracy.	
Long-term goal	By June 2023, Malcolm will produce at least 20 different CV.CVC words/ phrases (e.g., bottom; Hi, Mom) with phonemes within his repertoire independently with at least 80% accuracy over three consecutive sessions.
Benchmarks	By October 2023, Malcolm will produce at least 20 different CV words/phrases (e.g., hi, no, me) with phonemes within his repertoire independently with at least 80% accuracy over three consecutive sessions.
	By January 2024, Malcolm will produce at least 20 different CV.CV words/phrases (dino, bunny, no way) with phonemes within his repertoire independently with at least 80% accuracy over three consecutive sessions.
	By April 2024, Malcolm will produce at least 20 different VC and CVC words (on, put) with phonemes within his repertoire independently with at least 80% accuracy over three consecutive sessions.

Table 12–4. Setting Benchmarks by Establishing the Skill in More Challenging Environmental Contexts

Establishing the Skill in More Challenging Environmental Contexts (e.g., in different settings, with less familiar communicative partners)	
Present Level of Performance: Jacqueline is able to repeat simple "wh" and "yes-no" questions (e.g., Do you want a cookie? Where is the blue fish?) when given a clinician model during structured treatment session activities with 85% accuracy. *Note: Accuracy of production included using the interrogative reversal, correct word sequencing, and intelligible speech.*	
Long-Term Goal	By June 2024, Jacqueline will produce "wh" and "yes-no" questions without benefit of a model in the classroom with a peer during free play or game activities using a question cue card as needed with at least 80% accuracy over three data collection sessions.
Benchmarks	By October 2023, Jacqueline will repeat "wh" and "yes-no" questions during treatment sessions with the clinician during structured conversation or game activities given a model and using a question cue card as needed with at least 80% accuracy over three data collection sessions.
	By January 2024, Jacqueline will produce "wh" and "yes-no" questions without benefit of a model during treatment sessions with the clinician during structured conversation or game activities using a question cue card as needed with at least 80% accuracy over three data collection sessions.
	By April 2024, Jacqueline will produce "wh" and "yes-no" questions without benefit of a model during treatment sessions with a peer during structured conversation or game activities using a question cue card as needed with at least 80% accuracy over three data collection sessions.

Nobriga and St. Clair (2018) provide a tutorial about goal development that includes a goal-writing flowchart. The flowchart (p. 39) provides a nice illustration of the thought process used in developing and evaluating goals. For example, one question on the flowchart refers to whether the criterion for meeting the goal is clear (e.g., % correct, number of attempts, number of cues) and if a data sheet could be created for it. If not, the criterion for meeting the goal will need to be redetermined.

Other Considerations in Establishing Goals for Children With CAS

When developing goals for children with CAS, it is important to have a clear understanding about what you want the child to accomplish. Does the child need to increase vocal and verbal output, increase complexity of phonotactic repertoire, increase phonemic repertoire, increase vowel accuracy, improve accuracy of specific phonemes, improve speech prosody, reduce reliance on adult cueing, demonstrate greater flexibility in the number of contexts in which they can produce specific phonemes, or increase overall intelligibility and comprehensibility? Are the child's speech productions expected to be completely accurate or would intelligible approximations of target utterances be acceptable? Following are additional considerations when developing goals for children with CAS.

Goals That Reflect Accuracy of the Child's Productions

The most common way to measure a child's performance in a specific skill area is to measure the accuracy or consistency of the child's performance. The goal in Box 12–5 measures accuracy of production.

■ **Box 12–5.** Goal Reflecting Production Accuracy

> The child will accurately produce initial bilabial phonemes /b, m/ and alveolar phonemes /d, n/ in CV words with a model (as needed) in at least 8 of 10 trials for two consecutive sessions.

Goals That Reflect Expanding Flexibility of Coarticulation

Children with CAS may demonstrate limitations in the variety of contexts in which they can produce specific phonemes. For example, a child may only be able to produce the bilabials /p, b, m/ in syllables with central and high back vowels (e.g., puhpuh, boo, muh, moo). To support the establishment of these phonemes in a wider range of coarticulatory contexts, a benchmark goal that measures growth in coarticulatory flexibility may be developed, such as the goal in Box 12–6.

■ **Box 12–6.** Goal That Measures Increased Coarticulatory Flexibility

> The child will establish greater flexibility in production of words with initial bilabials /p, b, m/ by accurately producing 10 new CV, CV.CV and/ or CVC words in which the bilabial phoneme is followed by mid- and low-back vowels and front vowels (e.g., puppy, mom, mommy, baby, me, bow) with an adult model in 8 of 10 trials for two consecutive sessions.

Goals That Reflect Improvement in Comprehensibility

Children with CAS who exhibit reduced intelligibility may or may not use strategies effectively to increase the comprehensibility of their verbal communication. A child with limited speech intelligibility who takes advantage of a robust gestural system, reduces their rate of speech when needed, and introduces the topic about what they are going to discuss, will be easier to understand than a child with similar intelligibility challenges who does not use these strategies. A goal such as the sample goal in Box 12–7 could be drafted for a child who needs to work on improving comprehensibility.

■ Box 12–7. Goal Addressing Improved Comprehensibility

> During 5-min conversational interactions with a peer, the child will use two or more of the six previously practiced strategies for increasing comprehensibility (i.e., reducing rate of speech, pausing at phrase breaks, introducing the topic before giving specific and detailed information, using gestures, emphasizing key words, and repeating key words for clarification) with no more than one clinician cue in four of five opportunities over two consecutive sessions.

Goals That Reflect Specified Approximations of Target Utterances

During treatment, target utterances that are important for the child's social and linguistic development may be introduced that are not yet completely within the child's motor control. A goal may be to increase intelligible production of power phrases, with the understanding that some of the targeted phrases may include phonemes not yet within the child's repertoire. A goal may be written that supports the establishment of power phrases but allows for some flexibility in the definition of "accuracy" so the child can establish a wider range of functional phrases that support linguistic and social-emotional development. Box 12–8 shows a sample goal that sets specific elements of acceptable approximation.

■ Box 12–8. Goal Specifying Allowable Approximations

> The child will produce accurate or close, intelligible approximations of at least 10 new two- to four-syllable power phrases (e.g., Let me do it. Where is _____? Can I _____? What's that? I need a break. I don't know.) independently during structured play activities with at least 80% accuracy over three consecutive sessions. Specifically, "close approximations" may include liquid gliding or vowelization of /l/ and /r/ and cluster reduction.

Goals That Reflect Level of Speech Intelligibility

When writing goals that specify that a child will improve speech intelligibility, it is important to specify how the degree of intelligibility will be measured. The SLP may measure the level of intelligibility by marking the number of words in a language sample that were intelligible to the clinician. Another way to measure intelligibility is determining the percentage of the child's productions that were understood by a peer. Box 12–9 is an example of a goal that measures intelligibility by observing the peer's responses.

■ Box 12–9. Goal Measuring Speech Intelligibility

> The child will produce questions and comments during conversation that are understood by peers in at least 8 of 10 communication attempts over two consecutive sessions as measured by the peer responding in a way that is consistent with understanding the child's message (e.g., making an appropriate response, following the child's instruction, responding to the child's question).

Another way to measure growth in speech intelligibility is through the use of a word or sentence intelligibility task (see Chapter 2 for more detailed information on speech intelligibility measures). Box 12–10 would be appropriate when using these types of measures.

■ Box 12–10. Goal Measuring Speech Intelligibility

> The child will increase intelligibility of words in phrases of four to six words in length from 40% to 60% following 12 treatment sessions.

Goals That Reflect Quantity and Variety of Vocal/Verbal Output

It may be difficult to write goals that are extremely specific and prescriptive for children who demonstrate limited vocal and verbal output. Although children who have limited speech typically follow a progression of syllable shape development beginning with V, CV, or VC, and then moving on to increasingly complex syllable structures, it may be challenging for the clinician to anticipate the early phonemes that will be established in the child's repertoire. Defining the earliest phonemes in a child's vocal and verbal development may be limiting, as goals that are too specific may not reflect progress the child has made. For some children, it may be advisable to establish goals that measure increased vocalizations and verbal attempts, increased flexibility of productions, or increased use of a wider variety of different words, like those shown in Box 12–11.

■ Box 12–11. Goals for Increasing Number of Vocalizations Per Session

> 1. The child will produce at least 50 vocalizations and/or verbalizations during a 30-min session over two consecutive sessions.
>
> 2. The child will demonstrate an increase in consonant repertoire from the current repertoire of three consonant phonemes by producing at least four new consonant phonemes in at least five new words for each phoneme when provided with a model.
>
> 3. The child will spontaneously produce at least 15 <u>different</u> words or word approximations during play activities during a 30-min treatment session over two consecutive sessions.

Goals That Reflect Establishing Greater Spontaneity

Children with CAS can become rather cue dependent. That is, they may rely on the clinician providing direct models or other cues to facilitate production of target words. Parents often ask if the child will ever be able to say the target words without needing to hear the adult model first. For children who are dependent on adult cues, the goal in Box 12–12 may be appropriate.

Table 12–2 also provides examples of short-term objectives (benchmarks) that reflect faded cueing over time to reduce a child's reliance on modeling and other types of cues.

■ Box 12–12. Goal Reflecting Reduced Cue Dependency

> The child will reduce dependence on adult cues by accurately producing 20 different variegated CV.CV targets in the context of a game activity with 80% accuracy over two consecutive sessions without adult cues or models.

Goals That Reflect Increased Verbal Initiation

Some children are reticent to initiate any verbal interaction (e.g., requesting, greeting, commenting, negating). Box 12–13 would be appropriate for increasing verbal initiation in children who are reluctant communicators.

■ Box 12–13. Goal Reflecting Reduced Verbal Initiation

> The child will initiate greetings and requests in at least 8 of 10 opportunities during a 30-min session (when at least 10 clear opportunities to do so are made available, e.g., placing favorite toys on a high shelf, giving a child something to open that is difficult to open, and having the child say "bye" when being dropped off and "hi" when being picked up).

Measuring and Charting Progress

The way the goal is written will guide the type of charting that will be used for progress monitoring. The clinician will need to determine if a binary charting system (correct or incorrect) will provide enough information to show how the child is progressing toward the goal. More detailed data collection allows the clinician to recognize ways in which a child is making progress, even in children who may be making relatively slow progress. It may be beneficial to chart if the target utterance was correct or incorrect, but also to chart the conditions under which the child was able to produce target utterances (e.g., rate of speech, degree of cueing, fluidity of coarticulatory transitions, use of appropriate syllable stress, closeness of approximations).

Let's assume the child achieved 85% accuracy in production of target utterances with tactile cues, simultaneous production, and at a reduced rate during a session. In the following session, the child achieved 75% accuracy in production of target utterances with only a direct model and at a normal rate of production. If there was no indication or charting of the conditions of performance (reduced rate or normal rate, with or without cueing, and types of cueing provided), it may appear at face value that the child performed more poorly in the second session than the first session. In fact, the child is demonstrating important growth by reducing dependency on cueing and speaking closer to a habitual rate of speech, which supports generalization of the child's speech skills.

Another factor to consider when charting the child's performance is how closely the child's productions approximate the target utterances. Consider if one of the child's target words was "mommy," and the child produced the target utterance as [ba] during the first 2 weeks of treatment, [ma] during the next week of treatment, [mama] during the next week of treatment, and eventually attained accurate production by the fifth week of treatment. Using a binary scoring system, the clinician may chart each of the child's productions throughout the first 4 weeks of treatment as inaccurate. This simple "correct" or "incorrect" charting would not reflect the gains the child had made toward developing increasingly closer approximations of the target utterance. By transcribing the child's production, the child's progress toward the goal would be more apparent. Charting incremental progress also may be beneficial to substantiate speech production gains on a child's IEP or to an insurance company.

Strand (2020) recommends doing probe testing to monitor progress. Rather than charting each of the child's productions during a session, the clinician uses probe testing to rate production accuracy of the child's target utterances outside the treatment portion of the session. The child produces the target utterances five times each in random order either at the beginning or end of the session. The targets are produced either in response to a question or following a model, and the production accuracy is rated as either correct, close approximation, or incorrect, receiving scores of 2, 1, or 0, respectively. When the child achieves four of five correct productions of a target in two consecutive probe sessions, that target utterance is cycled out and replaced by a new target.

Tables 12–5, 12–6, and 12–7 are sample data collection charts that can be used during treatment. Choose a data collection system that helps reflect the child's progress in treatment. Table 12–5 is an example of a chart to show the level of cueing provided for the child and the child's accuracy with various levels of cueing.

An example of a chart that provides space for phonetic transcription of the child's productions is shown in Table 12–6.

The next data collection form, shown in Table 12–7 was designed to track percentage consonants correct (PCC), percentage vowels correct (PVC), percentage phonemes correct (PPC), correct sentential stress, and smooth coarticulation. This provides a finer-tune measure for tracking segmental and suprasegmental accuracy. Once the clinician knows the target utterances they will be working on, they can write the sentences in International Phonetic Alphabet in advance of collecting the data. Sounds that are omitted can be crossed out, distortions can be circled, and substitutions can be written in over the errored phoneme. This allows for efficient online data collection.

Blank data collection forms can be found in the online materials.

Table 12–5. Data Collection Incorporating Levels of Cueing

Name: _____ Date: _____

Goal: The child will increase accuracy of production of short phrases that include at least one closed syllable (consonant at the end of a syllable) with at least 80% accuracy without a model. Phonemes to consider in closed syllables because they may be facilitative include /p, t, m, n, f, s/

Key: | = correct   - = incorrect

Target Utterance	Elicited Without Model	Delayed Model	Direct Model	Simultaneous Production	Additional Cues (e.g., Tactile)
Hi mom	- - ||| - |||	- - |||	||||		
way up		- - -	||||	- - |||| - ||||	- |||
go in					
go home					
my house					
turn off					
my turn					

Table 12–6. Data Collection With Transcription

Name: _____ Date: _____

Goal: *The child will increase accuracy of production of CV and reduplicated CVCV target stimuli with maximal cueing (cueing may include direct models, simultaneous productions, tactile cues, reduced rate, and other types of cues) that incorporate phonemes in their phonetic repertoire in at least 15 new target utterances with 90% accuracy over two consecutive sessions.*

Target Utterances	Transcriptions Transcribe the child's productions and mark the number of instances of each of those productions.			
mama Percentage correct: 13/18 (72%)	/ba.ba/ |||	/ma.ba/ ||	/ma.ma/ |||| |||| |||	
dada				
me				

Table 12–7. Sample Data Collection Form for Tracking PPC, PCC, PVC, Prosody, and Coarticulation and Marking Levels of Cueing Provided

DATA SHEET FOR PHRASES-ARTICULATORY ACCURACY

CLIENT'S NAME _____ DATE _____

1-Direct imitation 2-Direct imitation with clinician miming the phrases simultaneously

3-Simultaneous without tactile cues 4-Simultaneous w/tactile cues

Target Phrase and Transcription Put your target phrase in IPA on lines one and two. Take data at the level the child is most successful or take data on direct imitation only and on the third line be dynamic and see what type of cueing facilitates the best accuracy and not level of support. For prosody and coarticulation, score with + or –.	Level of Cueing	PPC	PCC	PVC	Prosody	Coartic-ulation
1. Target Phrase: Go home now /goʊ hoʊm naʊ/						
Child's Production #1　/goʊ hoʊ nɑ/	2	5/7	3/4	2/3	–	–
Child's Production #2　/goʊ hoʊm naʊ/	4	7/7	4/4	3/3	+	–
2.						
3						
4.						
5.						

Note. PCC, percentage consonants correct; PPC, percentage phonemes correct; PVC, percentage vowels correct.

References

Doran, G. T. (1981). There's a S.M.A.R.T. way to write management's goals and objectives. *Management Review, 70*, 35–36.

Farquharson, K., Tambyraja, S. R., Justice, L. M., & Redle, E. E. (2014). IEP goals for school-age children with speech sound disorders. *Journal of Communication Disorders, 52*, 184–195. https://doi.org/10.1016/j .jcomdis.2014.09.005

Nobriga, C., & St. Clair, J. (2018). Training goal writing: A practical and systematic approach. *Perspectives of the ASHA Special Interest Groups SIG 11, 3,* 36–47. https://doi.org/10.1044/persp3.SIG11.36

Oklahoma State Department of Education. (2014). *SIR team improvement plan for special education.* https://sde .ok.gov/sites/ok.gov.sde/files/documents/files/SIR%20 Team%20Improvement%20Plan%20Template.pdf

Partnering With Parents to Maximize Treatment Outcomes

When working with children with known or suspected apraxia of speech, developing a collaborative relationship with the family can have a substantial impact on treatment success. Parents are in a unique position to reinforce skills learned in therapy in naturalistic ways during the course of the day and to provide opportunities for extra practice at home. Extending practice opportunities to other settings and reinforcing newly learned skills beyond the relatively short periods of time the child is receiving direct treatment help facilitate skill development, with greatest improvements observed when home practice is completed regularly (ASHA, 2020).

Building Successful Partnerships With Parents

Bringing parents into the treatment process can offer substantial benefits to children with severe speech disorders. The speech-language pathologist (SLP) can help facilitate greater parent knowledge and involvement in treatment in several ways.

Guide Parents Toward Accurate and Comprehensive Information Sources About Childhood Apraxia of Speech

Apraxia Kids is a nonprofit organization devoted specifically to the needs and interests of children with childhood apraxia of speech (CAS). Apraxia Kids is the leading nonprofit that strengthens the support systems in the lives of children with apraxia of speech by educating professionals and families, facilitating community engagement and outreach, and investing in the future through advocacy and research.

Apraxia Kids' primary goals include

- increasing awareness about CAS
- providing accurate and reliable information on CAS and related issues

- educating parents, professionals, and others about CAS
- supporting research on CAS

By forging partnerships between families, professionals, and researchers, Apraxia Kids works to accomplish these goals through a number of channels:

- a comprehensive website (http://www.apraxia-kids.org) that holds the largest online repository of high-quality information about all aspects of CAS including articles, resource guides, and brochures for printing and downloading
- Facebook pages and support groups to meet the needs and interests of families and professionals
- CAS online seminars and workshops throughout the year and one major, annual national conference
- multiple awareness-building events sponsored by Apraxia Kids, including walks, media articles, and columns on the topic of CAS
- opportunities for researchers to meet, network, and plan
- funding for treatment research studies
- intensive training for professionals on the evaluation and treatment of CAS
- SLP directory to connect families with therapists who have some knowledge and experience with assessing and treating children with CAS

Reduce Professional Jargon

When discussing evaluation and treatment information with parents, make an effort to use terminology more familiar to the nonprofessional. If you do introduce professional terminology to parents, take the time to define terms that may be confusing to parents, so the parents can develop greater understanding of the challenges facing their child. When writing reports, be sure to define professional terms (e.g., phoneme, phonological awareness, syllable shape, praxis, alveolar ridge, velum, lingual, labial) to make the reports meaningful to parents.

Coach Parents in Speech and Language Facilitation Strategies

Parents will benefit from learning strategies to support their child's speech and language development. In addition to *modeling* good strategies for facilitating communication, SLPs can provide *explicit instruction* to parents in ways that increase interaction and engagement with their children. Specific recommendations can be provided to parents for ways to elicit imitation at a level that is appropriate for the child, whether that be imitation of speech, environmental and animal sounds, or gross motor movements. Parents can be coached in ways to use play to increase babbling, sound exploration, and imitation of oral and facial movements. As children begin to imitate sounds and words, it is important to provide specific recommendations of ways to support practice of speech skills at home, and how to encourage their children to practice new speech targets in daily activities and play routines.

The same strategies SLPs use to facilitate a child's production of more complex utterances such as *modeling*, *expansion*, and *expatiation* can be taught to parents. Help parents learn to *model* utterances that match their child's language skill level. If the child is playing with a doll and covers the doll with a blanket, the parent may model, "Baby is sleeping" or "nigh nigh baby." Parents can use *expansion* by adding words or morphological markers that increase complexity without adding new information. If the child says, "Baby sleep," the parent could reply, "Yes, the baby is sleeping." Parents also can be encouraged to add new information to their child's utterances by using *expatiation*. In the "Baby sleep," example, the parent could reply, "Yes, the baby is sleeping. Let's put the baby to bed."

Parents can learn to use *focused stimulation* to provide their child with multiple exposures of desired linguistic forms or speech targets. Ellis Weismer and Robertson (2006) describe focused stimulation as when "the child is provided with concentrated exposures of specific linguistic forms/functions/uses within naturalistic communicative contexts" (p. 175). Providing multiple exposures of specific linguistic forms and phonemic targets can be beneficial for children with speech and language impairments. Clinicians can demonstrate focused stimulation during treatment and provide parents guidance and opportunities to practice using focused stimulation while modeling specific targets. Be sure that parents understand the importance of face-to-face interaction when modeling target utterances.

Explain your rationale for choosing specific toys and books that offer greater opportunities to expose the child to specific targets. Offer parents ideas for toys, games, books, and songs that can be used to elicit specific linguistic structures or phonetic targets. Model different ways the text from books can be modified to elicit specific targets and how books can be read in a more interactive manner.

Offer Guidance to Parents Regarding Simple Adaptations to the Home Environment

Hancock and Kaiser (2006) provide the following recommendations for ways the home environment can be engineered to expand opportunities for purposeful communication:

- selection of materials
  - suggest high interest materials that facilitate interaction
  - consider materials that have multiple parts to encourage labeling, requesting, and problem solving
  - use materials that require assistance to open or put together
  - integrate materials or activities that require a communicative partner
- arrangement of materials
  - have materials in view, but out of reach
  - limit the number of toys available to encourage more focused attention on one activity before moving on to another
- management of materials
  - encourage the mixing of toys and materials in interesting ways (e.g., making animals footprint cookies with animal toys and play dough)
  - create opportunities for requesting more pieces by controlling the child's access to materials
  - omit materials required to complete a project or a play scheme (e.g., a brush for painting, a blanket for a doll's bed)
  - encourage parents to do silly and unexpected things during play (e.g., put the doll's hat on her foot)

Provide Opportunities for Parents to Observe and Participate in Treatment Sessions

Even parents who have difficulty attending their child's speech therapy sessions should be provided with opportunities to observe their child's treatment at least periodically. If parents are unable to participate in the treatment sessions directly, consider sharing videos of treatment sessions. For children who become distracted or find it difficult to sustain effort when parents are in the treatment room, parents may be able to observe sessions through a two-way mirror (if available) or to join the session toward the end when the clinician and child can "show" the parent what was practiced during treatment. Recording portions of the session to share with the parents can also provide a way for the parents to actually see the treatment strategies being used.

Provide Regular Updates Regarding Treatment Progress

Regular progress monitoring can help provide parents with objective measures of growth and change. By explicitly stating the child's present levels of performance and developing clear and measurable goals and objectives, progress monitoring will be meaningful (see Chapter 12 for a more detailed discussion about writing goals and objectives and measuring progress). Table 13–1 provides samples of how initial assessments guide the development of measurable goals. The child's progress toward these goals can be monitored regularly, and the information obtained from periodic measurements can be shared with parents so measurable progress is recognized.

Table 13–1. Samples of Progress Measures

Initial Performance Date: 11/1/22	Measurable Goals	Update Measure Date: 2/1/23
Expressive vocabulary of 8 words	Increase number of words in expressive vocabulary to 50	Expressive vocabulary of 42 words
Consonant inventory: /b, m, h/ Vowel inventory: /u, ɑ, ʌ/	Add alveolar phonemes /t, d, n/ and voiceless bilabial /p/ to consonant repertoire Increase vowel repertoire from 3 to 6 vowels	Consonant inventory: /p, b, t, d, m, n, f, h/ Vowel inventory: /i, e, u, ʊ, o, ɑ, ʌ, aɪ/
Syllable shape inventory: V, CV, CVCV reduplicated	Increase syllable shape inventory by producing targets with the following syllable shapes: CVC, CVCV with consonant harmony, variegated CVCV	Syllable shape inventory: V, V.V, CV, CVC, consonant harmonized CVCV, variegated CVCV
Percentage Consonants Correct (PCC) in conversational speech: 42%	Increase PCC in conversational speech to 60%	PCC in conversational speech: 68%

When progress toward attaining goals is slow, it is important to show the small steps the child is achieving in speech development. Helping parents recognize small steps toward goal achievement will provide comfort and hopefulness to parents who are deeply concerned about their child's speech development.

Teach Parents the Cues Used in Treatment

SLPs become experts at helping children produce target utterances correctly, in part because they regularly provide valuable visual, auditory, tactile, and metacognitive cues to their clients. Children's productions during home practice are apt to be more accurate if the parents are aware of, and can provide, similar types of cues. Teach parents beneficial cues or provide videos illustrating the use of various cues, such as tactile cues, hand motions, or metaphors (described in Chapter 3) that benefit their child. Sharing this information can support parents in helping their children achieve greater success in settings outside of therapy. Hands-on practice in the use of the cues during therapy also serves as a valuable learning tool for parents.

Provide Home Practice Activities and Materials

Provide parents with clear and manageable home practice suggestions. This extra practice across settings can help facilitate carryover and generalization of new speech skills. Some parents may become overwhelmed if the expected amount of home practice is exhaustive. Practice is more likely to be extended into the home environment when certain conditions exist:

- home practice assignments can be incorporated easily into the daily routines of the family (bedtime, bath time, mealtime, storybook reading, car rides)
- targets to be practiced are those with which the child can be successful
- parents are provided with clear and specific recommendations for home practice

For children who have very limited expressive vocabulary, consider creating a picture book containing words that are within the child's motor control. Encourage the parents to be part of the creation of the practice book by gradually adding new pictures. The book can serve both as a home practice picture set and as a tangible recognition of accomplishment. The child should be encouraged to bring the book home after each session to show the family any new words that have been added to the book. When print is added to the photos, opportunities are provided to highlight various aspects of print awareness as a way to incorporate phonological and phonemic awareness goals into the practice (e.g., initial sounds of words, the concept of a word, sound-letter association). Box 13–1 provides samples of home practice activities that may be manageable for families.

Encourage Parents to Create Their Own Games and Activities for Home Practice

Parents bring their own style and creativity into their parent-child interactions. As parents begin to become more comfortable with reinforcing their child's speech efforts, they often

■ Box 13–1. Sample Homework and Naturalistic Practice Activities

- Encourage your child to say "buh buh" for *bubble* correctly at least five times each day during bath time.

- Review 10 pictures from your child's core vocabulary book each day.

- Take a little time each day to play with farm animals or read books about farm animals and practice making the animal sound noises your child has been practicing in therapy.

- Play the board game sent home in the home practice bag, and encourage your child to use functional phrases while playing the game, such as *"my turn," "your turn," "I got a _____"*) while taking turns during the game. Each time the child lands on a *star*, the child can practice one of the phrases attached to the game.

- Encourage your child to say "hi" using a good "h" sound as each family member comes down for breakfast each morning.

- Hide the five practice cards around the room and have your child search for them, practicing each phrase five times after they find it.

come up with unique ways to establish practice routines that their child will find enjoyable. The SLP should acknowledge and encourage the efforts by parents to make the practice activities work in the context of their family.

Solicit Input From Parents Regarding Target Utterance Selection

Ask parents to generate a list of words or phrases they would like their child to practice. It might not be possible to work on some items on the list immediately if the phonetic complexity is too high. Nevertheless, it is important to work on functional communication. Although we may have our own goals in mind, listening to parents can shed light on possible goals and targets we may not have considered. Encourage parents to provide a variety of targets, including names of family and friends, favorite toys, foods, and activities. Table 13–2 is a sample questionnaire for generating functional targets that can be copied and sent home to the family to complete. This questionnaire is available in the online materials. A more comprehensive questionnaire by Wilson and Gildersleeve-Neumann can be found on the Apraxia Kids website (http://www.apraxia-kids.org/wp-content/uploads/2018/12/Parent-Questionnaire.pdf).

Address Parents' Fears Related to Introducing Augmentative and Alternative Communication in Treatment

Parents may be concerned that teaching their child sign language or encouraging their child to point to a picture of a desired item on a picture board will have a negative impact on speech progress. Assure the parents that research studies have found that using Augmentative and Alternative Communication (AAC) does not deter, and often enhances, verbal communication in children with limited speech development (see Chapter 6). To incorporate AAC into a natural environment, parents can be provided with pictured sentence strips that can be used at mealtimes to help the child make requests with full sentences. Picture-assisted writing tools,

Table 13–2. Functional Target Utterance Parent Questionnaire

FUNCTIONAL TARGET UTTERANCE PARENT QUESTIONNAIRE	
Thank you for taking the time to complete this questionnaire. It will be immensely helpful when we plan your child's speech therapy sessions. *Please list some words or phrases that can help guide some of the target utterances your child can work on during speech therapy sessions. For instance, in the section for "People," write down the words your family uses to name family, friends, pets, etc., in your child's life whom he may want to talk about (e.g., "Papa" for grandpa; "Nona" for grandma; "Lulu" for Lucy).* *Think about the words your family traditionally uses to label people, things, and events in your lives. If your child says, "Lulu" for Lucy, but the rest of the family calls them "Lucy," you can include both versions in your list.*	
People (family, neighbors, friends, teachers/playmates, pets)	
Favorite toys (e.g., blocks, cars, puzzles)	
Favorite play activities (e.g., dress up, going to playground, art activities)	
Favorite foods (what your child typically eats at meals and snacks)	
Favorite books	
Functional words/phrases your child tries to say or would like to say if they could (e.g., no, mine, stop it, go home, all done, I want ____)	

continues

Table 13–2. *continued*

Things your child has tried to say to someone over the past few weeks that caused frustration when the listener was not able to understand them	
Any other things that come to mind that may be important for your child to be able to express what is important to them	

such as Pixwriter (https://www.attainmentcompany.com/pixwriter-software) can be used to quickly make these types of picture strips or topic boards to pass on to the families so they can begin to see the benefits of incorporating AAC into the environment.

Help Parents Recognize and Welcome the Changes in Treatment Structure That Evolve Over Time

Parents may have been advised that intensive, one-on-one treatment is the standard protocol for a child with CAS, so they may express concerns if the SLP suggests a dyad or group setting. In fact, some children benefit from treatment provided in dyads (two children to one clinician) as they may be more eager to practice their targets in the presence of a peer. Over the course of therapy, the structure of the child's treatment program may need to change. The child who required intensive treatment during the preschool years may have made substantial progress and may be ready for a modification to the treatment intensity. When the child has developed greater control over sensorimotor speech planning, the child's more substantial communication needs may be in the areas of language, literacy, or social communication, for which dyads or small-group treatment would be more beneficial. Reassure parents that the changes are being made in the best interests of their child.

Be Sensitive to the Parents' Emotions Around Learning the Nature and Extent of Their Child's Disability

When delivering evaluation results and sharing the diagnosis of CAS with parents, they may experience a wide range of emotions. Rusiewicz et al. (2018) reported that parents expressed concerns not only about their child's speech and ability to achieve intelligible speech, but also about their child's success in peer social interactions. Be thoughtful and empathic in the way these evaluation results are delivered, recognizing that this information may be upsetting and frightening for families. Do not stop at sharing the assessment findings but try to paint a clear picture of short- and long-term goals and how these immediate goals will be addressed.

Even when children demonstrate substantial communication challenges, it is important to describe the child's strengths as well as needs. Describe the strengths that are meaningful in building functional communication skills and capacities (e.g., "Serena perseveres, even when faced with difficult tasks. Some of the things she will be working on will be difficult, and her perseverance will serve her well." "Even though Joshua does not have any real words yet, he is using gestures and facial expressions that often make his messages quite clear to me. These are very important skills in overall communication, so we will continue to support and encourage these as we begin to work on his speech development.")

There are two documents provided in the appendix of this chapter (Appendix 13–A and Appendix 13–B) and in the online materials that can be copied and shared with parents and caregivers. The first document, "Supporting Your Child's Speech Therapy at Home," provides suggestions for ways to encourage home practice. The second document is titled, "Understanding Childhood Apraxia of Speech." It provides parents with an overview of CAS, its characteristics, and the role of the SLP in evaluating and treating the child with CAS.

References

American Speech-Language-Hearing Association. (2020). Completion of home program linked to greatest communication gains. *The ASHA Leader.* https://doi.org/10.1044/leader.NOMS.25032020.28

Ellis Weismer, S., & Robertson, S. (2006). Focused stimulation approach to language intervention. In R. J. McCauley & M. E. Fey (Eds.), *Treatment of language disorders in children* (pp. 175–202). Paul H. Brookes.

Hancock, T. B., & Kaiser, A. P. (2006). Enhanced milieu teaching. In R. J. McCauley & M. E. Fey (Eds.), *Treatment of language disorders in children* (pp. 203–236). Paul H. Brookes.

Rusiewicz, H. L., Maize, K., & Ptakowski, T. (2018). Parental experiences and perceptions related to childhood apraxia of speech: Focus on functional implications. *International Journal of Speech-Language Pathology, 20,* 569–580. https://doi.org/10.1080/17549507.2017.1359333

APPENDIX 13–A
Supporting Your Child's Speech Therapy at Home

Parents play an important role in the speech therapy process for children with childhood apraxia of speech (CAS). The more you can do at home to support the types of things your child is working on in speech-language therapy sessions, the more opportunities there will be for these new skills to be carried over into other settings. You do not need to spend hours each week doing speech therapy drills with your child; however, reinforcement of the therapy goals throughout the week and follow-through on speech homework can make a big difference for your child. You can support your child's learning in several ways.

Observe Your Child's Therapy Sessions. When possible, observe your child's speech therapy sessions. Your ability to participate in the treatment sessions may depend on clinician preference, work schedules, other children who require supervision, or your child's ability to put forth effort and maintain focus when you are in the therapy room. Observations can take a variety of forms:

- sitting through the treatment sessions
- joining your child for the last few minutes of the sessions to get a recap of what was learned or how to employ some of the strategies used by the therapist
- watching recorded segments of sessions

By observing sessions in real time or watching recordings taken during treatment sessions, you will see what sounds, words, or sentences your child is practicing, as well as the types of cues the speech-language pathologist (SLP) uses to help your child achieve success. Does the therapist model the words and ask your child to repeat, say the word at the same time as your child, or give a hand signal as a reminder? Perhaps the SLP is encouraging your child to produce the words without any cues. Knowing the types of cues your child needs will be beneficial when you try to reinforce your child's newly learned skills at home.

Communicate with Your Child's SLP. Maintain regular contact with your child's SLP regarding what your child is working on in therapy, as well as the types of things your child is struggling to communicate about at home or in other settings. When you are aware of what your child is working on in therapy, it will be easier for you to reinforce these skills at home. Likewise, if your child's SLP is aware of some of the things your child is struggling to communicate at home or in other settings, the therapist may be able to include these in your child's speech therapy sessions. For instance, if your child is becoming frustrated when friends or siblings take away toys during play activities, the SLP may be able to help your child learn to say, "That's mine," "Not yet," or "Wait a minute." An older child who is preparing for an oral presentation at school may benefit from spending time practicing the script during speech-language therapy sessions.

If your child is working with more than one SLP (e.g., private SLP and school SLP), be sure that the therapists have a plan to communicate regularly with one another. This could take the form of online or face-to-face team meetings, a notebook that travels between the home, the school SLP, and the private SLP, and regular email or text messaging. Also consider inviting the private SLP to your child's Individualized Education Program meeting.

Do not hesitate to ask your child's SLP questions. Here are some questions you may consider to gain a deeper understanding of your child's speech development and how to manage communication breakdowns when they occur:

- What goals are you currently addressing with my child?
- How is my child progressing on these goals?
- What target words/phrases/sentences should we be working on at home?
- When my child struggles to say the targets correctly, what cues can I use to encourage correct productions?
- What types of activities can I be doing at home to encourage my child to practice those targets?
- What can I do to motivate my child who is resistant to practicing at home?
- When I don't understand my child, what should I do or say?
- What can I do when other people don't understand my child?
- How can I reduce my child's frustration when my child is not able to make themself understood?

Encourage Your Child to Use Words or Phrases Being Targeted in Therapy. Ask your child's SLP what words or phrases your child should be practicing at home. Your child's speech-language pathologist may provide worksheets, picture books, or picture cards for home practice or may offer suggestions for ways to practice new words and phrases at home in the context of everyday activities. Taking a little time each day to review the take-home materials with your child will be more beneficial than one long practice session each week at home.

Provide Your Child's Speech-Language Pathologist With Information About Your Child's Interests and Things That Motivate Your Child. Speech-language therapy is very challenging for a child with CAS. Some children find this hard work to be frustrating and may not want to fully participate in the activities unless the activities are *highly* motivating. Because you know your child so well, you may be able to provide some insight as to the types of toys or activities that will motivate your child to participate more fully in the speech therapy sessions.

Learn What You Can About Childhood Apraxia of Speech. Apraxia Kids is an excellent source of information and support for parents of children with CAS. They maintain a website (http://www.apraxiakids.org) where you can obtain accurate information about all aspects of CAS, as well as Facebook support groups where you can reach out to other families who may be experiencing similar struggles.

APPENDIX 13-B
Understanding Childhood Apraxia of Speech

Childhood apraxia of speech (CAS) is a sensorimotor speech disorder that affects children. Speaking is a complex process that involves coordinating not only the muscles of the jaw, lips, and the tongue (articulation), but also the muscles that support breathing (respiration), turn on and off the voice (phonation), and move the soft palate up and down to direct the flow of air out the mouth or the nose (resonance). The muscle movements for speech are highly refined and require accurate timing of all these muscle groups to work in a coordination for clear and consistent speech production to occur. For a child with CAS, planning and coordinating these movements is challenging and affects the intelligibility of their speech.

Consider the child who is trying to say a fairly simple word such as, *"come."* What is required for the child to produce this word? Let's break it down.

Steps Involved in Saying the Word "Come"

1. The child has an *intention* to communicate an idea. This is a <u>cognitive/thinking skill</u>.

2. The child finds the word, "come," in his vocabulary "bank" to represent the idea he wants to express. This is a <u>language skill</u>.

3. The child plans out what his <u>speech systems</u> (respiration, phonation, resonance, articulation) and the muscles that make up these systems are going to do. This is the <u>sensorimotor planning phase</u> and the phase where speech breaks down in children with CAS.

   a. Inhale quickly to get ready to speak on the exhalation (respiration).

   b. Lift up the soft palate/velum (the soft tissue just at the back of the roof of your mouth) to close off the passageway between the pharynx and the nasal cavity, so the sound comes out the mouth and not the nose when making the /k/ sound (represented by the letter "c") (resonance).

   c. Raise up the back of the tongue to contact the soft palate to say the /k/ sound.

   d. Open the vocal cords (vocal folds) so the voice is not turned on when saying /k/ (otherwise it would sound like /g/).

   e. Get ready for the "uh" vowel sound, represented by the letter "o" in the word "come," by opening the jaw slightly and dropping the tongue to the mid-front position of the oral cavity and get ready to turn on your voice.

   f. Vibrate the vocal folds (phonation) while the tongue is in position for the "uh" vowel (articulation).

   g. Get ready to lower the soft palate to prepare for the /m/ sound.

   h. Keep your vocal folds vibrating (phonation) while the air flows into the nasal cavity (resonance) and close your lips to say the /m/ sound (articulation).

4. The child completes production of the word "come." This is the <u>motor execution phase</u>.

Children with CAS do not have significant weakness or paralysis of the muscles for speech. They have adequate strength to make speech sounds but have difficulty planning and coordinating the muscle movements for speech. These challenges with planning interfere with speech production and manifest themselves in different ways, depending on the child. Some children with CAS have tremendous difficulty imitating sounds and words, whereas others are speaking, but their speech is highly unintelligible.

Characteristics of Childhood Apraxia of Speech

Following are some of the characteristics associated with CAS. <u>Keep in mind that no child will demonstrate each characteristic listed</u>:

- inconsistent speech errors
  - producing the same word in different ways on different occasions (e.g., banana produced as "bana," "babana," and "nana")
  - producing specific speech sounds in different ways on different occasions (e.g., the child produces "s" correctly sometimes, but substitutes "b," "t," or "h" for "s" at other times)
- difficulty combining sounds and syllables (e.g., child can say "ma" and "me" but cannot say "mommy")
- pauses or breaks between sounds, syllables, or words (e.g., "Ha..ppy...birth..day")
- omitting sounds or syllables in words (e.g., 4-year-old says, "nana" for *banana* or "da-ee" for *daddy*)
- producing words in simpler ways beyond the age when these simplified versions would be expected (e.g., a 3-year-old who persists in saying "wawa" for *water*)
- greater difficulty saying longer words or phrases than shorter ones
- limited variety of consonant and vowel sounds
- possible history of limited babbling during infancy
- groping or struggling to speak (child appears to be searching for how to start the word by moving the mouth into different positions)
- monotonous or robotic-sounding speech
- placing stress on the incorrect syllable of a word (e.g., "bana**na**" for *ba**na**na*) or placing equal stress on each syllable of a word (e.g., "**di-no-saur**" for ***di**nosaur*)
- possible difficulty imitating and sequencing nonspeech movements of the lips and tongue (e.g., popping or rounding the lips, protruding, or lifting the tongue, moving the tongue from side to side)
- possible difficulty eating that is unrelated to muscular strength
- slow development of speech
- better ability to understand language than to use language expressively
- general clumsiness or poor fine and/or gross motor coordination
- possible difficulty in school learning literacy skills like reading, spelling, and writing

Assessing a Child With Suspected Childhood Apraxia of Speech

A speech-language pathologist (SLP) who has experience working with children with speech sound disorders, specifically sensorimotor speech disorders including CAS, is the appropriate person to evaluate and diagnose CAS. A hearing screening or evaluation should always be conducted to rule out any possible hearing loss impacting speech development. An audiologist is the professional who conducts the hearing evaluation. A thorough motor speech evaluation will need to be conducted to properly differentiate CAS from other speech disorders. During a motor speech evaluation, the SLP will evaluate the following areas:

- *Oral structure and function.* The muscle tone of the oral-facial area will be evaluated to rule out (or in) speech problems that are caused by significant muscle weakness or reduced muscle tone. Imitation of nonspeech movements (e.g., puckering the lips, smiling, moving the tongue from side to side, licking the lips) and sequencing these movements will be evaluated. Children who can imitate sounds will be asked to repeat syllables to assess the speed and rhythm of syllable production (e.g., saying "puh puh puh," "tuh tuh tuh," and "puh tuh kuh" repeatedly). The child's coordination during drinking, chewing, and swallowing may also be evaluated.

- *Speech sounds.* The SLP will make note of each consonant and vowel sound the child is able to produce. The types of speech sound errors the child makes also will be noted, including substitutions of one sound for another; omissions of sounds at the beginning, middle, and/or end of words; or distortions of sounds. In addition, the child's overall speech intelligibility will be described.

- *Syllable shapes.* The types of syllable shapes the child uses in terms of the sequences of consonant (C) and vowel (V) sounds will be described. Examples include CV (no, she), VC (up, ouch), CVC (hop, night), CV.CV (mama, daddy, bunny), CCVC (snap, black), CVC.CVC (cupcake, napkin). Syllable structures can be quite complex in the case of multisyllabic words like *refrigerator* or *encyclopedia.*

- *Prosody.* The melody of speech will be evaluated to determine if the child is using stress on the correct syllables of words (**bu**nny, to**ma**to) and on individual words within sentences ("Give THAT one to me." versus "Give that one to ME."), as well as appropriate and varied intonation, rhythm, and tone of voice.

In addition to a motor speech evaluation, the SLP may evaluate the following other areas, depending on the age and skill level of the child:

- *Voice and fluency.* If the SLP recognizes difficulties with voice quality (e.g., hoarseness, harshness, breathiness) or the fluency of the child's speech (stuttering more than would be expected for the child's age), these areas will be more thoroughly evaluated.

- *Language.* The SLP will evaluate the child's ability to understand spoken language (receptive language) and use language (expressive language). Areas of language assessment may include vocabulary, grammar, syntax, comprehension of questions and instructions, and the ability to use connected language to tell a story. In addition, the child's social language skills may be assessed to determine if the child is using language, gestures, and facial expressions appropriately, and using language for a wide range of social purposes (e.g., requesting an item or an activity, greeting, protesting, asking and answering questions, asking for assistance, sharing information).

- *Literacy.* The SLP may evaluate the child's phonological awareness skills. Phonological awareness refers to the ability to think about and manipulate the sounds of words as separate from the meaning of those words. Some phonological awareness skills include recognizing words that rhyme, blending syllables or sounds together to create a word (e.g., ba + na + na = banana; sh + i + p = ship), separating words into individual sounds (e.g., hats = h + a + t + s), associating sounds with the letters used to spell those sounds, and grouping words together with the same beginning or ending sounds. If the SLP suspects that the child's reading, spelling, writing, and/or phonological awareness skills are delayed, the SLP will consult with the child's teacher and other members of the educational team to request a more thorough evaluation of the child's learning.

Treatment for Childhood Apraxia of Speech

Children with CAS benefit from frequent and intensive treatment. Repetitive practice of speech movement sequences is essential for children to develop the ability to learn new speech movements and to make these movements more automatic. Therefore, individual therapy sessions are recommended, particularly earlier in the treatment process, when children are beginning to develop control of their sensorimotor speech skills. As children make progress, the amount of treatment may be reduced. Inclusion in small groups also may be beneficial so children can practice using their speech skills with peers.

Although therapists use somewhat different methods to support speech development in children with CAS, the common, underlying element of treatment should be to help children plan and program speech movement sequences. The most appropriate treatment programs are those that

- help the child learn to say **sequences of sounds**, not just individual sounds
- use **multisensory cueing techniques** (visual, auditory, tactile/touch cues) to increase speech accuracy
- encourage **repetitive practice** of words, phrases, and sentences so children develop greater ability to say words and sentences accurately and automatically, particularly when children are beginning to learn new words and sentences
- help the child develop normal **stress**, **rhythm**, and **intonation** patterns
- work on other areas of communication (e.g., receptive and expressive language, phonological awareness, social communication, etc.) to support the child's overall competence in communication

Some children with CAS may benefit from the use of augmentative forms of communication, including sign language, picture boards, or electronic communication devices. Sign language or picture boards may be used in conjunction with speech for younger children in the early stages of speech and language development or older children whose speech is difficult to understand. For some children, these augmentative modes of communication may be faded over time as speech intelligibility improves. For other children whose apraxia is quite severe, augmentative communication systems may become the primary mode of communication.

Parents play a critical role in the treatment process for children with CAS. Finding opportunities at home to practice the skills that are being worked on in speech therapy will help to reinforce the newly learned skills and provide increased practice opportunities to help your child achieve optimal progress. Children with CAS frequently require treatment for extended periods of time. This sustained effort can be challenging for both the child and the family. Care should be taken to be supportive of the gains the child is making in communication, even if these successes are gradual and slow in coming.

Glossary

Affricate: A phoneme that combines a plosive with a fricative, including /tʃ/ ("ch" sound) and /dʒ/ ("j" sound).

Aided communication: The use of some tangible object external to the body to express an idea (e.g., writing, pointing to a picture on a communication board).

Alliteration: The repeated use of an initial phoneme across words within a phrase/sentence (e.g., "Peter Piper picked a peck of pickled peppers.").

Allophone: Variation of a phoneme, while still recognizing it as the same phoneme, as in /o/ and /oʊ/.

Alveolar phonemes: Consonant sounds produced with the tongue tip making contact with the alveolar ridge, including /t/, /d/, /n/, /s/, /z/, /l/.

Assimilation: A phonological pattern in which one phoneme in a word becomes similar to another neighboring phoneme in the word (e.g., "lellow" for *yellow*; "nunny" for *money*).

Ataxic dysarthria: A type of dysarthria caused by damage to the cerebellum that causes poor coordination, imprecise speech production, inconsistency, and disordered prosody.

Auditory cues: Assistive cues that the learner can hear (e.g., verbal model).

Automatic speech: Producing speech without volitional control. Children with apraxia often are able to produce "automatic" or well-rehearsed words or phrases easily but have difficulty with less familiar or novel utterances requiring greater volitional control.

Autosomal dominant monogenic trait: Autosomal dominant refers to when one gene from a parent results in a particular trait or disorder; a monogenic trait is when a disorder involves a single gene.

Backward chaining: Building a target utterance from back to front in increasingly longer segments (e.g., can, rican, merican, American).

Basal ganglia: The group of structures deep within the cerebral hemispheres that impact initiation and execution of movement.

Bilabial phoneme: Consonant sounds produced with active participation of both lips, including /p/, /b/, /m/, /w/.

Blocked practice: A schedule of repetitive practice of the same motor skill in order to achieve accurate performance of a movement. After accurate performance is established, shifting to a *random practice* schedule is recommended to support generalization of the motor skill.

Bound morpheme: A morpheme that cannot stand alone—it can only occur meaningfully when attached to another part of a word (e.g., the "ed" in *waited*).

Canonical babbling: Consonant-vowel combinations produced in children's babbling that may be repetitive (e.g., [ba.ba.ba], [di.di.di]) or varied (e.g., [ba.di.e.ma]).

Carrier phrase: A phrase or sentence in which one part of the phrase remains stable and one (or more) words will vary (e.g., "More _____," "I want _____." or "Do you have a _____?").

Chunking: Grouping syntactic or semantic units of a sentence, followed by a brief pause (e.g., I am sick / so I can't go to school.).

Closed syllable: A syllable ending in a consonant (e.g., ba<u>ck</u>pa<u>ck</u>, bu<u>s</u>).

Coarticulation: The influence on one phoneme by the phonemes that precede or follow it.

Coarticulatory transitions: The shifts in articulatory movements from phoneme to phoneme that occur during speech.

Communication modes: The means by which a person communicates ideas (e.g., speech, writing, manual signs, gestures, picture communication boards, voice output communication devices, etc.).

Communicative functions: The function or purpose of any communicative act (e.g., requesting, demanding, greeting, apologizing, obtaining information).

Communicative intent: The use of speech (or other mode of communication) for the purpose of making something happen (e.g., pointing toward an object to generate shared interest with another person, saying "cookie" in order to obtain a treat from a caregiver).

Comorbid: Two or more medical or educational conditions that exist together, though typically independent of one another.

Complex neurobehavioral disorder: An umbrella term that includes neurobehavioral disorders related to acquired and congenital conditions (e.g., cerebral palsy, Down syndrome, autism spectrum disorder, 22q11.2 deletion syndrome).

Comprehensibility: The degree to which the listener understands the speaker in the communicative context based on factors not limited to the intelligibility of speech.

Constant practice: Producing the target utterances in a relatively constant manner or context.

Corticobulbar pathways: The motor neurons that go from the motor cortex to the cranial nerves to innervate muscles of the face, head, and neck.

Context variability: Variability in phoneme production when phonemes are produced correctly only in certain words or only in certain facilitating coarticulatory contexts.

Contrastive stress: Relative emphasis applied to certain words within sentences produced by increasing loudness, syllable duration, and/or pitch.

Decontextualized language: Language related to things that are not present, or to events in the past or future.

Delayed imitation: In speech, modeling a target utterance for a child, but adding a short (1–3 s) pause prior to the child's repetition of the utterance.

de novo genetic alteration: This is new variant of a gene due to a mutation that was not passed down from either parent.

Developmental phonological disorder: Difficulty learning the sound distinctions or phonemic rules of a language resulting in patterns of errors (e.g., deletion of final consonants, fronting of velar consonants, simplification of consonant clusters, etc.).

Diadochokinesis: The ability of a speaker to rapidly produce, alternate, and sequence repetitive articulatory movements (e.g., / pʌpʌpʌ /; / pʌtʌkʌ/).

Diffusion axon imaging: A brain imaging technique that uses magnetic resonance imaging (MRI) to provide a 3D reconstruction of the neural tracts.

Diphthongs: Vowels produced by combining two pure vowels in a gliding motion (e.g., /aɪ/ as in "hi").

Direct imitation: In speech, modeling a target utterance for the child's immediate repetition.

Discrete practice: Structuring opportunities for a learner to practice a selected target behavior.

Discrete trial approaches: Teaching selected target behaviors in a planned, controlled, and systematic manner.

Distributed practice: Less frequent sessions over a longer period of time.

Distribution of practice: How sessions are divided in terms of frequency of sessions and duration of sessions.

Dysarthria: Refers to a group of motor speech disorders that are caused by central or peripheral nervous system damage that results in weakness, paralysis, or incoordination of the speech muscles. Dysarthria may impact some or each of the speech subsystems, including respiration, phonation, articulation, and resonance.

Evidence-based practice: Integration of the best available research evidence, clinical expertise, and client/family values/preferences to guide clinical decision-making.

Evidence-informed decision-making: Integration of the three parts of evidence-based practice, along with internal evidence based on data collected from treatment to inform and guide clinical decision-making.

Excessive equal stress: The use of a pattern of intonation in which the same degree of stress is applied to each syllable or a word or sentence.

Expansion: Repeating back what the child said, but adding a word(s) to make the utterance more complete and/or grammatically correct.

Expository language: The use of language to inform or instruct.

Extrinsic feedback: Information provided by an outside source regarding the learner's performance of a motor skill.

Facilitating context: Coarticulatory contexts that facilitate accurate production of a target phoneme.

Feedback: In apraxia therapy, providing the learner with knowledge of performance (what was correct or not correct about the speech production) or knowledge of results (was the production correct or incorrect) as a way of influencing or modifying the learner's future performance.

Feedforward programs: Motor plans for speech targets that can be predicted based on the child's experience with production of that target utterance.

Focused attention: The learner's focus on the salient cues provided to support an understanding of the expectations of the task.

Forward chaining: Building a target utterance in increasingly longer segments from front to back of the utterance (e.g., an, ani, animal).

Fractional anisotropy: A brain imaging technique that allows the researcher measure connectivity in the brain.

Fricative: Consonants in which frication of the breath passes through a narrowed opening, including /f/, /v/, /θ/ (voiceless "th" as in *bath*), /ð/ (voiced "th" as in *bathe*), /s/, /z/, /ʃ/ ("sh"), /ʒ/ (similar to "sh" but with voice as the "g" in *beige*), /h/.

Glide phonemes: Consonant sounds produce with a vowel-type manner and having a vowel-type quality as in /w/ and /j/ ("y" sound).

Graphic cues: Written cues to bring the child's attention to specific aspects of the target utterance.

Groping: A behavior sometimes observed in childhood apraxia of speech in which the child moves the articulators in an apparent attempt to "find" the correct initial articulatory onset.

Heterogeneity: The quality of being diverse. For example, no two children with childhood apraxia of speech are exactly alike because it is a heterogeneous disorder.

Homonymy: Loss of lexical contrast between two or more words due to a phonological process or substitution, causing two or more different words to sound the same (e.g., the child substitutes /t/ for /k/, causing "coat" and "tote" to sound identical).

Hypernasal: The "nasal" resonance quality of speech when the speaker does not raise the velum, or the velum does not contact sufficiently the back wall of the pharynx during speech production. The cause of hypernasality may be behavioral (e.g., sound specific nasal emission, velar mislearning) or organic (e.g., velopharyngeal insufficiency due to cleft palate or submucous cleft or velopharyngeal impairment due to dysarthria).

Hyponasal: The "nasal" resonance quality of speech when the vibration of sound in the nasal cavity is reduced during production of phonemes that are typically nasal (/m/, /n/, /ŋ/). This can be due to obstruction in the nasal passage.

ICF–CY: International Classification of Functioning, Disability, and Health: Children and Youth version.

Idiopathic: This refers to when the cause of a disease or disorder is unknown.

Independent analysis: In speech analysis, a description of the child's capacities related to phoneme repertoire, syllable shape repertoire, syllable stress pattern repertoire, etc., without regard to whether the child's productions were accurate.

Interhemispheric: Refers to communication (pathways) that travel between the cerebral hemispheres.

Intonation: The modulation of pitch, duration, loudness, and/or quality to convey the mood or emotion of the speaker.

Intrahemispheric: Refers to when pathways travel within a hemisphere.

Intrinsic feedback: Sensory information obtained by the learner (not by an outside source) when performing a motor skill that is processed through the senses.

Jargon: A string of babble sounds produced by infants and toddlers that vary in prosody but have no meaning.

Juncture: Manner of moving between two successive syllables in speech by pausing, joining, or adding a phoneme.

Kinesthetic cues: Assistive cues that help the learner increase awareness of the body's internal sense of movement.

Knowledge of performance: Feedback from an outside source regarding a specific aspect of the motor skill that was performed correctly or incorrectly.

Knowledge of results: Feedback from an outside source regarding whether or not the motor skill was performed correctly.

Labial phonemes: Speech sounds produced with active participation of one or both lips (e.g., /p/, /b/, /m/, /f/, /v/, /w/).

Lax vowels: Vowels produced with less lingual tension and for a shorter duration than tense vowels, including /ɪ, ɛ, æ, ʊ, ɑ, ʌ, ə, ɚ/.

Levels of evidence: Hierarchy of evidence based on the quality of the research design.

Lexical: A term pertaining to the vocabulary or words of a language.

Lexical stress: Word-level stress in which greater relative stress is placed on a specific syllable of a word with 2+ syllables.

Linguistic stress: Relative emphasis applied to certain syllables within words produced by increasing loudness, syllable duration, and/or pitch.

Manual signs: Any of several manual/hand gesture systems of communication.

Massed practice: Frequent sessions over a shorter time frame.

Maximal performance: Refers to maximum repetition rate [MRR] during repetitions of syllables (e.g., /pə.tə.kə/).

Metacognitive cues: Assistive cues to help the learner think about movement by giving the movement a description or providing an association for the learner to connect to the movement.

Metaphor: An analogy that provides a cue regarding some salient aspect of a target phoneme (e.g., "s" shy snake sound).

Mime: Occurs when the clinician produces the word simultaneously with the child, using only mouth movements but no voice.

Minimal pair: Paired words with one phoneme variation (e.g., meat/mitt; cake/take) used to highlight the sound variations through meaningful semantic differences.

Monophthong: A vowel produced with a single articulatory movement, as in /i/, /e/, /o/.

Moto-kinesthetic: Treatment approaches (often used for speech therapy) in which tactile-kinesthetic cues are applied to specific muscles with varying degrees of pressure and specific durations to establish a greater sense of (a) which muscles need to move; (b) in which direction; (c) with what degree of muscle contraction; and (d) for how long, in order to accurately produce a movement.

Motor planning: In speech, the formulation of a spatial and temporal strategy for production of a sequence of speech sounds. Disruption in a child's ability to learn and control motor planning of speech results in childhood apraxia of speech.

Movement gestures: The coordination of articulatory movements to allow for a continuous flow of movement from one phoneme to another during production of an utterance.

Multidisciplinary evaluation: An evaluation completed by individuals from a variety of backgrounds to obtain a more complete understanding of a child's strengths and needs.

Multimodal communication: The use of more than one mode for communication (e.g., speech, gestures, manual signs, picture boards).

Narrative language: Language used for the purpose of sharing an account, story, or experience.

Nasal phonemes: Consonant sounds produced with air moving through the nasal (nose) openings including /m/, /n/, and /ŋ/ (ng).

Neurobehavioral disorders: Behavioral problems associated with brain disorders.

Neuromuscular: Pertaining to or affecting both nerves and muscles.

Onset: The portion of the syllable that precedes the vowel of the syllable (e.g., "sp" in the word spoon). Each syllable of a multisyllable word has an onset and a rhyme.

Open syllable: A syllable ending in a vowel sound (e.g., pr<u>o</u>gram; st<u>ay</u>).

Optimum challenge point: The point where the task is neither too easy nor too difficult.

Pathognomonic: A sign or symptom that is characteristic of a particular disease or disorder.

Phoneme error variability: Production of specific phonemes in different ways (e.g., /s/ produced as /s, p, t, h/). It can also be referred to as phonemic level inconsistency.

Phonetic accuracy: Referring to the accuracy of production of individual phonemes.

Phonetic inventory: Referring to the consonants, vowels, and word shapes produced in an individual's repertoire, regardless of accuracy.

Phonetic placement cues: Verbal descriptions regarding how the learner needs to move or position the articulators to accurately produce a phoneme or phoneme sequence.

Phonics: Sound/letter correspondence and the use of this correspondence to facilitate reading and spelling.

Phonological awareness: The ability to reflect on and manipulate the structure of an utterance (e.g., into words, syllables, or sounds) as distinct from the meaning of the utterance. Phonological awareness tasks may include rhyming, counting syllables in words, determining which two words in a set begin or end with the same sound, etc.

Phonological planning: The process of selecting and sequencing phonemes.

Phonotactics: An area of phonology that defines the restrictions within a given language of the ways in which phonemes are permitted to be combined.

Phrasal stress: The natural stress of a specific language.

Polysyllabic: Words containing more than one syllable.

Pre-practice: Use of strategies to facilitate initial skill acquisition (e.g., shaping, modeling).

Principles of motor learning: Principles from motor learning research that guide how we organize the treatment sessions in terms of conditions of practice and conditions of feedback.

Proprioceptive cues: Assistive cues that help the learner increase awareness of the amount of effort/force with which the body is moving, the speed of movement, and how the different body parts are moving in relation to one another in space.

Prosody: Referring to stress, intonation, rhythm, pitch, loudness, and rate in a person's speech.

Provisional diagnosis: A most likely diagnosis based on currently available information. A child who exhibits some features of childhood apraxia of speech but is unable to participate fully in a motor speech evaluation (due to age, level of cooperation, comprehension of test instructions, etc.), may be given a "provisional diagnosis" of childhood apraxia of speech until further information would be available to make a more certain diagnosis.

Pure vowel: *See monophthong*

Quasi-resonant nuclei: Phonated sounds with limited resonance.

Random practice: Practicing a number of different motor tasks in random order.

Rebus pictures: Simple drawings and/or letters that are combined to represent a specific word.

Reciprocity: A variety of back-and-forth actions between individuals for social purposes (e.g., conversations, play, gestures, sounds, etc.). Individuals with autism spectrum disorders frequently demonstrate deficits in social reciprocity.

Reflexive sounds: Early vocalizations produced in the first 2 months of life that are reflexive in nature, such as crying, fussing, coughing, and burping.

Reinforcer: A term used to describe a response that serves to strengthen the behavior that precedes it (e.g., gleefully pretending to be startled when the child says "boo" will increase the likelihood that the child will continue to produce that word).

Relational analysis: In speech analysis, a comparison of the child's capacities in phoneme, syllable shape, and stress pattern productions compared to the correct adult production of these.

Repetitive practice: Providing enough practice trials of a motor skill so that the motor skill becomes generalized, and the action can be produced more automatically.

Residual articulation errors: Articulation errors that have not resolved beyond an age when the speech sound should have been attained.

Resonance: The vibration of the pharynx, oral, and nasal cavities during speech that gives speech its characteristic quality. In speech, the lowering of the velum (soft palate) gives speech a "nasal" quality, since sound energy is allowed to vibrate within the nasal cavity.

Retention: Maintenance of a skill over time.

Rhotics: The "r"-colored phonemes and their variations (i.e., rhotic diphthongs and triphthongs).

Rhythm: A term related to the rhythmic timing of stressed and unstressed syllables in sentences.

Rime: The portion of the syllable that includes the vowel and any phonemes that come after it (e.g., "oon" in the word spoon). Each syllable of a multisyllable word has an *onset* and a rime.

Segmental: Pertaining to the discrete phonetic elements of speech, including vowels and consonants.

Semivowels: A term used to describe /w/ and /j/ "y sound" phonemes that have a vowel-like quality, but function as a consonant. Semivowels are also referred to as glides.

Shaping: Making gradual articulatory shifts to move progressively from a sound a child can produce to the accurate production of a target phoneme.

Simplifications: Making a motor task easier in some way in order for the learner to experience success.

Simultaneous production: Occurs when the learner is watching the clinician, and the learner and the clinician produce a target utterance at the same time.

Social-pragmatic approaches: Intervention approaches used in treatment for children with social communication challenges (e.g., autism, pervasive developmental disorder) that attempt to increase the child's capacities for improved initiation and spontaneous communication by focusing on the child's motivations and interests.

Spatiotemporal parameters: The limits or boundaries of the positioning and timing of the articulatory mechanism required to produce speech sounds and words accurately.

Stimuli: The target utterances practiced during the session.

Stops/plosive phonemes: Speech sounds produce by the speaker blocking the flow of air and then releasing it as in /p, b, t, d, k, g/.

Stress: Relative emphasis applied to certain syllables within words or words within sentences by using increased loudness, syllable duration, higher pitch.

Stressed syllable: The syllable of a word that receives the greatest relative stress.

Suprasegmental: Pertaining to features of speech such as stress, pitch, timing, and duration.

Syllable cues: Cues to reduce omission of syllables in a target utterance (e.g., tapping, clapping).

Syllable pictures: Picture cues for one or more syllables of a word to support accurate production of a whole word by separating syllables into separate words (e.g., pictures of "rain" and "bow" for "rainbow" or pictures of "cow" and the letter "V" for "movie").

Syllable segregation: Noticeable and longer than expected gaps between the syllables of a word.

Syllable shape: Phoneme sequences that comprise a syllable (e.g., CV "bow"; VC "up"; CVC "pot"; CCVC "spot"); sometimes referred to as *word shape*.

Tactile cues: Assistive cues that provide the learner with input to the skin.

Telepractice: The use of telecommunications technology that links the clinician with the client for delivery of diagnostic or treatment services.

Tense vowels: Vowels produced with greater lingual tension and for a longer duration than lax vowels, including /i, eɪ, u, oʊ, ɔ, ɝ/.

Token-to-token variability: Variability in repeated productions of the same word.

Transfer: Generalization of a skill to other contexts.

Triphthongs: Vowels produced by combining three vowels (a diphthong and a rhotic vowel) in a gliding motion (e.g., /aɪr/ as in "fire").

Ultrasound biofeedback: In speech therapy, technology that utilizes real-time visual feedback in the form of ultrasound images to facilitate accurate production of certain lingual phonemes.

Unaided communication: Expressing ideas communicatively without the use of any tangible objects external to the body (e.g., speech, gestures, manual signs).

Variable practice: producing target utterances in varied manners or contexts.

Velar phonemes: Speech sounds produced by lifting the back part of the tongue to or near the back part of the roof of the mouth near the velum (soft palate) as in /k/, /g/, /ŋ/ ("ng"), /w/.

Velopharyngeal insufficiency: Occurs when the velopharyngeal mechanism is not sufficient to separate the oral cavity from the nasal cavity during speech, resulting in increased hypernasal resonance quality.

Video modeling: Use of videos to model the correct target utterances.

Visual cues: Assistive cues that the learner can see.

Vocant: Vowel-like sounds produced in infancy that cannot be transcribed as adult vowel sounds on the vowel quadrilateral.

Volitional control: Conscious awareness and focused effort on specific aspects of a movement.

Volitional speech: Speech produced under voluntary control.

Vowel quadrilateral: The diagram representing the tongue position (front, central, back) and tongue height (high, mid, low) for each pure vowel in a language.

Weak syllable: The syllable(s) of a word receiving less relative stress.

Word shape: Phoneme sequences that can be combined to create single-syllable and multisyllable words (e.g., CVC "cat"; CVCC "cats"; CV.CV "mommy"; CV.CVC "peanut"). Often used interchangeably with *syllable shape*.

WHO: World Health Organization.

Index

Note: Page numbers in **bold** reference non-text material.